The Interplay of Microbiome and Immune Response in Health and Diseases

The Interplay of Microbiome and Immune Response in Health and Diseases

Special Issue Editors

Amedeo Amedei
Gwendolyn Barceló-Coblijn

MDPI • Basel • Beijing • Wuhan • Barcelona • Belgrade

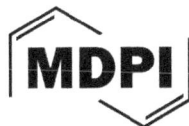

MDPI

Special Issue Editors

Amedeo Amedei
University of Florence
Italy

Gwendolyn Barceló-Coblijn
Research Unit—Hospital Universitari Son Espases
Spain

Editorial Office
MDPI
St. Alban-Anlage 66
4052 Basel, Switzerland

This is a reprint of articles from the Special Issue published online in the open access journal *International Journal of Molecular Sciences* (ISSN 1422-0067) from 2018 to 2019 (available at: https://www.mdpi.com/journal/ijms/special_issues/microbiome_immune)

For citation purposes, cite each article independently as indicated on the article page online and as indicated below:

LastName, A.A.; LastName, B.B.; LastName, C.C. Article Title. *Journal Name* **Year**, *Article Number*, Page Range.

ISBN 978-3-03921-646-8 (Pbk)
ISBN 978-3-03921-647-5 (PDF)

Contents

About the Special Issue Editors vii

Amedeo Amedei and Gwendolyn Barceló-Coblijn
Editorial of Special Issue "The Interplay of Microbiome and Immune Response in Health
and Diseases"
Reprinted from: *Int. J. Mol. Sci.* **2019**, *20*, 3708, doi:10.3390/ijms20153708 1

Amedeo Amedei and Federico Boem
I've *Gut* A Feeling: Microbiota Impacting the Conceptual and Experimental Perspectives of
Personalized Medicine
Reprinted from: *Int. J. Mol. Sci.* **2018**, *19*, 3756, doi:10.3390/ijms19123756 6

Devinder Toor, Mishi Kaushal Wasson, Prashant Kumar, G. Karthikeyan,
Naveen Kumar Kaushik, Chhavi Goel, Sandhya Singh, Anil Kumar and Hridayesh Prakash
Dysbiosis Disrupts Gut Immune Homeostasis and Promotes Gastric Diseases
Reprinted from: *Int. J. Mol. Sci.* **2019**, *20*, 2432, doi:10.3390/ijms20102432 19

Ivana Milosevic, Ankica Vujovic, Aleksandra Barac, Marina Djelic, Milos Korac,
Aleksandra Radovanovic Spurnic, Ivana Gmizic, Olja Stevanovic, Vladimir Djordjevic,
Nebojsa Lekic, Edda Russo and Amedeo Amedei
Gut-Liver Axis, Gut Microbiota, and Its Modulation in the Management of Liver Diseases:
A Review of the Literature
Reprinted from: *Int. J. Mol. Sci.* **2019**, *20*, 395, doi:10.3390/ijms20020395 33

Elena Gianchecchi and Alessandra Fierabracci
Recent Advances on Microbiota Involvement in the Pathogenesis of Autoimmunity
Reprinted from: *Int. J. Mol. Sci.* **2019**, *20*, 283, doi:10.3390/ijms20020283 49

Andrea Picchianti-Diamanti, Concetta Panebianco, Simonetta Salemi, Maria Laura Sorgi,
Roberta Di Rosa, Alessandro Tropea, Mayla Sgrulletti, Gerardo Salerno, Fulvia Terracciano,
Raffaele D'Amelio, Bruno Laganà and Valerio Pazienza
Analysis of Gut Microbiota in Rheumatoid Arthritis Patients: Disease-Related Dysbiosis and
Modifications Induced by Etanercept
Reprinted from: *Int. J. Mol. Sci.* **2018**, *19*, 2938, doi:10.3390/ijms19102938 77

Rossella Cianci, Laura Franza, Giovanni Schinzari, Ernesto Rossi, Gianluca Ianiro,
Giampaolo Tortora, Antonio Gasbarrini, Giovanni Gambassi and Giovanni Cammarota
The Interplay between Immunity and Microbiota at Intestinal Immunological Niche: The Case
of Cancer
Reprinted from: *Int. J. Mol. Sci.* **2019**, *20*, 501, doi:10.3390/ijms20030501 88

Giovanni Brandi and Giorgio Frega
Microbiota: Overview and Implication in Immunotherapy-Based Cancer Treatments
Reprinted from: *Int. J. Mol. Sci.* **2019**, *20*, 2699, doi:10.3390/ijms20112699 104

Valentina Zuccaro, Andrea Lombardi, Erika Asperges, Paolo Sacchi, Piero Marone,
Alessandra Gazzola, Luca Arcaini and Raffaele Bruno
The Possible Role of Gut Microbiota and Microbial Translocation Profiling During Chemo-Free
Treatment of Lymphoid Malignancies
Reprinted from: *Int. J. Mol. Sci.* **2019**, *20*, 1748, doi:10.3390/ijms20071748 120

Loris Riccardo Lopetuso, Maria Ernestina Giorgio, Angela Saviano, Franco Scaldaferri, Antonio Gasbarrini and Giovanni Cammarota
Bacteriocins and Bacteriophages: Therapeutic Weapons for Gastrointestinal Diseases?
Reprinted from: *Int. J. Mol. Sci.* **2019**, *20*, 183, doi:10.3390/ijms20010183 . . . . **130**

Clovis Bortolus, Muriel Billamboz, Rogatien Charlet, Karine Lecointe, Boualem Sendid, Alina Ghinet and Samir Jawhara
A Small Aromatic Compound Has Antifungal Properties and Potential Anti-Inflammatory Effects against Intestinal Inflammation
Reprinted from: *Int. J. Mol. Sci.* **2019**, *20*, 321, doi:10.3390/ijms20020321 . . . . **142**

Rogatien Charlet, Boualem Sendid, Srini V. Kaveri, Daniel Poulain, Jagadeesh Bayry and Samir Jawhara
Intravenous Immunoglobulin Therapy Eliminates *Candida albicans* and Maintains Intestinal Homeostasis in a Murine Model of Dextran Sulfate Sodium-Induced Colitis
Reprinted from: *Int. J. Mol. Sci.* **2019**, *20*, 1473, doi:10.3390/ijms20061473 . . . . **156**

Fang Liu, Zhaojie Li, Xiong Wang, Changhu Xue, Qingjuan Tang and Robert W. Li
Microbial Co-Occurrence Patterns and Keystone Species in the Gut Microbial Community of Mice in Response to Stress and Chondroitin Sulfate Disaccharide
Reprinted from: *Int. J. Mol. Sci.* **2019**, *20*, 2130, doi:10.3390/ijms20092130 . . . . **169**

Maria Gabriella Torcia
Interplay among Vaginal Microbiome, Immune Response and Sexually Transmitted Viral Infections
Reprinted from: *Int. J. Mol. Sci.* **2019**, *20*, 266, doi:10.3390/ijms20020266 . . . . **184**

About the Special Issue Editors

Amedeo Amedei graduated with full marks and honors in Biology from Florence University in 1996. He started his scientific career studying the role of Th1/Th2 lymphocytes in GVHD, atopic dermatitis, and kidney rejection. Afterwards, he examined the role of *Helicobacter pylori*-specific immune response in gastric diseases. In 2003, he began his doctorate degree in Clinical and Experimental Medicine. In 2005, he began as Researcher at the Department of Experimental and Clinical Medicine (University of Florence), where he was appointed Associate Professor in 2015. Recently, Prof. Amedei's scientific interests have been focused on cancer immunology and the role of the microbiome. His scientific production is a testament to his prestigious international profile: 141 peer-reviewed articles (5904 citations), 8 book chapters, and one patent. Prof. Amedei is serving on the editorial board of various international journals and is a scientific reviewer for numerous international research projects of private and public entities. He has been serving on the Scientific Council of "Toscana Life Sciences" (TLS) since 2016.

Gwendolyn Barceló-Coblijn graduated with full marks and honors in Biology from the University of Szeged (Hungary) in 2003. She has been continuously involved in the study of fatty acid and membrane lipid metabolism in different biological contexts, covering topics like nutrition or cancer treatment. After two postdoctoral positions at the University of North Dakota (USA, 2004–2006) and the University of the Balearic Islands (Spain, 2006–2012), in 2013, she founded the group "Lipids in Human Pathology" of the Health Research Institute of the Balearic Islands (IdISBa, Palma, Spain). As Full Researcher since 2019, her main research is focused on the detection of lipid biomarkers for diseases such as cancer or inflammatory bowel disease using cutting-edge analytical techniques, such as imaging mass spectrometry, while investigating how changes in membrane lipid metabolism account for the changes in the lipidome. In recent years, her research has incorporated study of the role of the microbiota in colorectal cancer, IBD, and infections by *Clostridium difficile*. She has published 38 peer-reviewed articles, three book chapters, and two patents. She also serves on the editorial board of numerous international journals.

International Journal of
Molecular Sciences

MDPI

Editorial

Editorial of Special Issue "The Interplay of Microbiome and Immune Response in Health and Diseases"

Amedeo Amedei [1,2,*] and Gwendolyn Barceló-Coblijn [3]

1   Department of Experimental and Clinical Medicine, University of Florence, 50134 Florence, Italy
2   SOD of Interdisciplinary Internal Medicine, Azienda Ospedaliera Universitaria Careggi (AOUC), 50134 Florence, Italy
3   Lipids in Human Pathology, Health Research Institute of the Balearic Islands (IdISBa, Institut d'Investigació Sanitària Illes Balears), 07120 Palma, Balearic Islands, Spain
*   Correspondence: amedeo.amedei@unifi.it

Received: 22 July 2019; Accepted: 25 July 2019; Published: 29 July 2019

Increasing data suggests and supports the idea that the gut microbiota (GM) modulates different host pathways, playing a crucial role in human physiology and consequently impacting in the development of some pathologic conditions. Explorations of how the microscopic communities might contribute to health or disease have moved from obscure to ubiquitous. Recently, studies have linked our microbial settlers to inflammatory bowel diseases (IBD)s, obesity, asthma, autism spectrum disorders, stroke, diabetes, and cancer. In agreement with Hanage, who suggested a scepticism dose about the predominant role of microbiota [1], we have edited this special issue with the aim to publish manuscripts respecting this spirit of scientific rigor to the detriment of enthusiasm (which often characterizes GM studies).

However, there is no doubt that microbial metabolites bridge various, even distant, areas of the organism by way of the hormone and immune system, contributing to the development of different pathologies, such as the autoimmune disorders, as discussed by Gianchecci et al. [2]. The impact of a GM imbalanced in autoimmunity pathogenesis has been suggested by different experimental evidence, and physiological mechanisms, (i.e., the establishment of immune homeostasis) are influenced by commensal bacteria. Microbiota alterations generate effects in the immune system, such as intestinal inflammation, enhanced gut permeability, and defective tolerance to food antigens. In particular, early findings reported differences in the gut microbiome of subjects affected by several autoimmune conditions, including prediabetes.

In addition, the microbiota seen also have implications in the therapeutic approaches of lymphoid malignancies and immunotherapy-based cancer treatments. Zuccaro et al. [3], discussed the microbiota impact during chemo-free treatment of lymphoid malignancies. To date, no studies have been planned to evaluate the GM composition in patients with lymphoproliferative disorders (and treated with chemo-free therapies), and the probable association between GM, treatment outcome, and immune-related adverse events has never been analysed. The authors remark the necessity of additional studies to make opportunities for a more personalized approach in the patients' subset.

During the last few years, the GM has gained increasing attention as a consequence of its immunomodulator role. In particular, with the introduction of checkpoint inhibitors' immunotherapy and adoptive cell transfer in oncology, these findings became of primary relevance in light of experimental data that suggested microbiota involvement as a credible predictor of responsiveness. These impacting themes have been discussed by Brandi et al. [4], who reviewed the GM implication in anti-cancer immunotherapy strategies, remarking the need to identify the specific GM actions and develop innovative strategies to favourably edit its composition.

It is important to link microbiota alterations (dysbiosis) and intestinal-correlated diseases. In this regard, the manuscript of Lopetuso et al. [5] is interesting, since it explores the role of bacteriocins and bacteriophages in the most recurrent gastrointestinal disorders, speculating on their potential therapeutic application. The bacteriocins are bactericidal peptides (produced by both gram+ and gram-bacteria) with an inhibitory activity against diverse groups of undesirable microorganisms. Conversely, the bacteriophages are viruses that are able to infect bacteria, forcing them to produce viral components. Bacteriocins and bacteriophages can influence both human health and diseases because they modulate the intestinal microbiota and regulate the relationships between different microorganisms, strains, and cells living in the human gut.

However, one of the most important messages that this special issue conveys is that we are still far from understanding the full extent of GM actions on human health and the impact of its manipulation. Cianci et al. [6] systematically reviewed these advances, linking gut microbiota not only to colorectal cancer, but also to oesophageal, stomach, and pancreatic cancer, and hepatocellular carcinoma. Hence, the GM action appears to go beyond the direct effect on the intestines, reaching those districts that may not be directly colonized by the various microbial species. This is crucially important when designing new therapies, including surgery and radiotherapy, aiming to restore the damaged microbiome during assessment of their impact on a patient's health. This concept is extensively covered by Toor et al. [7] in which the authors stressed their concerns on the impact of the microbiome on the uncontrolled use of antibiotics (which is also a current major concern for the Public Health Authorities), chemotherapeutic drugs, or even changes in dietary patterns. The authors not only summarized state-of-the-art strategies to study gut microbiomes, but they also included new strategies to manage dysbiosis through diet, bile acids, and immune pharmaceutics.

It is clear that one of the major concerns in the field is how immunotherapy may affect the delicate equilibrium existing in the microbiome ecosystem, and vice versa. Picchianti–Diamanti et al. [8] addressed this question in the context of rheumatoid arthritis (RA). In a pilot study, the authors demonstrated that in addition to oral microbiota dysbiosis, gut dysbiosis was also detected. Hence, the comparison of the impact of intestinal microbiota in three groups of RA patients and patients receiving methotrexate and/or etanercept (a biotechnological agent targeting TNF-alpha) led the authors to conclude that part of the benefits of this treatment is related to the partial restoration of the beneficial microbiota.

However, the scenario gets more complex when considering the connections established by distant organs, such as gut-associated lymphoid tissue (GALT, explained by Toor et al. [7]) or the gut-liver axis reviewed by Milosevic et al. [9]. Milosevic et al. evaluated another GM aspect, the so called "gut-liver axis", which has attracted great attention in recent years. GM communication is bi-directional and involves endocrine and immunological mechanisms. In this way, gut-dysbiosis and composition of "ancient" microbiota could be linked to the pathogenesis of numerous chronic liver diseases, such as chronic hepatitis B and C, alcoholic liver disease, development of liver cirrhosis, and finally the hepatocellular carcinoma. The authors discussed the current evidence supporting a GM role in the management of these different chronic liver diseases and potential novel therapeutic GM targets, such as fecal microbiota transplants, antibiotics, and probiotics.

Detecting the microbial interactions is essential to understand the GM structure and function. In a mouse model, Liu et al. [10] inferred the microbial co-occurrence patterns using a random matrix theory-based approach in the GM in response to chondroitin sulfate disaccharide (CSD) under healthy and stressed conditions. A total of 34 operational taxonomic units (OTU) were identified as module hubs and connectors, likely acting as generalists in the microbial community. In particular, *Mucispirillum schaedleri* acted as a connector in the stressed network in response to the CSD supplement and may play a crucial role in bridging intimate interactions between the host and its microbiome. In addition, several modules correlated with physiological parameters were detected. A positive correlation between node connectivity of the proteobacteria with superoxide dismutase activities under stress suggested that proteobacteria can be developed as a potential pathological marker. These results provided novel insights into GM interactions and may facilitate future endeavours in microbial community engineering, directly influencing some molecular pathways.

The GM role is being extensively studied in the context of chronic inflammatory diseases, in particular in inflammatory bowel diseases (IBDs), which have a multifactorial etiology (not firmly established yet). The fact that IBD incidence is steadily increasing in developed and developing countries clearly suggests that lifestyle changes are key players in the onset of these diseases. Many studies have established that the GM biodiversity is frequently altered in IBD patients, in particular because of the reduction in firmicutes and an increase in proteobacteria. In this situation, IBD patients are highly vulnerable to any opportunistic pathogen, such as *Candida (C) albicans*, a serious clinical problem due to the high associated morbidity and mortality. Consequently, the *C. albicans* infection complicates the IBD treatment, as the anti-inflammatory compounds most commonly prescribed do not have antifungal activity. With the aim to identify new compounds showing this dual effect, i.e., compound having simultaneously antifungal and anti-inflammatory properties, Bortolus et al. [11] investigated the antifungal properties of a novel compound, 2,3-dihydroxy-4-methoxybenzaldehyde (DHMB). Using in vitro and in vivo models (murine DSS-induced colitis model), the authors demonstrated the great potential this aromatic molecule has as an antifungal agent with anti-inflammatory properties. On the other hand, Charlet et al. [12] investigated an alternative approach widely used in the management of various inflammatory and autoimmune diseases: Immunotherapy with intravenous immunoglobulin (IVIg). Using the same murine model, the authors demonstrate that this treatment has a clear impact on GM composition, decreasing the content in *Escherichia coli*, *Enterococcus faecalis*, and *C. albicans* populations. Conversely, the beneficial effects of IVIg were associated with the suppression of inflammatory cytokine IL-6 and the enhancement of IL-10 and PPAR-gamma (involved in inflammation resolution). Hence, it seems that the beneficial effects of IVIg in infectious diseases goes beyond a simple neutralization of microbes, acting actively on anti-inflammatory pathways, which turned out to be critical for protection against infection.

Importantly, all the basic concepts and general approaches developed while studying gut microbiota may also apply, to a greater or lesser degree, to other biological systems. such as the vaginal or skin ecosystems. This special issue contains a comprehensive review by Torcia [13] on the interplay among vaginal microbiome, immune response, and sexually transmitted infections (STIs). In addition to the role that the cervico-vaginal microbiota has during egg fertilization and pregnancy, its maintenance is key in the prevention of infectious pathogens, particularly during the transmission of the human immunodeficiency virus (HIV), the human papilloma virus (HPV), and the herpes simplex virus 2 (HSV2). Furthermore, an increased risk of STI acquisition is clearly associated to vaginal dysbiosis. Torcia [13] described the current knowledge on how the immune system, epithelial cells, and microbiota are interconnected and discussed different prevention strategies. The latter has become a worldwide health issue due to the high incidence of STIs in low- and middle-income countries and due to their resurgence in developing countries.

Finally, Park et al. [14] discussed the GM role in the largest organ in the human body: The skin. As in the gut, liver, or vagina, the pathological alteration of the microbiome system often leads to inflammation. Interestingly, the authors described the opposite impact on the skin health of two members of the same genus, *Staphylococcus (S) aureus* and *S. epidermidis* and they warn about the importance of understanding how these two species can modulate the cutaneous-immune response prior to manipulating their levels as part of a treatment. It is clear that this warning should be issued for any microbiome ecosystem.

In other words, the different studies and data presented and discussed in this special issue suggest the microbiota centrality in the development and maintenance of the "health" and in favouring (those cases in which the microbiota's complex relational architecture is dysregulated) the onset of pathological conditions. The intricate relationships between the microbiota and human beings, which invest core notions of biomedicine, such as "health" and "the individual," concern not only problems of an empirical nature, but seem to require the need to adopt new concepts and novel perspectives in order to be properly analysed and utilized, especially for their therapeutic implementation. In this context, it is very adequate the contribution of Amedei et al. [15], which illuminates the discussion of the theoretical proposals and innovations (from the ecological component to the notion of the polygenomic organism) aimed at producing this perspective change. In conclusion, the authors analysed what impact and what new challenges these novel approaches might have on personalized medicine.

Conflicts of Interest: The authors declare no conflict of interest.

References

1. Hanage, W.P. Microbiology: Microbiome science needs a healthy dose of scepticism. *Nature* **2014**, *512*, 247–248. [CrossRef] [PubMed]
2. Gianchecchi, E.; Fierabracci, A. Recent Advances on Microbiota Involvement in the Pathogenesis of Autoimmunity. *Int. J. Mol. Sci.* **2019**, *20*, 283. [CrossRef] [PubMed]
3. Zuccaro, V.; Lombardi, A.; Asperges, E.; Sacchi, P.; Marone, P.; Gazzola, A.; Arcaini, L.; Bruno, R. The Possible Role of Gut Microbiota and Microbial Translocation Profiling During Chemo-Free Treatment of Lymphoid Malignancies. *Int. J. Mol. Sci.* **2019**, *20*, 1748. [CrossRef] [PubMed]
4. Brandi, G.; Frega, G. Microbiota: Overview and Implication in Immunotherapy-Based Cancer Treatments. *Int. J. Mol. Sci.* **2019**, *20*, 2699. [CrossRef] [PubMed]
5. Lopetuso, L.R.; Giorgio, M.E.; Saviano, A.; Scaldaferri, F.; Gasbarrini, A.; Cammarota, G. Bacteriocins and Bacteriophages: Therapeutic Weapons for Gastrointestinal Diseases? *Int. J. Mol. Sci.* **2019**, *20*, 183. [CrossRef] [PubMed]
6. Cianci, R.; Franza, L.; Schinzari, G.; Rossi, E.; Ianiro, G.; Tortora, G.; Gasbarrini, A.; Gambassi, G.; Cammarota, G. The Interplay between Immunity and Microbiota at Intestinal Immunological Niche: The Case of Cancer. *Int. J. Mol. Sci.* **2019**, *20*, 501. [CrossRef] [PubMed]
7. Toor, D.; Wsson, M.K.; Kumar, P.; Karthikeyan, G.; Kaushik, N.K.; Goel, C.; Singh, S.; Kumar, A.; Prakash, H. Dysbiosis Disrupts Gut Immune Homeostasis and Promotes Gastric Diseases. *Int. J. Mol. Sci.* **2019**, *20*, 2432. [CrossRef] [PubMed]
8. Picchianti-Diamanti, A.; Panebianco, C.; Salemi, S.; Sorgi, M.L.; Di Rosa, R.; Tropea, A.; Sgrulletti, M.; Salerno, G.; Terracciano, F.; D'Amelio, R.; et al. Analysis of Gut Microbiota in Rheumatoid Arthritis Patients: Disease-Related Dysbiosis and Modifications Induced by Etanercept. *Int. J. Mol. Sci.* **2018**, *19*, 2938. [CrossRef] [PubMed]
9. Milosevic, I.; Vujovic, A.; Barac, A.; Djelic, M.; Korac, M.; Radovanovic Spurnic, A.; Gmizic, I.; Stevanovic, O.; Djordjevic, V.; Lekic, N.; et al. Gut-Liver Axis, Gut Microbiota, and Its Modulation in the Management of Liver Diseases: A Review of the Literature. *Int. J. Mol. Sci.* **2019**, *20*, 395. [CrossRef] [PubMed]
10. Liu, F.; Li, Z.; Wang, X.; Xue, C.; Tang, Q.; Li, R.W. Microbial Co Occurrence Patterns and Keystone Species in the Gut Microbial Community of Mice in Response to Stress and Chondroitin Sulfate Disaccharide. *Int. J. Mol. Sci.* **2019**, *20*, 2130. [CrossRef] [PubMed]
11. Bortolus, C.; Billamboz, M.; Charlet, R.; Lecointe, K.; Sendid, B.; Ghinet, A.; Jawhara, A. Small Aromatic Compound Has Antifungal Properties and Potential Anti-Inflammatory Effects against Intestinal Inflammation. *Int. J. Mol. Sci.* **2019**, *20*, 321. [CrossRef] [PubMed]
12. Charlet, R.; Sendid, B.; Kaveri, S.V.; Poulain, D.; Bayry, J.; Jawhara, S. Intravenous Immunoglobulin Therapy Eliminates *Candida albicans* and Maintains Intestinal Homeostasis in a Murine Model of Dextran Sulfate Sodium-Induced Colitis. *Int. J. Mol. Sci.* **2019**, *20*, 1473. [CrossRef] [PubMed]
13. Torcia, M.G. Interplay among Vaginal Microbiome, Immune Response and Sexually Transmitted Viral Infections. *Int. J. Mol. Sci.* **2019**, *20*, 266. [CrossRef] [PubMed]

14. Park, Y.J.; Kim, C.W.; Lee, H.K. Interactions between Host Immunity and Skin-Colonizing Staphylococci: No Two Siblings Are Alike. *Int. J. Mol. Sci.* **2019**, *20*, 718. [CrossRef] [PubMed]

15. Amedei, A.; Boem, F. I've *Gut* A Feeling: Microbiota Impacting the Conceptual and Experimental Perspectives of Personalized Medicine. *Int. J. Mol. Sci.* **2018**, *19*, 3756. [CrossRef] [PubMed]

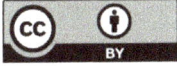

International Journal of
Molecular Sciences

MDPI

Review

I've *Gut* A Feeling: Microbiota Impacting the Conceptual and Experimental Perspectives of Personalized Medicine

Amedeo Amedei [1,2,*] and Federico Boem [1]

[1] Department of Experimental and Clinical Medicine, University of Florence, Largo Brambilla, 03 50134, Firenze, Italy; federico.boem@gmail.com
[2] Department of Biomedicine, Azienda Ospedaliera Universitaria Careggi (AOUC), Largo Brambilla, 03 50134, Firenze, Italy
* Correspondence: amedeo.amedei@unifi.it

Received: 21 September 2018; Accepted: 16 November 2018; Published: 27 November 2018

Abstract: In recent years, the human microbiota has gained increasing relevance both in research and clinical fields. Increasing studies seem to suggest the centrality of the microbiota and its composition both in the development and maintenance of what we call "health" and in generating and/or favoring (those cases in which the microbiota's complex relational architecture is dysregulated) the onset of pathological conditions. The complex relationships between the microbiota and human beings, which invest core notions of biomedicine such as "health" and "individual," do concern not only problems of an empirical nature but seem to require the need to adopt new concepts and new perspectives in order to be properly analysed and utilized, especially for their therapeutic implementation. In this contribution we report and discuss some of the theoretical proposals and innovations (from the ecological component to the notion of polygenomic organism) aimed at producing this change of perspective. In conclusion, we summarily analyze what impact and what new challenges these new approaches might have on personalized/person centred/precision medicine.

Keywords: microbiome; health; precision medicine; genomics

---

1. Introduction

A famous metaphor to describe "life" is the tree. The tree enables to express two life aspects, that might appear somehow in contrast. On the one hand, each leaf stands for a species, highlighting a particular unique form according to which "life" manifests itself, thus showing the differences among living things and justifying the need for classification. On the other hand, each branch, connecting species, represents the historical trajectory (roughly saying: the phylogeny) recalling the fact that all living creatures share a common descent and reminding us that our partition of the living world is not so cutting as we would like. The tension between the necessity to order the living world and the awareness of its "ramified" unity, is a key feature of biological sciences since their origin [1]. Biological species are surely grasped and described as distinct one from each other, however not sharply as the categories that we usually adopt to classify them. Species boundaries are, in many cases, fuzzy rather than sharp. Indeed, biological species do not exist (in the real world) in the isolation of taxonomical hierarchies. They are rather intimately connected to each other. Sometimes the nature of this relation is so intrinsic that is labelled as symbiosis or the reciprocal interdependence of different organisms (either parasitic or mutualistic). So, human beings and their microbial community can be seen as a clear example of symbiosis.

However, the fuzziness of biological borders can be considered also from a different angle. New findings, also made possible by a new theoretical perspective, challenge the notion of *symbiosis* as such and push towards a radical change in the organization of the living world. Life is less linear and far more intricate than we thought. Recent evidence indicate that *horizontal gene transfer*, which is a form of transfer of genetic material that does not occur vertically (from parents to offspring) but horizontally and therefore it is also called *lateral gene transfer* [2], can be widespread and a broader phenomenon than thought (not confined to prokaryotes and thus including eukaryotes). Phylogeny is no longer only a vertical trajectory and of note, evolution can operate also horizontally. Maybe, a more suitable metaphor than the *tree*, describing this aspect of life is constituted by the *web*. According to some researchers, individuals belonging to plant or animal species should no longer be considered as such, that is, as single, distinctive biological forms, but rather as networks of biomolecular interactions, whose nodes are represented by the host and its associated microorganisms. These networks, to all effects new categories of biological organization, are called *holobionts*. Given the nature of these relationships, the holobionts' genomes should be treated together and not separately, thus constituting a *hologenome*. Such intergenomic associations become so essential that previous models of animal and plant biology, without this dimension, should be considered, at least, partial and sketchy [3].

The consequences of such a change, that is conceptual before being experimental, have the potential to radically transform not just the way we use to understand various biomedical phenomena (such as certain physiological functions or dysfunctions) but also the modalities through which we could interfere with the very same phenomena (*e.g.*, which therapies).

Given such a new perspective, it should not be surprising that human *microbiota* (usually meant the variety of "microbial taxa associated with humans" [4]) has become the pivot of an intense investigation. The nature and the modalities of these association might vary, depending on the functions and mechanisms considered, but it is now widely recognized that the relationship between microbial communities and their host is fundamental both for basic and applied research (especially biomedical) [5].

New evidence highlight how microbiota plays a key role in human physiology, directly affecting metabolic pathways, spanning from intestinal to brain activities [6,7]. Indeed, recent findings indicate how an imbalance in the architecture of intestinal microbial populations might be directly involved in the development of different medical conditions (from metabolic to mood disorders) shedding new light on the aetiology of different diseases (such as obesity, asthma, autism spectrum disorders, stroke, diabetes and cancer) [6] (Figure 1).

Increasing studies suggest that microbiota contributes, in different ways and through different modalities, to the thin "red line" that separates physiological conditions from pathological ones. Recently, some researchers have acknowledged the central role of different bacterial populations and strains in modulating the adaptive immune response, thus affecting, for example, cancer development [8]. Moreover, a more precise understanding of general microbiota composition, imbalance among and within bacterial populations and their different localizations (*e.g.*, either gut residents or oral ones) may offer new hints to understand the origin and the progression of certain disease and thus new potential tools for a more specific diagnosis [9].

This situation is also due to the magnitude (both functionally and structurally) of microbiota itself, given that microbial cells in the gut outnumber cells of the host [6]. Microbiota metabolites and especially SCFAs (Short-Chain Fatty Acids) connect different areas of the organism, through the mediation of the immune and hormone system, such as the so called *gut-brain axis* [6,10,11] suggesting that the crosstalk between the organism and its microbial residents is a crucial factor for the sustenance of physiological and health conditions. In addition to that, it is imperative to recall that these microorganisms are no longer localized just in the gut. This can explain why the transition, within scientific terminology, from "gut flora" to "microbiota" does not coincide just with the need of a more precise or less restrictive, semantics. Rather, as words count for concepts, such a shift mirrors the fact that commensal, non-commensal and pathogenic organisms populate (beyond the intestinal tract) the skin, oral mucosa, lungs and other organs and tissues of the so-called "host organism" [12].

In addition, resident microorganisms are not just bacteria: fungi, phages and even viruses definitely belong to the microbiota broadly intended and constitute some of its new genuine subdivisions.

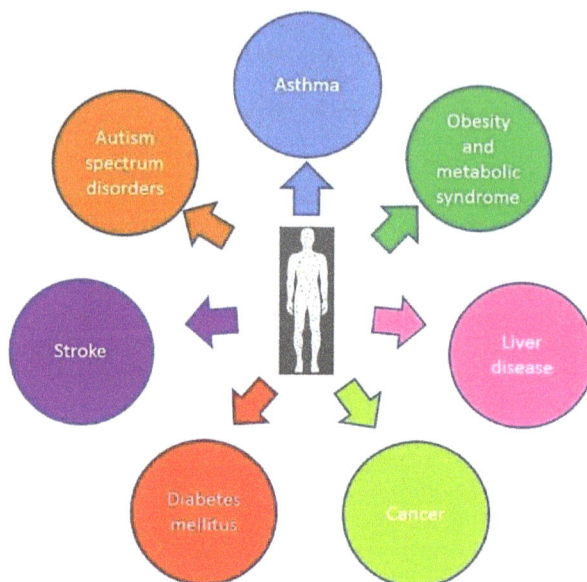

Figure 1. Different Human diseases correlated with the gut microbiome. We have reported some of the medical conditions where the experimental data suggest a direct involvement of gut microbiome in development.

Finally an important caveat. The growing number of studies on the microbiota has generated many hopes, expectations but also a sort of *explanatory hype*, that would make the microbiota the new keystone for the understanding of otherwise unexplainable phenomena [13]. This vision is not only simplistic and reductive but also dangerous. The difficulty in establishing causal directions and priorities in biology suggests caution and urges us to consider the growing impact of studies on the microbiota in another light. Microbiota is indeed central but is a pivotal element among others. Therefore, in describing and reporting the theoretical proposals concerning the study and understanding of the microbiota, it is necessary to remember how the increasing interest on it should not be taken as privileged one compared to others. Rather, new perspectives on it should be seen as a way to build new systemic approaches (in which, for example, human and microbial genetics are considered more closely related). Hopefully, these systemic approaches would provide a more refined and adequate basis for personalized medicine

2. Composition and Microbiota Status

Due to computational methods, such as metagenomic sequencing [14], it is now possible to assess the genetic contribution of bacteria to host's activities and to obtain a better (although still not exhaustive and incomplete) estimation of microbial population. To the most recent status of knowledge, microbial community is constituted by a biomass of 1.5–2.0 kg, mainly composed by anaerobic *Bacteria* [6]. According to recent reviews [6,15] the most represented phyla are *Actinobacteria, Bacteroidetes, Firmicutes, Proteobacteria* and *Verrucomicrobia*. The composition diversity and the balance between different phyla and populations (among and within phyla) may differ from the different subjects. Nevertheless, these differences, maybe in distinct ways and by distinct means, see some key functions preserved (such as degradation of some chemicals) in order to display and maintain "normal and physiological conditions." However, it is always very hard to determine what is "normal" in a biological sense. A thing that might be unfeasible for an individual, could be on average for another one. As a matter of fact, the complex relationship existing between microbial interactions and composition and other factors (such as, among the others, the human immune system) is a key factor to determine not just a more adequate notion of *health* in general but, also, a more adequate notion of *"personal health"* (*i.e.*, its unique conditions). Moreover, as already mentioned, microbiota cannot be reduced or restricted to anaerobic Bacteria. The very same development of sequencing technologies revealed that other organisms, less investigated, might have a (more or less impactful) role in this complex network of interactions. For instance, the term "Mycobiota" [16] has been then coined to address the fungal component (most of the time composed by not culturable strains) of the general microbiota. Similar studies have started to be conducted concerning *viral* genomes [17], sometimes defined as "Virome").

In addition, one must not forget that biological landscapes as such are shaped by the interaction with the environment. This does not refer just to general, external conditions (*e.g.*, the pH) but of course, involve both dietary and life style habits of the "host" and its genome/epigenome. Both commensal and non-commensal organisms (among the same or different population and phyla) can either collaborate or compete to niche construction/shape creating a true, intricate *ecosystem*. If we embrace the perspective of the human body as an "ecosystem," then ecological/relational categories and new theoretical tools [18,19] will be needed to correctly address this picture (potentially modifying or updating the notion of health itself).

As a consequence of the microbiota importance in all the aforementioned aspects of humans biology, several scholars and scientists have elaborated new ways and proposals to adequately address this archetype. In this review we want to examine these different proposals (from the *missing organ hypothesis* to the *polygenomic organism*), which have been developed with the purpose of elaborating conceptual tools that could account for the current developments of scientific investigations. In fact, some of the last recent research directions have highlighted that central concepts of contemporary biology such as organism, organ, symbiosis and so forth, seem to be no longer perfectly adequate, given the time of their formulation, to account for the latest findings and discoveries produced by experimental work. This set of theoretical elaborations, which we will briefly present here, appears central and actually responds to a twofold movement. On the one hand, as mentioned, new concepts are necessary in order to be able to describe and substantiate, more accurately, the new types of phenomena that research discovers. On the other hand, a new conceptual and theoretical equipment is precisely what makes the discovery and classification of new phenomena possible.

3. Microbiota: the Missing Organ

Due to its relevance for human health and physiology, some researchers have proposed to refer to microbiota as a "missing organ" of human body [20–23]. Far from being just an analogy or a working metaphor, these authors declare that there are strong reasons to look at microbiota as a true organ. From a functionalist perspective, it is argued that human constitution is already made by interactions with cells of different types (and subtypes), displaying diverse, type-associated, activities.

Moreover, the investigation into the formation of eukaryotic cells strongly suggests a relationship with *mitochondrial* origin and evolution. Famously, mitochondria are sub-cellular organelles essentially to provide chemical energy (in the form of ATP) to eukaryotic cells. Nevertheless, in recent years, it has been shown that mitochondria are also involved in other, crucial, cellular activities, such as metabolism of both amino acids and nucleotides, fatty-acid assimilation, protein synthesis, forms of programmed cell death (*e.g.,* apoptosis) and the regulation of various homeostatic factors [24]. However, the fascinating detail is that phylogenetic analyses indicate mitochondria having a prokaryotic origin, thus showing that a fundamental eukaryotic cell compartment has an endosymbiotic provenance. The presence of elements, once exogenous, in the constitution of eukaryotic organisms, should make us reflect on the notions of "identity" and "unity" of biological entities. Accordingly, it should not be strange to look at microbiota as a legitimate part of "humans" as organisms (this somehow implies that if we want to adopt the elusive notion of "human nature," the microbiota would definitely contribute to it).

The property of being an *organism* (a central notion in biology [25] is generally associated with the capacity of reproducing within a given specific lineage. *Homo sapiens* (whose genome includes also mitochondrial genome) lineage is notoriously transmitted by vertical descent. However, as recently highlighted, the transmission of the human microbiota to the progeny can also occur through other modalities, less specific but still reproducible. In this way there is the possibility of inheriting a microbiota constituted by a coherent base, specified into inter-individual variations, which are preserved throughout the generations inside a parental line [20]. From this perspective, the various forms of physical-chemical interactions between microbiota and its "host" are so deep-rooted and integrated, that considering microbiota as merely external, just because of the genomic differences, seems, at least, questionable. First, the human genome itself displays the *vestiges* (now fully part of what we call "human") of past infections and interactions with other organisms (such as the famous Human Endogenous Retro Viruses - HERVs) [26]. Second, the magnitude of activities of the microbiota itself can be genuinely seen comparable to those of a traditional organ [23]. This is also why other authors [27] have proposed to classify (with an eye towards possible manipulation/modification for biomedical purposes in the light of health problems) microbial populations according to *functional criteria* (rather than just phylogenetical). This type of move, not free of problems [28], is somehow motivated by the need of finding how (*e.g.*, in which ways and how much) microbial activity contributes to host functionality despite the distinct genomic origins.

If this is the case, further studies might have the potential to revolutionize entire areas of clinical investigations and the rationale of many health-care strategies. Indeed, certain future therapeutic interventions could be directed to the "new physiological" pathways. Drugs could be designed to address interactions within the "missing organ" itself or with the other ones. As some researchers argue, if medicine has historically been developed through specialties based on organs or organ systems (think of cardiology, pneumology or gastroenterology), it would not be strange to think of a future development of a specific branch such as "microbiomology" or "clinical microbiology." Such a specialty, starting from the consideration of the structure of the microbiota as an actual organ, would study its physiology and pathology, keeping an eye to its relevance both in diagnostics and preventive medicine. [20].

4. Beyond the Symbiosis and The Missing Organ: the "Holobiont"

By considering the countless interactions between the host and its microbiota (however differently composed) either as a symbiosis or as a relationship between an organism and one of its organs is still far from a radical conceptual change that some scientists are proposing in addressing these issues.

As already mentioned in the introduction, a completely distinct view that challenges both the theoretical and the experimental side is constituted by the notions of *holobiont* and *hologenome*. According to this perspective [3], we should stop at seeing symbiosis as an interaction (no matter how complex or peculiar) of different organisms (such as the "host" and its commensal associated species) but rather as a complex unity of biological organization (as much as the organism itself) that should be considered as the privileged one. The specificity of this viewpoint is that, contrary to the traditional notion of symbiosis, which is basically an extension of the current understanding concerning these phenomena, the notions of *holobiont* and *hologenome* challenge the contemporary conceptual view. They do so by offering not just a different angle from which one should look at these phenomena but a deconstruction of the categories according to which we consider those "things," precisely our phenomena on interest (*i.e.*, the system we want to investigate). Moreover, such a change of prospect will inevitably provide different categories and, as a consequence of that, a different experimental possibilities. As François Jacob famously argued, the work of the biologist necessarily starts with the choice of an operative framework, defined as the "experimental system." According to

Jacob, all depends from this initial decision: the type of experiments that can be conducted but also the type of legitimate hypotheses that can be formulated and therefore also the type of answers the scientist can obtain [29]. According to this sense, due to their hybrid nature (in between organisms and communities) [30], holobionts and hologenomes might have the potential to become a "New System."

Bordenstein and Theis [3] also provide a list of key points in order to clarify the holobiont perspective and to avoid misconceptions about it.

First, as already mentioned, holobionts and hologenomes can be seen as units of biological organization. This immediately embeds an ecological perspective in the study of molecular interactions. Being a unit of biological organization means to understand that organisms do not exist in isolation. From a functional point of view, their existence, development, evolution are intrinsically shaped by the reciprocal interaction and by the relation with the environment (both organic and not organic). For instance, one can see a virus as simply as a sequence of either DNA or RNA within a protein capsid. But from a different viewpoint, let us call it a *processual view*, the perspective of biological organization around units formed by different organisms and their genomes, that virus is now a part of interconnected system to which it will contribute in terms of physiology, development, function or dysfunction.

Second, it is important not to mistake holobionts and hologenomes for organs, super-organisms or metagenomes. Indeed, on one hand, organs and super-organisms both share the same genomes, while on the other, the term metagenome simply states that there is something more than the genome but clearly does not take into account the interactive/organismic/ecological perspective, which is at the core of holobiont and hologenome conceptualization (as the "disunity" of the holobiont brings important features as much as its unity [30]).

Third, the netlike nature of hologenome suggests that all the genomes involved should be considered. Moreover, being hologenomes a multiplicity of genomes (nuclei, organelles, bacteria, fungi and viruses), variations and mutations can occur at any level of the network and might have an impact on the entire organizational unit. In addition, since such units could be the target of evolutionary change, this change in perspective might also affect our perception and conceptualization of the evolutionary process itself. This should not be taken in a radical, superficial or simplistic way, meaning that we need to abort the *evolutionary theory*. Rather, both hologenomes and holobionts challenge a particular interpretation of evolutionary change, the so-called "neo Darwinian framework," which neglects any form of plasticity or porosity within the genome itself. On the contrary, by adopting a view closer to, the so called, "extended synthesis" [31,32], both inheritance and different forms of genetic transmissions such as horizontal gene transfer [2] (which is now documented also between prokaryotes and eukaryotes) as well as the incorporation of environmental elements, should be now fully considered.

5. Holobionts, Faecal Transplantation and Bacteriotherapy.

The holobiont perspective is particularly intriguing (and challenging) when specific therapeutic interventions concerning the microbiota are considered. Nowadays, Faecal Microbiota Transplantation (FMT) is a quite established therapeutic intervention, famously adopted to treat infection with *Clostridium difficile* [33,34] In the wake of this success, it has been suggested that the microbiota could be seen and adopted as a real therapy, a *bacteriotherapy* [33], also in other pathological conditions. Again, from a conceptual point of view, this approach poses this type of intervention as a hybrid, in between "organ transplantation" and "immunotherapy."

From the holobiont perspective the possibility to use microbiota as a therapy (and a personalized one, see also section 8) can be seen as a way to re-establish/reinforce either the structure or the efficiency of a network whose functionality and shape are at core of the global health of the system. Thus, several approaches may be adopted to pursue this scope (mimicking traditional strategies). On the one hand, dietary and lifestyle interventions (*e.g.* probiotics, prebiotics, other nutraceutical compounds) can directly modulate the composition and the functionality of microbiota [35–38]. Other approaches involve a genetic manipulation of microbiota itself [36,39,40]. In this case the idea is to use genetically modified strains of bacteria in order not only to act as ad hoc therapy but also in the preventive phase, as tools to diagnose specific pathologies. By trying to intervene on the network (*i.e.*, intervening on the holobiont), this approach has the potential of being more effective, more coordinated and, at the same time, less invasive and less expensive compared to current methods [39].

However, despite the coherence of the hypothesis, the novelty of the field and the consequent lack of knowledge both pose some difficulties that cannot be forgotten. As a matter of fact, an increasing number of studies do suggest that the microbiota is directly involved in the metabolic syndrome, showing a role in determining key factors such as insulin resistance or blood pressure [33]. Nonetheless, at the moment, only few researches show sufficiently robust data to legitimize a direct causal link (on which researchers and clinicians might operate). Therefore, some researchers have highlighted the need to investigate these relationships through new studies (including RTCs) that require greater attention to the specific bacterial strains involved, to the changes in their metabolites, trying to clarify how the genetic and epigenetic aspects of the microbiota and the host will influence each other (of course the relationship with the immune system is central here) [10,13,33].

Moreover, as recently reported and coherently with the holobiont perspective, the microbiota appears to be deeply personalized, showing a high inter-variability among different subjects (also, due to dietary diversities, showing variations among cultures and geographical regions) and important fluctuations during diverse phases of the day [13]. In addition, in case of genetically engineered microbiota, despite their designed precision, the impact of their introduction on the entire network (with possible unwanted effects) still needs to be fully addressed and evaluated.Nevertheless, these difficulties should not discourage further scientific investigations. In the recent years we have understood that the interactions between the elements and the components of that system that is our organism (and on this see also section 6) are more complex than we thought. At the same time, this awareness shows us the need for a new systemic viewpoint (and the limitation of purely reductionist approaches). The fact that many aspects of this perspective are still obscure is precisely a reason to conduct more research into it.

6. The Polygenomic Organism

The increasing interest towards microbiota and its interactions (whose modalities are still widely unknown) and the rise of new concepts such as holobionts and hologenomes (to deal with the netlike nature of these phenomena) urge us to critically address the notion of organism itself which was already at the centre of conceptual change in biology [25,41]. However, this is not because of a highly theoretical, speculative exercise (that, nevertheless, will be interesting in itself). Rather, by reconsidering fundamental notions at the core of the theoretical apparatus we adopt to deal with disease and health we might find new ways to approach issues that really matter from a practical point of view.

A first way to challenge the current concept of organism is the assumption of individual *genetic homogeneity*. According to some scholars this idea is decidedly deceptive. In fact, such a view constitutes the basis of a series of misunderstandings concerning the characteristics of those systemic entities, usually called as "organisms [42].

The first critical element of genetic homogeneity is understanding that in both natural and artificial processes we see a significant degree of chimerism and mosaicism in many, not to say almost all, multicellular organisms, including humans. The degree of similarity in this context seems to be fuzzier than previously described. Therefore one may argue that the hypothesis according to which every cell of an organism has the same genome of another one could be, at least, an oversimplification of a more intricate picture [42].

A second layer is constituted by *epigenetics*. Epigenetics has shown that, even if genomes of cells within an organism will be somehow homogeneous in their constitution, the way in which genes and other functional elements of a genome are expressed is far from being the same. Rather, such a diversity in expression and regulation provides also an explanation of different cell types [42].

By following these suggestions, it is possible to conceive that entities we classify as living unities might not be those identified by our traditional notion of species and organisms. For instance, the phenomenon of chimerism challenges our ideas about the consistency of organisms themselves. Moreover and maybe more dramatically, the profound interactions and interconnections among living beings normally considered members of the different species or lineages. Of course, the change of perspective is not meant to determine which should be the right way to divide and classify the living world. Rather, it suggests that different approaches might reveal connections and causal relations that may result intrinsically hidden, according to other ways of partitioning the living world.

As is well argued by Dupré, the different elements of a cell can "co-operate" in a rather complex way. In some cases, the combination of different communities of different species of microorganisms gives rise to real diversified and separate lineages (such as mitochondria). In other cases, the cooperation characterizes phenomena of even higher complexity (the case of multicellular organisms) and we face real *systemic units*, composed of different entities, interacting together in a synergistic way. A situation so complex and articulated between cooperative and competitive processes, will also require that different research interests, bearers of different questions, would be and should be prosecuted. It is not bizarre to think that such research directions will produce new ways of delimiting and distinguishing biological individuals and their boundaries, or at least to believe they will deeply question those currently employed [42].

7. Microbiota and Health: the Ecological Perspective and New Research Directions

If we take all these perspective seriously, it is hard not to believe that they are going to affect other notions, central to both research and clinical investigation. If the notion of biological individual will be modified (or at least updated), also the concept of health itself may face a radical change. In other words, if we move from the conception of individuals as *punctiform units* to the view that what we call individuals are rather *peculiar intertwined networks*, or sophisticated micro-ecosystems, the idea of health seems to acquire a more ecological nuance [43], also suggesting a complex system of *health levels* in which that individual health cannot be fully detached from "healthy conditions" of other layers into play.

This is not just in theory. In the last years, several promising, interdisciplinary approaches have been developed to translate an ecological perspective into research and clinical practices. For instance, in the case of cancer, increasing studies suggest how it should be considered as a multifactorial disease [44,45]. This is due to the fact that a large number of endogenous and exogenous factors (such as diet, exposure to certain environments, lifestyles) and their peculiar (most of the time *personalized*) combination, can give rise to the conditions for the development of the disease.

In this respect, immunotherapy represents a promising action line. However, if the microbiota is actually considered as a functional part of the immune system itself and thus, the immune response is a network-based, environmental feature, the ecological perspective becomes central in analyzing the immune response in the tumour microenvironment [45]. Moreover, if we embrace a network perspective on health (such as the holobiont view) the distinction of exogenous and endogenous becomes less neat and less sharp.

The emerging field of *molecular pathological epidemiology* (MPE) constitutes a promising research agenda in this direction, by creating a hybrid field between pathology and data science [46,47]. This approach promotes a view that combines various potential risk factors (the epidemiological point of view) with molecular pathology [47]. Accordingly, any disease can be phenotyped, based on pathogenic mechanisms. A research based on MPE can determine a better understanding of pathogenic landscape and evaluate how an association is depth and intense for given subtypes. Unlike traditional epidemiological research, this approach may help detecting causal connections [46]. This is particularly relevant, given that microbiota's activities and functions, by playing potential diverse (protective or risk) factors, can be finally seen in the web of causal connections, thus determining the overall health status of the network.

Given the current scope of personalized/precision biomedicine in treating the individual, rather than disease, the transformation foreseen here may also change the strategies we adopt in dealing with a various number of pathologies, still not fully curable or treatable.

8. Precision Medicine/Personalized Medicine: the Individual and the System

In the last years, the health care system has rapidly changed. Both newspapers and specialized press report and hail the new era of personalized, stratified, person-centred, precision medicine (Figure 2). Indeed, these expressions are often used interchangeably [48]. This semantic blurriness [49] mirrors economic, institutional solutions and approaches, aiming at the establishment of a new paradigm for health care systems.

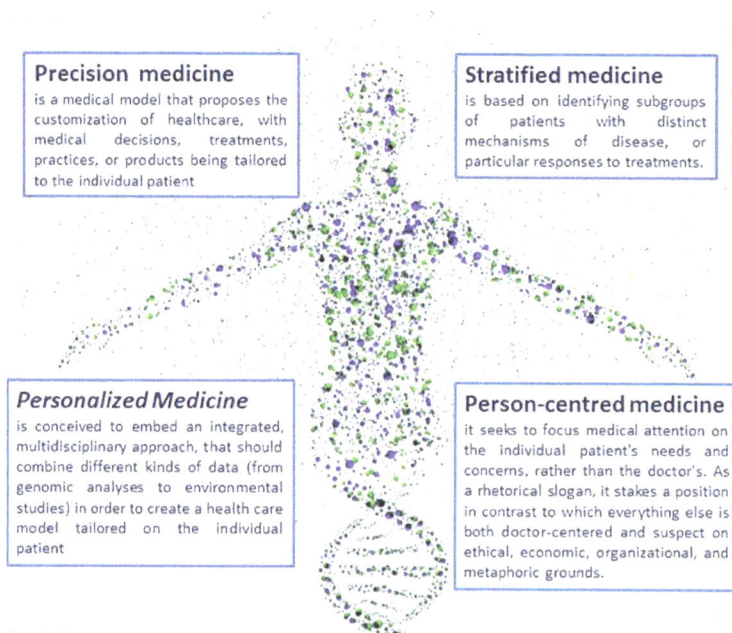

Precision medicine
is a medical model that proposes the customization of healthcare, with medical decisions, treatments, practices, or products being tailored to the individual patient

Stratified medicine
is based on identifying subgroups of patients with distinct mechanisms of disease, or particular responses to treatments.

Personalized Medicine
is conceived to embed an integrated, multidisciplinary approach, that should combine different kinds of data (from genomic analyses to environmental studies) in order to create a health care model tailored on the individual patient

Person-centred medicine
it seeks to focus medical attention on the individual patient's needs and concerns, rather than the doctor's. As a rhetorical slogan, it stakes a position in contrast to which everything else is both doctor-centered and suspect on ethical, economic, organizational, and metaphoric grounds.

Figure 2. Definition of personalized, stratified, person-centred, precision medicine. We have fine defined these expressions that are often used interchangeably.

Spanning from the molecular understanding of biological phenomena to the implement of computational resources to study the general behaviour of living systems, *precision medicine* is normally conceived to embed an integrated, multidisciplinary approach, that should combine different kinds of data (from genomic analyses to environmental studies) in order to create a health care model tailored on the individual patient [50]. On the other hand, new approaches and techniques have fostered the division of population into many subgroups, which eventually need different and specific treatments (the so-called stratified medicine), thus paving the way to the decomposition of the universality of human kind, into a myriad of unique variants that will be able to detect individual specificities and therapeutically address them: personalized medicine.

Despite this terminological struggle, what is at stake here is the individuation of those features that contribute to the creation of medical model that should be more *predictive*, more *preventive* and more *personalised* (also in the sense of paying more attention to those aspects, cultural, ethical and psychological, often neglected by the clinic dimension). Therefore, a Predictive, Preventive and Personalised Medicine (PPPM) [50] will try to focus on diverse layers and aspects that contribute to dissect the notions of individual, health and disease and relative interventions. Thus, according to this perspective, both genetics and epigenetics, life style and related activities (such as diet and sport), socio-economic conditions, cultural belonging and psychological setting (all elements on which the impact of microbiota can be critical and cannot be mistreated) should all receive full consideration in a commonly framed manner [50]. Moreover, other aspects such as translational research, information technology and public dissemination of scientific and clinical results, biolaw and education will take part into the new model.

At first glance big data analyses granted by computational/omics methods seem to go in the direction of fostering this approach through the capacity to deal with data and information coming from various sources. However the situation might not be so optimistic. The case of precision oncology is somehow emblematic. In a recent issue on Nature, the haemato-oncologist Vinay Prasad has revealed that a large number of cancer patients has not benefited from the so-called precision medicine. Although the genome of a large number of patients (tens of thousands) has been already sequenced, the number of interesting or significative cases remains extremely low. Moreover, this approach does not seem to have shown that it can improve the results in controlled studies. Therefore precision oncology remains, as such, an approach still waiting to be corroborated and established [51]. How is it so?

Here of course we cannot and should not provide a technical answer. However it seems that profiling patients, in the light of precision/personalized medicine approaches, does not provide what has been thought to promise, probably due to the fact that the "complexity" of a patient's individuality (affecting also its clinical condition) may not and cannot be simply reduced to the collection of its data (or represented by it), no matter how much precise and rigorous such analysis can be. This is not to say that computational strategies employed by precision-oncology are useless. On the contrary, beside the information they provide concerning human genetic variants and stratification, they were also extremely important in revealing that personalization of healthcare (both in terms of precision and consideration of specific patient needs) cannot be done simply by enlarging the amount of data nor the sources of data. The determinants of individual health, which contribute to the specific identity of a single patient, cannot be fully and correctly understood just in terms of omics analysis.

By considering what has been said, it seems that biomedicine is facing a sort of paradox. On the one hand, both scientific understanding and patients' needs push towards a focus on the individual. On the other hand, research findings suggest that the decomposition of biological phenomena and their (so-called) reductionist analysis are only methodological and require more and more a systemic perspective in order to be adequately addressed and explained [52]. In addition, not only does traditional medical taxonomy (organ based) seem no longer suitable to fully appreciate the novelties of current scientific understanding of disease and health (and thus the potential therapies) [53] but the patient themselves, the biological entities that are the biomedicine focus, cannot longer be seen just as single units or "monads," bottom-layers of individualization.

In this respect, we propose that the advancement of the studies on the microbiota (both conceptual and empirical) may suggest a way to reconcile diverse perspectives and somehow to "solve" the paradox. Indeed, by looking at individual patients as networks of different but nevertheless fundamental, components it could be possible to start thinking and designing new systemic approaches for therapy that will be tailored but not reductionist. By forcing us to see human beings as ecosystems, these studies will help, somehow surprisingly, to better understand the individual patient and, at the same time, they will fully acknowledge that those individuals are also, by some means, a "multitude."

Author Contributions: A.A. and F.B. equally contributed to the article's conception and design; F.B. drafted the manuscript and A.A. revised it critically and gave the approval of the version to be published.

Funding: This research was funded by Toscana Region grant number: FAS2014 and Foundation 'Ente Cassa di Risparmio di Firenze: ex60%2017."

Acknowledgments: The research was founded with a grant from the regional contribution of "The Programma Attuativo Regionale (Toscana)" funded by FAS (now FSC) - MICpROBIMM and the Foundation 'Ente Cassa di Risparmio di Firenze.' The authors thank the Edda Russo for the support on the realization of figures.

Conflicts of Interest: The authors declare no conflict of interest.

References

1. Dupré, J. In defence of classification. *Stud. Hist. Phil. Biol. Biomed. Sci.* **2001**, *32*, 203–219. [CrossRef]
2. Husnik, F.; McCutcheon, J.P. Functional horizontal gene transfer from bacteria to eukaryotes. *Nat. Rev. Microbiol* **2018**, *16*, 67–79. [CrossRef] [PubMed]
3. Bordenstein, S.R.; Theis, K.R. Host biology in light of the microbiome: Ten principles of holobionts and hologenomes. *PLoS Biology* **2015**, *13*, 1–23. [CrossRef] [PubMed]
4. Ursell, L.K.; Metcalf, J.L.; Parfrey, L.W.; Knight, R. Defining the human microbiome. *Nutrition Reviews* **2012**, *70*, 69–82. [CrossRef] [PubMed]
5. Cani, P.D. Human gut microbiome: Hopes, threats and promises. *Gut* **2018**, *0*, 1–10. [CrossRef] [PubMed]
6. Schroeder, B.O.; Bäckhed, F. Signals from the gut microbiota to distant organs in physiology and disease. *Nat. Med.* **2016**, *22*, 1079–1089. [CrossRef] [PubMed]
7. Tremlett, H.; Bauer, K.C.; Appel-Cresswell, S.; Finlay, B.B.; Waubant, E. The gut microbiome in human neurological disease: A. review. *Ann. Neurol.* **2017**, *81*, 369–382. [CrossRef] [PubMed]
8. Russo, E.; Taddei, A.; Ringressi, M.N.; Ricci, F.; Amedei, A. The interplay between the microbiome and the adaptive immune response in cancer development. *Therap. Adv. Gastroenterol* **2016**, *9*, 594–605. [CrossRef] [PubMed]
9. Russo, E.; Bacci, G.; Chiellini, C.; Fagorzi, C.; Niccolai, E.; Taddei, A.; Ricci, F.; Ringressi, M.N.; Borrelli, R.; Melli, F.; et al. Preliminary comparison of oral and intestinal human microbiota in patients with colorectal cancer: A. pilot study. *Front Microbiol* **2018**, *8*, 2699. [CrossRef] [PubMed]
10. Belkaid, Y.; Hand, T.W. Role of the microbiota in immunity and inflammation. *Cell* **2014**, *1*, 15–24. [CrossRef] [PubMed]
11. Johnson, K.V.A.; Foster, K.R. Why does the microbiome affect behaviour? *Nat. Rev. Microbiol.* **2018**, *16*, 647–655. [CrossRef] [PubMed]
12. Schwiertz, A. Microbiota of the Human Body. A. Schwiertz, 1st ed. Springer International Publishing Switzerland; 2016.
13. Zmora, N.; Zeevi, D.; Korem, T.; Segal, E.; Elinav, E. Taking it Personally: Personalized Utilization of the Human Microbiome in Health and Disease. *Cell. Host. Microbe.* **2016**, *19*, 12–20. [CrossRef] [PubMed]
14. Qin, J.; Li, R.; Raes, J.; Arumugam, M.; Burgdorf, K.S.; Manichanh, C.; Nielsen, T.; Pons, N.; Levenez, F.; Yamada, T.; Mende, D.R.; et al. A human gut microbial gene catalogue established by metagenomic sequencing. *Nature* **2010**, *464*, 59–65. [CrossRef] [PubMed]
15. Tap, J.; Mondot, S.; Levenez, F.; Pelletier, E.; Caron, C.; Furet, J.P.; Ugarte, E.; Muñoz-Tamayo, R.; Paslier, D.L.; Nalin, R.; et al. Towards the human intestinal microbiota phylogenetic core. *Environ Microbiol.* **2009**, *11*, 2574–2584. [CrossRef] [PubMed]
16. Sam, Q.H.; Chang, M.W.; Chai, L.Y.A. The fungal mycobiome and its interaction with gut bacteria in the host. *Int. J. Mol. Sci.* **2017**, *18*, 330. [CrossRef] [PubMed]
17. Grasis, J.A. The intra-dependence of viruses and the holobiont. *Front. Immunol.* **2017**, *8*, 1501. [CrossRef] [PubMed]
18. Costello, E.K.; Stagaman, K.; Dethlefsen, L.; Bohannan, B.J.M.; Relman, D.A. The application of ecological theory toward an understanding of the human microbiome. *Science* **2012**, *336*, 1255–1262. [CrossRef] [PubMed]
19. Swiatczak, B.; Cohen, I.R. Gut feelings of safety: Tolerance to the microbiota mediated by innate immune receptors. *Microbiol Immunol.* **2015**, *59*, 573–585. [CrossRef] [PubMed]
20. Baquero, F.; Nombela, C. The microbiome as a human organ. *Clin. Microbiol Infect* **2002**, *18*, 2–4. [CrossRef] [PubMed]
21. Clarke, G.; Stilling, R.M.; Kennedy, P.J.; Stanton, C.; Cryan, J.F.; Dinan, T.G. Minireview: Gut Microbiota: The Neglected Endocrine Organ. *Mol. Endocrinol* **2014**, *28*, 1221–1238. [CrossRef] [PubMed]
22. Evans, J.M.; Morris, L.S.; Marchesi, J.R. The gut microbiome: The role of a virtual organ in the endocrinology of the host. *J. Endocrinol* **2013**, *218*, 37–47. [CrossRef] [PubMed]
23. O'Hara, A.M.; Shanahan, F. The gut flora as a forgotten organ. *EMBO Rep.* **2006**, *7*, 688–693. [CrossRef] [PubMed]

24. Roger, A.J.; Muñoz-Gómez, S.A.; Kamikawa, R. The Origin and Diversification of Mitochondria. *Curr. Biol.* **2017**, *27*, 1177–1192. [CrossRef] [PubMed]

25. Nicholson, D.J. The return of the organism as a fundamental explanatory concept in biology. *Philosophy Compass* **2014**, *9*, 347–359. [CrossRef]

26. Herrera, R.J.; Lowery, R.K.; Alfonso, A.; McDonald, J.F.; Luis, J.R. Ancient retroviral insertions among human populations. *J. Hum. Genet.* **2006**, *51*, 353–362. [CrossRef] [PubMed]

27. Rosen, C.E.; Palm, N.W. Functional Classification of the Gut Microbiota: The Key to Cracking the Microbiota Composition Code: Functional classifications of the gut microbiota reveal previously hidden contributions of indigenous gut bacteria to human health and disease. *BioEssays* **2017**, *39*, 1–12. [CrossRef] [PubMed]

28. Inkpen, S.A.; Douglas, G.M.; Brunet, T.D.P.; Leuschen, K.; Doolittle, W.F.; Langille, M.G.I. The coupling of taxonomy and function in microbiomes. *Biology Philosophy* **2017**, *32*, 1225–1243. [CrossRef]

29. Jacob, F. *La statue intérieure*; Editions Odile Jacob: Paris, 1987.

30. Skillings, D. Holobionts and the ecology of organisms: Multi-species communities or integrated individuals? *Biology Philosophy* **2016**, *31*, 875–892. [CrossRef]

31. Müller, G.B. Why an extended evolutionary synthesis is necessary. *Interface Focus* **2017**, *7*, 20170015. [CrossRef] [PubMed]

32. Pigliucci, M.; Müller, G.B. *Evolution, the extended synthesis*; MIT Press: Cambridge, MA, 2010.

33. de Groot, P.F.; Frissen, M.N.; de Clercq, N.C.; Nieuwdorp, M. Fecal microbiota transplantation in metabolic syndrome: History, present and future. *Gut Microbes* **2017**, *8*, 253–267.

34. Gupta, S.; Allen-Vercoe, E.; Petrof, E.O. Fecal microbiota transplantation: In perspective. *Therapeutic Advances Gastroenterology* **2016**, *9*, 229–239. [CrossRef] [PubMed]

35. Catinean, A. Neag, M.A. Muntean, D.M. Bocsan, I.C.; Buzoianu, A.D. An overview on the interplay between nutraceuticals and gut microbiota. *Peer J.* **2018**, *6*, e4465. [CrossRef] [PubMed]

36. Fuentes, S.; de Vos, W.M. How to Manipulate the Microbiota: Fecal Microbiota Transplantation. In *Microbiota of the Human Body. Advances in Experimental Medicine and Biology*; Springer: New York, NY, USA, 2016.

37. Marchesi, J.R.; Adams, D.H.; Fava, F.; Hermes, G.D.A.; Hirschfield, G.M.; Hold, G.; Hart, A. The gut microbiota and host health: A new clinical frontier. *Gut* **2016**, *65*, 330–339. [CrossRef] [PubMed]

38. Varankovich, N.V.; Nickerson, M.T.; Korber, D.R. Probiotic-based strategies for therapeutic and prophylactic use against multiple gastrointestinal diseases. *Frontiers Microbiology* **2015**, *6*, 1–14. [CrossRef] [PubMed]

39. Landry, B.P.; Tabor, J.J. Engineering Diagnostic and Therapeutic Gut Bacteria. *Microbiology Spectrum* **2017**, *5*, 1–22. [CrossRef] [PubMed]

40. Takiishi, T.; Cook, D.P.; Korf, H.; Sebastiani, G.; Mancarella, F.; Cunha, J.P.M.C.M.; Mathieu, C. Reversal of diabetes in NOD Mice by clinical-grade proinsulin and IL-10′secreting lactococcus lactis in combination with low-dose Anti-CD3 depends on the induction of Foxp3-Positive, T. Cells. *Diabetes* **2017**, *66*, 448–459. [CrossRef] [PubMed]

41. Nicholson, D.J. The machine conception of the organism in development andevolution: A. critical analysis. *Stud. Hist. Phil. Biol. Biomed Sci.* **2014**, *48*, 162–174. [CrossRef] [PubMed]

42. Dupré, J. The Polygenomic Organism. *The Sociological Review.* **2010**, *58*, 19–31. [CrossRef]

43. Mallee, H. The evolution of health as an ecological concept. *Curr. Opin. Environ Sustain* **2017**, *25*, 28–32. [CrossRef]

44. Olsen, J.; Overvad, K. The Concept of Multifactorial Etiology of Cancer. *Pharmacology Toxicology* **1993**, *72*, 33–38. [CrossRef] [PubMed]

45. Ramón y Cajal, S.; Capdevila, C.; Hernandez-Losa, J.; de Mattos, L.; Ghosh, A.; Lorent, J.; Topisirovic, I. Cancer as an ecomolecular disease and a neoplastic consortium. Biochimica et Biophysica Acta. *Rev. Cancer.* **2017**, *46*, 159–165.

46. Ogino, S.; Nowak, J.A.; Hamada, T.; Milner, D.A.; Nishihara, R. Insights into Pathogenic Interactions Among Environment, Host and Tumor at the Crossroads of Molecular Pathology and Epidemiology. *Annual Rev. Pathology* **2018**, *2018*, 83–103.

47. Ogino, S.; Nowak, J.A.; Hamada, T.; Phipps, A.I.; Peters, U.; Milner, D.A.; Song, M. Integrative analysis of exogenous, endogenous, tumour and immune factors for precision medicine. *Gut* **2018**, *67*, 1168–1180. [CrossRef] [PubMed]

48. Jameson, J.L.; Longo, D.L. Precision Medicine — Personalized, Problematic and Promising. *N Engl. J. Med.* **2015**, *372*, 2229–2234. [CrossRef] [PubMed]

49. De Grandis, G.; Halgunset, V. Conceptual and terminological confusion around personalised medicine: A. coping strategy. *BMC Medical Ethics* **2016**, *17*, 1–12. [CrossRef] [PubMed]

50. Golubnitschaja, O.; Baban, B.; Boniolo, G.; Wang, W.; Bubnov, R.; Kapalla, M.; Krapfenbauer, K.; Mozaffari, M.S.; Costigliola, V. Medicine in the early twenty-first century: Paradigm and anticipation - EPMA position paper 2016. *EPMA J.* **2016**, *7*, 1–13. [CrossRef] [PubMed]

51. Prasad, V. The precision-oncology illusion. *Nature* **2016**, *537*, S63. [CrossRef] [PubMed]

52. Federoff, H.J.; Gostin, L.O. Evolving from reductionism to holism: Is there a future for systems medicine? *JAMA* **2009**, *302*, 302,994–996. [CrossRef] [PubMed]

53. Baumbach, J.; Schmidt, H.H.H.W. The End of Medicine as We Know It: Introduction to the New Journal, Systems Medicine. *Systems Medicine* **2018**, *1*, 1–4. [CrossRef]

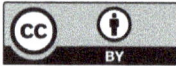

International Journal of
Molecular Sciences

MDPI

Review

Dysbiosis Disrupts Gut Immune Homeostasis and Promotes Gastric Diseases

Devinder Toor [1,†], Mishi Kaushal Wasson [1,†], Prashant Kumar [1], G. Karthikeyan [1], Naveen Kumar Kaushik [1], Chhavi Goel [1], Sandhya Singh [2], Anil Kumar [3] and Hridayesh Prakash [1,*]

[1]   Amity Institute of Virology and Immunology, Amity University, Sector 125,
Noida 201313, Uttar Pradesh, India; dtoor@amity.edu (D.T.); mwasson@amity.edu (M.K.W.);
pkumar18@amity.edu (P.K.); gkarthikeyan@amity.edu (G.K.); nkkaushik@amity.edu (N.K.K.);
cgoel@amity.edu (C.G.)
[2]   Department of Animal Biology, School of Life Sciences, University of Hyderabad,
Hyderabad 500046, Telengana, India; sandhya_singh1@yahoo.com
[3]   National Institute of Immunology, Aruna Asaf Ali Marg, New Delhi 110067, India; anilk@nii.ac.in
*   Correspondence: hprakash@amity.edu; Tel.: +(0)91-120-4392961
†   These authors contributed equally.

Received: 26 March 2019; Accepted: 19 April 2019; Published: 16 May 2019

Abstract: Perturbation in the microbial population/colony index has harmful consequences on human health. Both biological and social factors influence the composition of the gut microbiota and also promote gastric diseases. Changes in the gut microbiota manifest in disease progression owing to epigenetic modification in the host, which in turn influences differentiation and function of immune cells adversely. Uncontrolled use of antibiotics, chemotherapeutic drugs, and any change in the diet pattern usually contribute to the changes in the colony index of sensitive strains known to release microbial content in the tissue micromilieu. Ligands released from dying microbes induce Toll-like receptor (TLR) mimicry, skew hypoxia, and cause sterile inflammation, which further contributes to the severity of inflammatory, autoimmune, and tumorous diseases. The major aim and scope of this review is both to discuss various modalities/interventions across the globe and to utilize microbiota-based therapeutic approaches for mitigating the disease burden.

Keywords: gut microbiota; macrophages; TLR mimicry; immune epigenetics; metabolism; sterile inflammation

1. Introduction

An organism is not just an organism but a niche of a large number of communities. The harmony between these communities or biosis determines the health of that organism. From a bacterium, a unicellular system, to the most sophisticated and successful animal of the ecosystem, Homo sapiens are obliged to various other ecological partners on which they depend for a healthy life. The human body harbors a large number of microbiota—on skin, gut, genitals, and other tissues—which are beneficial and are involved in a variety of vital functions. They protect the body from the penetration of pathogenic microbes. These beneficial microbial colonies compete with one another for space and resources. Among various partners, it is human and bacteria which have evolved together during the course of evolution, and symbiosis among them, in the gut, is vital for overall health of an individual. These microbiota contribute to the metabolism and nutrition which are important for human health and, therefore, a balance in the composition of these commensal organisms [1] is crucial to maintain the homeostasis. Intestinal or gut microbes also assist with endogenous turnover of vitamin B complex and other nutrients like minerals and amino acids metabolism and turnover.

The exact composition of the human microbiome, which is important for the homeostasis, still remains largely elusive. The best studied gastrointestinal tract (GI tract) microbiota, which comprises viruses, bacteria, fungi, and protozoa, is estimated to be nearly 100 trillion in numbers [2]. Recent studies have provided compelling evidence demarcating good and bad microbiota. Good microbiota interacts with the immune system and keeps their activity at bay contributing to the homeostatic mechanism. However, bad gut microbiota interacts with the immune system differentially and promotes non immunogenic hyper inflammatory reactions which disturb the homeostasis and promote various gastric diseases. Frequent or uncontrolled use of antibiotics, chemotherapeutic drugs, and change in dietary pattern have shown to disrupt the microbiome, leading to disturbance in microbiota or dysbiosis or dysbacteriosis [3] characterized with an imbalance of life-supportive microbes. Among various organs, the gastrointestinal tract, being the most populous, is the most sensitive to being affected by dysbiosis.

A recent meeting of WHO has suggested that degree of dysbiosis can control the severity of various diseases including metabolic, obesity, malnutrition, diabetes, and chronic inflammatory diseases such as inflammatory bowel disease (IBD), and encompassing ulcerative colitis (UC) and Crohn's disease (CD) [4]. Although various advanced technology platforms like high-throughput sequencing technologies (HTS) as well as genomic techniques have enabled us to understand the influence of the gut microbiome on human health and disease, our knowledge regarding dysbiosis-driven pathogenesis of gastric disease is still in infancy. In view of this, it is important to explore various molecular and immunological aspects of dysbiosis to better understand the clinical relevance of gut microbiome and disease pathogenesis. In this review, we uncovered the state-of-the-art tools that can be exploited to study the gut microbiome with special emphasis on gastrointestinal (GI) diseases, and also put forward therapeutic strategies involving manipulation of gut microbiota by probiotics and various immunoregulatory mechanisms [5] for the management of dysbiosis.

2. Eco-Physiological Balance of Gut Microbiota with Gut-Associated Tissues

The gastrointestinal tract in human beings acts as an interface between the host body and antigens/environmental factors. The number of bacterial cells inhabiting the GI tract is almost equal to the total number of cells in the human body, and their genomic content is approximately 10 times more than the human genome [6]. The data generated by Human Microbiome Project and MetaHIT reveals the presence of approximately 2200 different microbial species in the human gut which are divided into 12 bacterial phyla and 1 archaean taxon [7]. Most of these species belong to *Proteobacteria, Firmicutes, Actinobacteria,* and *Bacteroidetes* phylum, and their distribution varies with age of individual [7].

Normal gut microbiota comprises mostly several genera of Gram-positive Firmicutes and many different Gram-negative bacteroidetes like *Bacteroides, Prevotella, Parabacteroides,* and *Alistipes*. In addition, several other phyla, including the *Proteobacteria, Actinobacteria, Fusobacteria, Verrucomicrobia,* methanogenic archaea, Eukarya (protists and fungi), and other more transient colonizers, are found to be part of the human GI microbiome. Claesson et al. reported that younger individuals between 28 and 46 years of age show higher Firmicutes-to-Bacteroidetes ratio than elderly individuals above 65 years of age [8]. It is further reported that 386 of the identified species are anaerobic and, hence, are located in mucosal regions like the oral cavity and GI tract [7]. Besides exhibiting diversity in composition, the gut microbiota also shows region-/country-specific microbial signatures which further signify that the microbiome is greatly affected by diet as well as the host genetics including age, race, and sex of individuals (Figure 1). However, possibility of functional redundancy between different compositions of gut microbiota cannot be ruled out [9,10]. The host body gets several benefits from these microbes viz. strengthening of gut integrity, food metabolism, protection against virulent pathogens, and regulation of innate immunity [11–14]. However, if the composition of gut microbiota is altered (dysbiosis), these mechanisms may be disrupted, leading to several inflammatory and other diseases and infections.

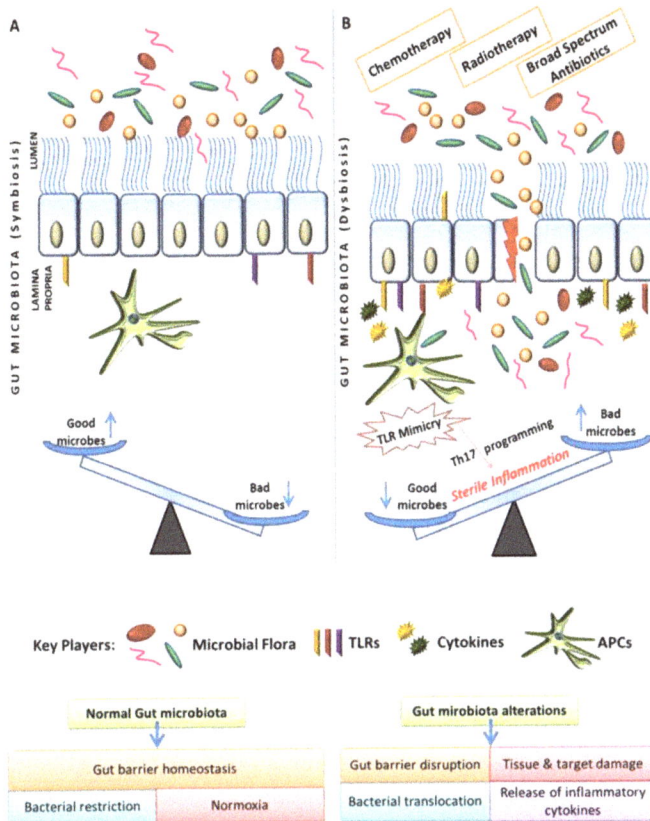

Figure 1. Disruption of normal gut tissue micromilieu including intestinal villi and gut epithelium (**A**) during dysbiosis (**B**) perturb gut immune homeostasis and GI colony index, which is manifested by TLR mimicry, Th17 programming, and hypoxia, which sensitizes normalized gut tissue micromilieu (**A**) for the progression of gastric inflammatory and tumor diseases.

The GI tract is colonized by commensal bacteria shortly after birth and the simple bacterial community gradually develops into a complex ecosystem which then starts showing symbiotic relationship with the host [15]. Commensal bacteria, including species of *Bacteroides, Lactobacilli, Bifidobacterium*, and so forth, maintain energy homeostasis by digestion of food components which otherwise cannot be digested by the stomach and intestine of germ-free individuals [16,17]. The gut microbiota also produce a significant amount (~100mM/L per day) of short-chain fatty acids (SCFAs) which act as an energy source for intestinal epithelium and also help regulate gut motility, glucose homeostasis, and inflammation [18,19]. These SCFAs have the capacity to inhibit the growth of enteropathogenic bacteria viz. *S. typhimurium*, enterohaemorrhagic *E. coli*, or *C. rodentium* in the intestine [20]. These commensal microbes also contribute some of the essentially vital vitamins such as cobalamin, vitamin K, riboflavin, biotin, and folates to the host [21].

3. Gut Microbiota Plays Critical Role in the Maintenance of Mucosal Immune Homeostasis

The gut microbiota plays an important role in the development of the normal mucosal immune system (humoral and cellular), including the development of gut-associated lymphoid tissues [22,23]. The signaling molecules and metabolites released by commensal microbes are recognized by hematopoietic as well as nonhematopoietic cells of innate immune system which further drive several physiological responses [24]. Reports also indicate that function of gut dendritic cells is largely modulated by tolerogenic response produced by gut microbiota which also inhibits the Th17 anti-inflammatory pathway [25]. Other protective mechanisms of commensal bacteria against invading pathogens include their ability to out-compete pathogens for nutrients and also to produce antimicrobial peptides. Human commensal bacteria like *Bacteroides fragilis* express commensal colonization factors which are required for penetrating the colonic mucus and colonizing the intestinal crypts while another commensal bacterium, *Bacteroides thetaiotaomicron*, expresses corrinoid transporters which help in the uptake of corrinoids that are available in the intestine in limited amount. Competition among these commensal bacteria deprives the invading pathogens of the essential nutrients required for their survival [26,27]. Antimicrobial peptides include bacteriocins like Thuricin CD, which is derived from a commensal bacterium, *Bacillus thurigiensis*, and has the potential to target bacterial pathogens without affecting other commensal bacteria [28]. Commensal bacteria also harbor bacteriophages which confer growth advantage over pathogenic bacteria which do not harbor these bacteriophages [29]. Some other commensal bacteria (e.g., Clostridia species) and the SCFAs produced by them promote proliferation of colonic Treg cells which limit inflammation and maintain intestinal homeostasis [30,31]. However, slight imbalance in the composition of gut microbiota may disturb immune homeostasis, leading to various inflammatory diseases and infections.

Under normal physiological conditions, symbiotic association of gut microbiota with gut-associated lymphoid tissue (GALT) contributes to immune homeostasis. Both macrophages and M cells of Peyer's patches play an important role in sensing antigens and transport to mucosal lymphoid nodes for immune responses [32]. Interestingly, gut microbiota colony index contributes to the overall health of the host by promoting the maturation and activation of myeloid cells of GALT, involved in patrolling, to restrict invaders in the gut, thus preventing disease progression. Changes in the composition of microbial communities disrupt gut homeostasis, which promotes leaky gut, inflammatory bowel disease, and allergic inflammation predisposing the affected individuals and making them more sensitive to developing cancer. Intake of broad-spectrum antibiotics efficiently depletes/changes the composition of faecal microbiota and impairs GALT architecture and functions [33]. Gut microbiota also secrete several immunogenic substances such as complex lipopolysaccharides present on the cell surface of Gram-negative bacteria involved in gut immune homeostasis maintenance. *Bacteroides fragilis* represents one class of bacteria found in the human intestine that contributes to immune homeostasis by promoting Foxp3+T cell activity in GALT [34].

Studies in *Bacteroides* have revealed multiple biochemical mechanisms involved in change of gut microbiota index to overcome several challenges posed by the dysbiosis. This may range from variable pH of GI tract to differential oxygen gradients and host immune surveillance. *Bacteroides* depend on other microbes, especially *Ruminococcus obeum*, in the gut to fulfill their need for corrinoid (Vitamin B12 class like cofactors) for their survival, suggesting that corrinoid producers seem to determine the diversity of the gut microbial community, particularly Bacteroides. Germ-free mice, exhibiting immune defects like imbalanced Th1/Th2 response and reduced serum levels of IgA in the gut, are ameliorated by colonization with *Bacteroides* [35], suggesting that host–microbiome interaction has important health implications.

4. Change in the Gut Microbiome Triggers Sterile Inflammation and Promotes Gastric Inflammatory Disease

Chronic and recurrent inflammation in the gut triggers oxidative stress which depletes sensitive microbes, leaving resistant strains unaffected. This dysbiosis continuously and adversely agitates GALT to promote sterile inflammatory response and sensitizes the host for chronic gastric disease. Various evidence [36–39] suggests that changes in intestinal microbiota drive changes in the intercellular tight junctions like desmoglins, facilitate the leaky gut, and enhance the interaction of various danger signals (like) released from the dying bacterial cells with immune cells, thus promoting sterile inflammation. Increasing evidence suggests that dysbiosis is associated with inflammatory bowel disease and a wide range of malignancies. Peyer's patches (PPs) are surrounded by follicle-associated epithelium (FAE), which forms the interface between the microenvironment of the lumen and the GALT. The FAE consists of specialized M cells that transport antigens and pathogens from the lumen towards underlying immune cells to regulate the immune response. The type of immune response depends upon the interactions between the immune cells located in the FAE and the lymphoid follicle. Immunological tolerance is developed against nonpathogenic normal microflora whereby generation of antigen-specific T cells suppresses activation of the immune system, thus protecting the mucosa from unnecessary inflammation. The gut microbiota and mucosal immunity constantly interact with each other to maintain intestinal homeostasis. However, if this balance is disturbed, dysfunction of the intestinal immune system occurs that further triggers a variety of diseases including IBD. Several studies indicated that intestinal dysbiosis causes an abnormal immune response leading to IBD inflammation and destruction of the gastrointestinal tract. Dysbiosis-driven chronic inflammatory and autoimmune diseases are associated with altered expression of pattern-recognition receptors (e.g., TLRs) and downstream signaling. Both innate immune and non-immune cells, such as intestinal epithelial and stromal cells, sense the pathogen-associated molecular patterns on microbial components mediated by their TLRs. Innate immune cells, such as dendritic cells and macrophages, sense pathogen-associated molecular pattern (PAMP) through TLRs, initiating rapid and effective inflammatory responses against microbial invasion.

Next-generation sequencing technology has enabled us to decipher information about the changes in the microbiome composition of intestinal microflora genome associated with development of the disease. Dysbiosis plays an important role in the development of inflammatory bowel disease (IBD), mainly due to decline in *Firmicutes* and *Bacteroidetes*, and an increase in detrimental bacteria such as *Proteobacteria* and *Actinobacteria* [40]. Due to altered microbial index in IBD, the ability of microbiota to adapt to environmental changes and defend against natural disturbances has been impaired. Therefore, manipulation of intestinal microflora has been a powerful preventive and therapeutic intervention for the management of this disease. These responses may be used as markers for immunomodulation in therapeutic intervention in IBD. A deficiency in IL-10 has been observed with cases of early-onset IBD [41].

Decrease in dietary fibers containing short-chain fatty acids (SCFAs) which are produced by the fermentation of gut bacteria [42] in the fecal samples from IBD patients [43] provides a correlation of dysbiosis with the onset and progression of IBD. The SCFAs are known to regulate inflammatory responses in different ways, such as binding of SCFA receptors (GPR43) and regulation of colonic Treg cell homeostasis [44] by restoring the colonic size and the functioning of the Treg cell pool in germ-free mice.

Altered composition of *Bacteroides* and *Firmicutes* has been reported in both animal models and in human subjects under disease conditions. Abundance of *Bacteroides* has been found in Estonian and Finnish children suffering from type 1 diabetes (T1D) as compared with Russian children who have lower T1D prevalence [45] but, however, were shown to have abundance of *Bifidobacterium*. This study also demonstrated that lipopolysaccharide (LPS) from *Bacteroides dorei*, the most common *Bacteroides* sp. in Finnish cohorts, promoted immune tolerance and failed to protect nonobesediabetic (NOD) mice from developing T1D as compared with LPS of *E. coli* origin. Metabolism of gut microbiota can also have adverse consequences, as shown by the facilitation of growth of enterohemorrhagic *E. coli* (EHEC), by *Bacteriodes*, especially *B. thetaiotamicron* and *B. vulgatus*, which cleave fucose and sialic acid moieties and other sugars from mucosal glycoproteins that are then consumed by EHEC, leading to enhanced expression of its virulence genes [46].

5. Change in the Gut Microbiome Triggers TLR Mimicry and Promotes Cancer-Related Inflammation

The pathogen recognition receptors (PRRs) present on the immune cells recognize the PAMPs on the commensal and pathogenic bacteria and execute immune response. PRRs like the Toll-like receptors (TLRs) and the nucleotide oligomerization domain (NOD) are expressed on follicle-associated epithelial or dendritic cells.

NOD2 regulates the size, number, and T-cell composition within PPs in response to the gut flora. NOD2 contributes in the immunologic tolerance towards gut microflora and plays an important role in the function of CD4+ T-cells, which in turn are able to modulate the para- and transcellular permeabilities. NOD2 influences the development of the GALT and is also able to modulate the immune response towards bacteria by limiting the development of a Th1 immune response. In wild-type mice DCs, there is proliferation of naïve CD4+ T-cells with a Th2-like cytokine profile, whereas DCs carrying NOD2 mutations promote the development of Th1-orientated cells. In the absence of NOD2, PPs present a higher rate of CD4+ T cells and M cells in the FAE and increase the results into increased levels of Th1 (IFN-γ, TNF-α, and IL-12p70) and Th2 (IL-4) cytokines. These immune alterations are associated with an increase of paracellular permeability and yeast/bacterial translocation [47]. Indeed, PPs from NOD2 −/− mice exhibit an elevated translocation of Escherichia coli, *Staphylococcus aureus*, and *Saccharomyces cerevisiae* [47].

Since gut microbiota lives in close proximity with colonic mucosa, dysbiosis not only influences inflammatory response but also the digestion and other vital functions of the gut. Dysbiosis-driven breakage of tolerance mechanism often leads to chronic inflammation and sensitizes the gut for chronic diseases other than IBD, like cancer, which actually depends upon the desmoplastic reactions mimicked by various microbial products. During dysbiosis, commensal bacteria are remodeled toward pathogenic bacteria which are accompanied by Th17 immune response which promotes pathogenic inflammation as observed in colorectal cancer (CRC).

Pathogenic bacteria like Enterotoxigenic *B. fragilis* promotes inflammation and produces genotoxins, which leads to cell proliferation and mutations, and enhances the colonization of bacterial species like *Fusobacterium* species that promote tumor progression [48]. All these processes are facilitated by the increased permeability of mucosal surfaces which allows bidirectional movement of the gut microbiota and their interaction with immune cells like CD169+/TCR-1+ lumen macrophages, type-2 neutrophiles, and regulatory T cells. This special interaction of these gut microbiota with refractory immune cells promotes desmoplastic reactions which further enhance sterile inflammation and sensitize the host for cancer progression. Most of these events are reported to promote epigenetic changes in neighboring cells.

Activation of PRRs like TLRs (especially TLR2 and TLR4) and NLRs, both by specific and nonspecific mechanisms, leads to TLR mimicry which confers chemo/radio resistance in tumor cells, influenced by the presence of pathogen-derived genotoxic factors like cyclomodulins which favor cellular proliferations and differentiation. During dysbiosis, activation of M1 macrophages contributes to the production of genotoxins in the form of ROS/RNI having toxic properties [48]. The *Fusobacterium* species that promotes the upregulation of noncanonical NF-κB-driven inflammatory genes has also been found in rich amounts in colonic tumors. Most of these mechanisms are similar to the pathogenesis of *H. pylori*-driven gastric cancer, including methylation of lysyl oxidase tumor suppressor gene which promotes tumor generation. Dysbiosis promotes not only bacterial but also virus-associated cancer. The expression of cancer-causing E6 and E7 protein of HPV is affected by estrogen and it has been shown that gut microbiota greatly modulates the blood estrogen level, thus contributing to tumor development [49,50]. Accumulated data suggests that dysbiosis-induced carcinogenesis is multifactorial in nature. Gut microbiota can pervasively dictate cancer progression by inducing desmoplastic reaction which includes sterile inflammation, epigenetic modification of DNA, and subsequent genomic instability of host cells [51].

We [52] and others [53–55] have previously demonstrated that many pathogenic microbes which are associated with cancer reprogram macrophages immunologically and metabolically during persistency. Apart from this, many pathogenic bacteria/viruses like *Helicobacter pylori*, *Fusobacterium nucleatum*, and *Chlamydia* sp. in the microbiota potentially alter the cell cycle progression and also inhibit apoptosis [56], thus conferring cancer-like phenotype in persistently infected tissue micromilieu. Moreover, cross-reactivity of gut microbiome or its metabolites with PRRs/TLRs is anticipated to promote TLR mimicry [57] and is believed to influence sterile inflammatory response for promoting cancer progression, as shown in Figure 1. In the same line, *F. nucleatum* can alter chemotherapeutic response in colorectal cancer.

Recent studies have illustrated that several bacteria species, such as members of *Proteobacteria*, *Firmicutes*, *Actinobacteria*, and *Fusobacteria* phyla, have been detected in gastric cancer biopsies [58] which may serve as a prognostic factor, thus reinforcing the association of dysbiosis with cancer.

Evidence illustrates that many bacteria like *H. pylori* modulate the host genome, altering different signaling pathways such as TLRs. The TLRs categorized as transmembrane proteins recognize PAMPs which are critical for innate and adaptive immunity. Lipids, nucleic acids, and proteins from dying bacterial, viral, or fungal cells are potent ligands or PAMPS and they interact preferentially with TLR-2,4, 5, and 9 [57] to trigger TLR mimicry and activate distinct signaling pathways. *H. pylori* upregulates TLR4 to facilitate its adherence to gastric epithelial cells and activates NF-κB via TLR5 interaction along with AP-1 and MAP kinases, resulting in expression and secretion of proinflammatory cytokines. Interestingly, hyperactivation of MAPK signaling has been associated with polarization of regulatory macrophages toward cancer-promoting phenotype. Besides altering regulatory pathways, numerous studies proposed that host genetic makeup can influence the interaction of various microbiota with host cells. For instance, genetic variants rs1640827 and rs17163737 of TLR5 lead to enhanced interactions with *H. pylori*, therefore increasing gastric cancer susceptibility [59]. A similar mechanism during dysbiosis is anticipated to lead to a similar response in various diseases. Many bacterial species like *S. bovis*, *Bacteroides fragilis*, *Escherichia coli*, *Enterococcus*, *Shigella*, *Klebsiella*, *Streptococcus*, *Peptostreptococcus*, and so forth, which are present in human gut microbiota, have been associated with progression of colorectal cancer (Table 1). Approximately, 25–80% of patients with *S. bovis* bacteremia exhibit CRC-like [60] symptoms and their stool samples have shown a higher population of bacteria belonging to the Bacteroides–Prevotella group.

Intragastric infiltration of Th17 cells like CD169+/TCR-1+ myeloid cells, CD4/fOXp3 Treg, and macrophages and immature DCs skew sterile inflammatory responses which potentially promote neoplastic transformation of infected or inflamed gut (Figure 1) during development of cancer. Thus, it is intriguing to understand the molecular/immunological mechanism and the causal relationship between the immune system and microflora in development of CRC. Studies using cyclophosphamide suggest that selective enrichment of the gut with Gram-positive bacteria can enhance Th1 immune responses and offer therapeutic benefits, indicating that the gut microbiota might promote anticancer immune responses [61].

Table 1. Overview of bacteria which are associated with different types of diseases.

Microorganism	Epigenetic Modifications	Disease
Enterococcus faecalis	Extracellular superoxide causing DNA breaks	CRC [62]
Shigella	Inflammation	CRC [63]
Escherichia coli	Syntheses of toxins	CRC [64]
Bacteroidesfragilis	Toxin production Inflammatory response by Th17/IL-17	CRC [65]
Streptococcus bovis	Inflammation	CRC [66]
Helicobacter pylori	Syntheses of toxins, DNA damage, p53 degradation	CRC [67]
Fusobacterium nucleatum	Modulates the tumor immune microenvironment	CRC [68]

Table 1. *Cont.*

Microorganism	Epigenetic Modifications	Disease
Bifidobacterium	Decreases b-glucuronidase activity	CRC [69]
Eubacterium rectale	Butyrate inducer	CRC [70]
Clostridium septicum	Secondary bile acids synthesis	CRC [71]
Faecalibacterium prausnitzii	Induces butyrate	CRC [72]
Lactobacillus	Decreases lactic acid; activation of Toll-like receptors	CRC [73]
Bacteroides fragilis	TLR2 ligand, orchestrates anti-inflammatory immune responses, stimulatesFoxp3C Treg cells	Colitis [74]
Faecalibacterium prausnitzii	Inhibits NF-kB activation	Crohn's disease [75]
B. thetaiotaomicron	Attenuates proinflammatory cytokine expression	Colitis [76]
Salmonella enteric	Flagellin is recognized by TLR5 which activates proinflammatory pathways in response to infections	Decreased susceptibility to IBD [77]
Escherichia coli	NOD2 mutation	Crohn's disease [78]
Staphylococcus aureus	Binds TLR2, inhibits proinflammatory cytokines TNF, IL-12, and IL-6	IBD [79,80]
Eubacterium rectale, Eubacterium hallii, and Roseburia	Natural HDAC inhibitors epigenetically activate p21, bax or suppress Cox-2	Cancer [81]

6. Immune Pharmaceutics as Next-Generation Modalities for Breaking Dysbiosis

Diet and geographical location play a major role in determining the microbial diversity in the gut. Uncontrolled use of antibiotics (both prescribed and indiscriminate usage) often kills a broad variety of sensitive gut microbes and leads to dysbiosis which warrants the inclusion of pro- and/or prebiotics to repopulate the gut and modulate the gut microbiome [82]. More than 1200 clinical trials investigating the effect of probiotics either alone or in combination, for various diseases, are listed in the clinical trials database, with several studies completed and in the data analysis stage [83,84]. Probiotics are live microorganisms generally belonging to the genera most commonly found in fermented foods. Probiotics modulate the gut micromilieu mainly by modulating intestinal epithelial signaling pathways, influencing the titer of sIgA and other Th2 effector cytokines, and by enhancing the intestinal epithelial barrier function by virtue of their increased mucin secretion [85]. It is interesting to note that every probiotic follows a particular mechanism for promoting balance or reconstituting health. Certain probiotics like *Lactobacilli* and *Bifidobacterium* have shown to compete with cariogenic species like *Streptococcus mutans*. In a clinical trial, twice daily oral or once weekly intravaginal administration of *Lactobacillus rhamnosus* GR-1 and *Lactobacillus reuteri* has shown to reduce recurrences of UTI and restore a normal lactobacilli-dominated vaginal flora over anaerobes in patients [86]. This is due to their potential to produce more lactose, which is an important nutrient that gets metabolized to glucose and galactose in most neonates. However, intolerance tolactose and its metabolism leads to the alterations in colonic microbiota. In such cases, probiotic supplementation could alleviate lactose intolerance. Such intervention is quite effective in preventing diseases like Eczema, diarrhea, upper RTI, necrotizing enterocholitis, and pulmonary exacerbation in children. Recently, a randomized, double-blind, placebo-controlled trial of *Lactobacillus acidophilus* and Inulin has shown the efficacy in reducing free and LDL bound cholesterol by 7.84 and 9.27%, respectively, in a cohort of obese patients [87]. It is becoming evident that the gut microbiome can actually have a role in obesity and irritable bowel syndrome (IBS) as well. A study reported that if mice are reared in a germ-free environment and have no microorganisms in their gut, such mice are protected from obesity and metabolic disorders like insulin resistance and glucose intolerance even when fed with a western-style diet loaded with high fat or high calories. Along similar lines, another recent study has established the link of specific gut microbiota on the therapeutic efficacy of metformin in the cohort of obese patients over lean cohort [88]. This is what is anticipated to be due to immune metabolic programming of M1 or Th1 macrophages [89] of obese patients towards M2 and/or scavenging macrophages by metformin which is believed to change the specific gut microbiota in obese people, contributing to the outcome.

7. Role of Bile Acids and Gut Microbiome

It is becoming increasingly clear that the gut microbiome utilizes the host food/nutrients for synthesizing bioactives that activate the cellular signaling mediated by cognate receptors on human cells. One important class of cholesterol-derived bioactives is the bile acids produced by host liver released into the duodenum after a meal which have been shown to be metabolized further by the resident microbiomes. These bile acid metabolites activate cellular receptors, in the GI tract as well as in the periphery, regulating several host metabolic process. Gut microbiota not only regulates bile acid synthesis, but also its reuptake, thus contributing to the available bile acid pool of the host [71].

Human liver produces cholic acid (CA) and chenodeoxycholic acid (CDCA), while murine liver produces CA and muricholic acid (MCA) which in turn are conjugated to aminoacids [90]. The amphipathic structure of bile acids gives them detergent-like properties that facilitate emulsification and absorption of dietary lipids and fat-soluble vitamins.

Further, it poses a challenge to the resident microbes, and these organisms have evolved a variety of ways to thrive in this environment. Several of these have bile-acid-inducible (BAI) genes. Metagenomics analysis has revealed that bile salt hydrolase (BSH) activity is present in many bacterial species which are the members of *Lactobacilli, Bifidobacteria, Clostridium*, and *Bacteroides* [90]. In reality, BSH activity is enriched in the gut microbiota and is probably responsible for increased resistance to bile toxicity. Another major microbial biotransformation of bile acids is by the hydroxysteroid dehydrogenases (HSDHs) which are present in *Actinobacteria, Proteobacteria, Firmicutes*, and *Bacteroidetes* [91].

Regulation of Bile Acid Synthesis via FXR: Role of Gut Microbial Metabolites

Synthesis of bile acids is regulated tightly by negative feedback inhibition through the nuclear receptor FXR, expressed at fairly high levels in the liver and ileum. The most potent ligand for FXR is CDCA, followed by CA, DCA, and LCA. Gut microbes have been demonstrated not only to metabolize bile acids but also to effect signaling throughFXR. The microbiota deconjugates the naturally occurring FXR antagonist taurine-conjugated MCA (TMCA) and thus promotes FXR signaling in mice and is also required for the production of secondary bile acids acting as ligands for TGR5 [92]. Bile acids can shape the gut microbiota community by promoting the growth of bile-acid-metabolizing bacteria and by inhibiting the growth of other bile-sensitive bacteria. It suggests that the interaction between the microbiota and bile acids is not unidirectional. Semisynthetic bile acids like obeticholic acid have shown to have clinically meaningful benefit in nonalcoholic fatty liver (NAFLD) patients in clinical trials. In addition, it is now evident that bile acids not only have direct antimicrobial effects, by destroying bacterial membranes due to their detergent properties, but also have indirect effects through FXR, by inducing transcription of antimicrobial agents (e.g., iNOS and IL-18) that affect the gut microbiota via the immune system [91].

8. Future Perspective

Although numerous animal and human studies so far have acclaimed the safety and health benefits of probiotics, this area of research is still in its infancy and warrants more rigorous studies to claim its impact on its expected outcome on health. Utilization of microbial-based strategies is expected to afford help in the management of large numbers of haemolytic/metabolic diseases. Industrial application of Microcins, Colicins, plantaricin, vibriocin, and so forth, which are bacteriocins toxins and produced by *E. coli, Lactobacillus* sp. have been explored against various bad gut microbiota associated with many diseases. Fecal material transplantation (FMT) represents one such intervention which is explored for the management of various infections and cancer. Transplantation of gut microbiota of "normal" mice into such germ-free mice led to significant weight gain even in the face of a normal diet, suggesting that the microbiome is contributing to this weight gain.

This approach has decisive influence on cancer-directed immune therapies, thus certainly representing a novel biological entity for affording better treatment options. Finally, it would be essential to identify the set of gut microbiota which is responsible in promoting gut immune homeostasis, mainly deciphering their immunomodulatory impact on the gut on the component of innate and adaptive immunity for homeostasis.

Author Contributions: H.P. was involved in conceptualization and writing. DT and MW were involved in writing and editing while P.K., G.K., N.K.K., C.G., S.S. and A.K. were involved in writing.

Funding: This research received no external funding.

Acknowledgments: Authors acknowledge Anuradha Vashisth, Indian Institute of Technology, New Delhi, India for language and grammatical corrections.

Conflicts of Interest: The authors declare no conflict of interest.

References

1. Eloe-Fadrosh, E.A.; Rasko, D.A. The human microbiome: From symbiosis to Pathogenesis. *Annu. Rev. Med.* **2014**, *64*, 145–163. [CrossRef] [PubMed]

2. Leblanc, J.G.; Milani, C.; Giori, G.S.; De Sesma, F.; Van Sinderen, D.; Ventura, M. Bacteria as vitamin suppliers to their host: A gut microbiota perspective. *Curr. Opin. Biotechnol.* **2013**, *24*, 160–168. [CrossRef] [PubMed]

3. Gareau, M.G.; Sherman, P.M.; Walker, W.A. Probiotics and the gut microbiota in intestinal health and disease. *Nat. Rev. Gastroenterol. Hepatol.* **2010**, *7*, 503–514. [CrossRef] [PubMed]

4. Kamada, N.; Seo, S.U.; Chen, G.Y.; Núñez, G. Role of the gut microbiota in immunity and inflammatory disease. *Nat. Rev. Immunol.* **2013**, *13*, 321. [CrossRef] [PubMed]

5. Fraser, C.M.; Ringel, Y.; Sanders, M.E.; Sartor, R.B.; Sherman, P.M.; Versalovic, J.; Young, V.; Finlay, B.B. Perspective Defining a Healthy Human Gut Microbiome: Current Concepts, Future Directions, and Clinical Applications. *Cell Host Microbe.* **2012**, *12*, 611–622.

6. Sender, R.; Fuchs, S.; Milo, R. Revised Estimates for the Number of Human and Bacteria Cells in the Body. *PLoS Biol.* **2016**, *14*, e1002533. [CrossRef] [PubMed]

7. Hugon, P.; Dufour, J.C.; Colson, P.; Fournier, P.E.; Sallah, K.; Raoult, D. A comprehensive repertoire of prokaryotic species identified in human beings. *Lancet Infect. Dis.* **2015**, *15*, 1211–1219. [CrossRef]

8. Stanton, C.; Cusack, S.; O'Mahony, D.; O'Connor, K.; Henry, C.; Greene-Diniz, R.; Claesson, M.J.; Fitzgerald, A.P.; Fitzgerald, G.; de Weerd, H.; et al. Composition, variability, and temporal stability of the intestinal microbiota of the elderly. *Proc. Natl. Acad. Sci. USA* **2010**, *108*, 4586–4591.

9. Rodriguez, J.M.; Murphy, K.; Stanton, C.; Ross, R.P.; Kober, O.I.; Juge, N.; Avershina, E.; Rudi, K.; Narbad, A.; Jenmalm, M.C.; et al. The composition of the gut microbiota throughout life, with an emphasis on early life. *Microb. Ecol. Heal. Dis.* **2015**, *26*, 26050. [CrossRef]

10. Manichanh, C.; Bork, P.; Hansen, T.; Brunak, S.; Xu, X.; Zhong, H.; Prifti, E.; Chen, W.; Sunagawa, S.; Zhang, W.; et al. An integrated catalog of reference genes in the human gut microbiome. *Nat. Biotechnol.* **2014**, *32*, 834–841.

11. Natividad, J.M.M.; Verdu, E.F. Modulation of intestinal barrier by intestinal microbiota: Pathological and therapeutic implications. *Pharmacol. Res.* **2013**, *69*, 42–51. [CrossRef]

12. Van Eunen, K.; den Besten, G.; Groen, A.K.; Reijngoud, D.; Venema, K.; Bakker, B.M. The role of short-chain fatty acids in the interplay between diet, gut microbiota, and host energy metabolism. *J. Lipid Res.* **2013**, *54*, 2325–2340.

13. Bäumler, A.J.; Sperandio, V. Interactions between the microbiota and pathogenic bacteria in the gut. *Nature* **2016**, *535*, 85–93. [CrossRef] [PubMed]

14. Gensollen, T.; Iyer, S.S.; Kasper, D.L.; Blumberg, R.S.; Medical, H. How colonization by microbiota in early life shapes the immune system. *Science* **2016**, *352*, 539–544. [CrossRef] [PubMed]

15. Kaetzel, C.S.; Frantz, A.L.; Stromberg, A.J.; Rogier, E.W.; Bruno, M.E.C.; Cohen, D.A.; Wedlund, L. Secretory antibodies in breast milk promote long-term intestinal homeostasis by regulating the gut microbiota and host gene expression. *Proc. Natl. Acad. Sci. USA* **2014**, *111*, 3074–3079.

16. Larsbrink, J.; Rogers, T.E.; Hemsworth, G.R.; Mckee, L.S.; Tauzin, A.S.; Spadiut, O.; Klinter, S.; Pudlo, N.A.; Urs, K.; Koropatkin, N.M.; et al. Inhibitors of Apoptosis Protein Antagonists (Smac Mimetic Compounds) Control Polarization of Macrophages during Microbial Challenge and Sterile Inflammatory Responses. *Nature* **2015**, *506*, 498–502. [CrossRef]

17. Goh, Y.J.; Klaenhammer, T.R. Genetic Mechanisms of Prebiotic Oligosaccharide Metabolism in Probiotic Microbes. *Annu. Rev. Food Sci. Technol.* **2014**, *6*, 137–156. [CrossRef]

18. Cani, P.D. Gutmicrobiota and obesity: Lessons from the microbiome. *Brief. Funct. Genomics* **2013**, *12*, 381–387. [CrossRef]

19. Valdes, A.M.; Walter, J.; Segal, E.; Spector, T.D. Role of the gut microbiota in nutrition and health. *BMJ* **2018**, *361*, 36–44. [CrossRef]

20. Bohez, L.; Boyen, F.; Timbermont, L.; Ducatelle, R.; Gantois, I.; Pasmans, F.; Haesebrouck, F.; van Immerseel, F. Oral immunisation of laying hens with the live vaccine strains of TAD Salmonella vac®E and TAD Salmonella vac®T reduces internal egg contamination with Salmonella Enteritidis. *Vaccine* **2006**, *24*, 6250–6255.

21. Koutmos, M.; Kabil, O.; Smith, J.L.; Banerjee, R. Structural basis for substrate activation and regulation by cystathionine beta-synthase (CBS) domains in cystathionine –synthase. *Proc. Natl. Acad. Sci. USA* **2010**, *107*, 20958–20963. [CrossRef]

22. Cebra, J.J. Influences of microbiota on intestinal immune system development. *Am. J. Clin. Nutr.* **1999**, *69*, 69–1046. [CrossRef]

23. Round, J.L.; Mazmanian, S.K. The gut microbiota shapes intestinal immune responses during health and disease. *Nat. Rev. Immunol.* **2014**, *9*, 25.

24. Malitsky, S.; Rothschild, D.; Moresi, C.; Kuperman, Y.; Elinav, E.; Rozin, S.; Harmelin, A.; Thaiss, C.A.; Halpern, Z.; Levy, M.; et al. Persistent microbiome alterations modulate the rate of post-dieting weight regain. *Nature* **2016**, *540*, 544–551.

25. Magrone, T.; Perez de Heredia, F.; Jirillo, E.; Morabito, G.; Marcos, A.; Serafini, M. Functional foods and nutraceuticals as therapeutic tools for the treatment of diet-related diseases. *Can. J. Physiol. Pharmacol.* **2013**, *396*, 387–396. [CrossRef]

26. Lee, S.M.; Donaldson, G.P.; Mikulski, Z.; Boyajian, S.; Ley, K.; Mazmanian, S.K.; Engineering, B.; Jolla, L. Bacterial colonization factors control specificity and stability of the gut microbiota. *Nature* **2014**, *501*, 426–429. [CrossRef]

27. Marrow, B.; Secreted, S.; Protect, C. Vitamin B12 as a modulator of gut microbial ecology. *Cell Metab.* **2014**, *71*, 3831–3840.

28. Vederas, J.C.; Ross, R.P.; Rea, M.C.; Hill, C.; Sit, C.S.; Zheng, J.; Clayton, E.; O'Connor, P.M.; Whittal, R.M. Thuricin CD, a posttranslationally modified bacteriocin with a narrow spectrum of activity against Clostridium difficile. *Proc. Natl. Acad. Sci. USA* **2010**, *107*, 9352–9357.

29. Rollins, D.; Clements, C.V.; Rodrigues, J.L.M.; Duerkop, B.A.; Hooper, L.V. A composite bacteriophage alters colonization by an intestinal commensal bacterium. *Proc. Natl. Acad. Sci. USA* **2012**, *109*, 17621–17626.

30. Atarashi, K.; Tanoue, T.; Oshima, K.; Suda, W.; Nagano, Y.; Nishikawa, H.; Fukuda, S.; Saito, T.; Narushima, S.; Hase, K.; et al. Treg induction by a rationally selected mixture of Clostridia strains from the human microbiota. *Nature* **2013**, *500*, 232–236. [CrossRef]

31. Arpaia, N.; Campbell, C.; Fan, X.; Dikiy, S.; Liu, H.; Cross, J.R.; Pfeffer, K.; Coffer, P.J.; Rudensky, A.Y.; Donald, B.; et al. Metabolites produced by commensal bacteria promote peripheral regulatory T-cell generation. *Nature* **2014**, *504*, 451–455. [CrossRef]

32. Da Silva, C.; Wagner, C.; Bonnardel, J.; Gorvel, J.; Lelouard, H. The Peyer's Patch Mononuclear Phagocyte System at Steady State and during Infection. *Front. Immunol.* **2017**, *8*, 1254. [CrossRef]

33. Chemouny, J.M.; Gleeson, P.J.; Abbad, L.; Lauriero, G.; Bredel, M.; Bex-coudrat, J.; Boedec, E.; Le Roux, K.; Daugas, E.; Vrtovsnik, F.; et al. Modulation of the microbiota by oral antibiotics treats immunoglobulin A nephropathy in humanized mice. *Nephrol. Dial. Transplant.* **2018**. [CrossRef]

34. Telesford, K.M.; Yan, W.; Ochoa-reparaz, J.; Pant, A.; Kircher, C.; Christy, M.A.; Begum-haque, S.; Kasper, D.L.; Kasper, L.H.; Telesford, K.M.; et al. A commensal symbiotic factor derived from Bacteroidesfragilis promotes human CD39 C Foxp3 C T cells and T reg function. *Gut Microbes* **2015**, *6*, 234–242. [CrossRef] [PubMed]

35. Kozakova, H.; Schwarzer, M.; Tuckova, L.; Srutkova, D.; Czarnowska, E.; Rosiak, I.; Hudcovic, T.; Schabussova, I.; Hermanova, P.; Zakostelska, Z.; et al. Colonization of germ-free mice with a mixture

of three lactobacillus strains enhances the integrity of gut mucosa and ameliorates allergic sensitization. *Cell. Mol. Immunol.* **2015**, *13*, 180–190. [CrossRef] [PubMed]

36. Conlon, M.A.; Bird, A.R. The Impact of Diet and Lifestyle on Gut Microbiota and Human Health. *Nutrients* **2015**, *7*, 17–44. [CrossRef] [PubMed]

37. Arrazuria, R.; Pérez, V.; Molina, E.; Juste, R.A.; Khafipour, E. Diet induced changes in the microbiota and cell composition of rabbit gut associated lymphoid tissue (GALT). *Sci. Rep.* **2018**, *8*, 14103. [CrossRef] [PubMed]

38. Thanabalasuriar, A.; Koutsouris, A.; Hecht, G.; Gruenheid, S. The bacterial virulence factor NleA's involvement in intestinal tight junction disruption during enteropathogenic E. coli infection is independent of its putative PDZ binding domain. *Gut Microbes* **2010**, *1*, 114–118. [CrossRef] [PubMed]

39. Capaldo, C.T.; Powell, D.N.; Kalman, D. Layered defense: How mucus and tight junctions seal the intestinal barrier. *J. Mol. Med.* **2017**, *95*, 927–934. [CrossRef]

40. Mohan, M.; Chow, C.T.; Ryan, C.N.; Chan, L.S.; Dufour, J.; Aye, P.P.; Blanchard, J.; Moehs, C.P.; Sestak, K. Dietary Gluten-Induced Gut Dysbiosis Is Accompanied by Selective Upregulation of microRNAs with Intestinal Tight Junction and Bacteria-Binding Motifs in Rhesus Macaque Model of Celiac Disease. *Nutrients* **2016**, *11*, 684. [CrossRef]

41. Hamilton, X.M.K.; Boudry, G.; Lemay, D.G.; Raybould, H.E. Changes in intestinal barrier function and gut microbiota in high-fat diet-fed rats are dynamic and region dependent. *Am. J. Physiol. Gastrointest. Liver. Physiol.* **2018**, *308*, G840–G851. [CrossRef]

42. Inohara, N.; Nun, G. Mechanisms of inflammation-driven bacterial dysbiosis in the gut. *Mucosal. Immunol.* **2017**, *10*, 18–26.

43. Salzer, E.; Kansu, A.; Sic, H.; Dogu, F.E.; Prengemann, N.K.; Santos-valente, E.; Pickl, W.F.; Demir, A.M.; Ensari, A.; Colinge, J.; et al. Early-onset inflammatory bowel disease and common variable immunodeficiency—like disease caused by IL-21 deficiency. *J. Allergy Clin. Immunol.* **2014**, *133*, 1651–1659. [CrossRef]

44. Desai, M.S.; Seekatz, A.M.; Koropatkin, N.M.; Stappenbeck, T.S.; Martens, E.C. A Dietary Fiber-Deprived Gut Microbiota Degrades the Colonic Mucus Barrier and Enhances Pathogen Article A Dietary Fiber-Deprived Gut Microbiota Degrades the Colonic Mucus Barrier and Enhances Pathogen Susceptibility. *Cell* **2016**, *167*, 1339–1353. [CrossRef] [PubMed]

45. Vatanen, T.; Kostic, A.D.; Hennezel, E.; Cullen, T.W.; Knip, M.; Xavier, R.J.; Huttenhower, C.; Gevers, D.; Cullen, T.W.; Szabo, S.J.; et al. Variation in Microbiome LPS Immunogenicity Contributes to Autoimmunity in Humans Article Variation in Microbiome LPS Immunogenicity Contributes to Autoimmunity in Humans. *Cell* **2016**, *165*, 842–853. [CrossRef] [PubMed]

46. Wexler, A.G.; Goodman, A.L. An insider's perspective: Bacteroides as a window into the microbiome. *Nat. Microbiol.* **2017**, *2*, 1–11. [CrossRef]

47. Barreau, F.; Meinzer, U.; Chareyre, F.; Berrebi, D.; Niwa-Kawakita, M.; Dussaillant, M.; Foligne, B.; Ollendorff, V.; Heyman, M.; Bonacorsi, S.; et al. CARD15/NOD2 Is Required for Peyer's Patches Homeostasis in Mice. *PLoS ONE* **2007**, *13*, e523. [CrossRef] [PubMed]

48. Sheflin, A.M.; Whitney, A.K.; Weir, T.L. Cancer-Promoting Effects of Microbial Dysbiosis. *Curr. Oncol. Rep.* **2014**, *16*, 406. [CrossRef] [PubMed]

49. Spurgeon, M.E.; Den Boon, J.A.; Horswill, M.; Barthakur, S.; Forouzan, O.; Rader, J.S. Human papillomavirus oncogenes reprogram the cervical cancer microenvironment independently of and synergistically with estrogen. *Proc. Natl. Acad. Sci. USA* **2017**, *114*, E9076–E9085. [CrossRef] [PubMed]

50. Chen, K.L.; Madak-erdogan, Z. Estrogen and Microbiota Crosstalk: Should We Pay Attention? *Trends Endocrinol. Metab.* **2016**, *27*, 752–755. [CrossRef]

51. Bhat, M.I.; Kapila, R. Dietary metabolites derived from gut microbiota: Critical modulators of epigenetic changes in mammals. *Nutr. Rev.* **2017**, *75*, 374–389. [CrossRef] [PubMed]

52. Nadella, V.; Mohanty, A.; Sharma, L.; Yellaboina, S.; Mollenkopf, H.-J.; Mazumdar, V.B.; Palaparthi, R.; Mylavarapu, M.B.; Maurya, R.; Kurukuti, S.; et al. Inhibitors of Apoptosis Protein Antagonists (Smac Mimetic Compounds) Control Polarization of Macrophages during Microbial Challenge and Sterile Inflammatory Responses. *Front. Immunol.* **2018**, *8*, 1–21.

53. Karpiński, T. Role of Oral Microbiota in Cancer Development. *Microorganisms* **2019**, *7*, 20. [CrossRef]

54. Xiong, Y.B.; Zhu, H.R.; Cheng, Y.L.; Yu, Z.H.; Chai, N. Gut microbiome and risk for colorectal cancer. *World Chin. J. Dig.* **2014**, *22*, 5653–5658. [CrossRef]

55. Nagy, K.N.; Sonkodi, I.; Szöke, I.; Nagy, E.; Newman, H.N. The microflora associated with human oral carcinomas. *Oral Oncol.* **1998**, *34*, 304–308. [CrossRef]

56. Gagnaire, A.; Nadel, B.; Raoult, D.; Neefjes, J.; Gorvel, J. Collateral damage: insights into bacterial mechanisms that predispose host cells to cancer. *Nat. Rev. Microbiol.* **2017**, *15*, 109. [CrossRef] [PubMed]

57. Frosali, S.; Pagliari, D.; Gambassi, G.; Landolfi, R.; Pandolfi, F.; Cianci, R. How the Intricate Interaction among Toll-Like Receptors, Microbiota, and Intestinal Immunity Can Influence Gastrointestinal Pathology. *J. Immunol. Res.* **2015**, *2015*, 1–12. [CrossRef]

58. Coker, O.O.; Dai, Z.; Nie, Y.; Zhao, G.; Cao, L.; Nakatsu, G.; Wu, W.K.K.; Wong, S.H.; Chen, Z.; Sung, J.J.Y. Mucosal microbiome dysbiosis in gastric carcinogenesis. *Gut* **2018**, *67*, 1024–1032. [CrossRef]

59. Xu, T.; Fu, D.; Ren, Y.; Dai, Y.; Lin, J.; Tang, L.; Ji, J. Genetic variations of TLR5 gene interacted with Helicobacter pylori infection among carcinogenesis of gastric cancer. *Oncotarget* **2017**, *8*, 31016–31022. [CrossRef]

60. Zou, S.; Fang, L.; Lee, M. Dysbiosis of gut microbiota in promoting the development of colorectal cancer. *Gastroenterol. Rep.* **2018**, *6*, 1–12. [CrossRef]

61. Viaud, S.; Saccheri, F.; Mignot, G.; Yamazaki, T.; Hannani, D.; Enot, D.P.; Pfirschke, C.; Engblom, C.; Pittet, J.; Schlitzer, A.; et al. The intestinal microbiota modulates the anticancer immune effects of cyclophosphamide. *Science* **2013**, *342*, 971–976. [CrossRef] [PubMed]

62. Boonanantanasarn, K.; Gill, A.L.; Yap, Y.; Jayaprakash, V.; Sullivan, M.A.; Gill, S.R. Enterococcus faecalis Enhances Cell Proliferation through Hydrogen Peroxide-Mediated Epidermal Growth Factor Receptor Activation. *Infect. Immun.* **2012**, *80*, 3545–3558. [CrossRef]

63. Gao, Z.; Guo, B.; Gao, R.; Zhu, Q.; Qin, H. Microbiota disbiosis is associated with colorectal cancer. *Front. Microbiol.* **2015**, *6*, 1–9. [CrossRef]

64. Nougayrède, J.P.; Homburg, S.; Taieb, F.; Boury, M.; Brzuszkiewicz, E.; Gottschalk, G.; Buchrieser, C.; Hacker, J.; Dobrindt, U.; Oswald, E. Escherichia *coli* induces DNA double-strand breaks in eukaryotic cells. *Science* **2006**, *313*, 848–851. [CrossRef]

65. Boleij, A.; Hechenbleikner, E.M.; Goodwin, A.C.; Badani, R.; Stein, E.M.; Lazarev, M.G.; Ellis, B.; Carroll, K.C.; Albesiano, E.; Wick, E.C.; et al. The bacteroidesfragilis toxin gene is prevalent in the colon mucosa of colorectal cancer patients. *Clin. Infect. Dis.* **2015**, *60*, 208–215. [CrossRef] [PubMed]

66. Biarc, J.; Nguyen, I.S.; Pini, A.; Gossé, F.; Richert, S.; Thiersé, D.; Van Dorsselaer, A.; Leize-Wagner, E.; Raul, F.; Klein, J.P.; et al. Carcinogenic properties of proteins with pro-inflammatory activity from Streptococcusinfantarius (formerly *S. bovis*). *Carcinogenesis* **2004**, *25*, 1477–1484. [CrossRef]

67. Blot, W.J. Helicobacter pylori protein-specific antibodies and risk of colorectal cancer. *Ann. Intern. Med.* **2013**, *86*, 517.

68. Kostic, A.D.; Chun, E.; Robertson, L.; Glickman, J.N.; Gallini, C.A.; Michaud, M.; Clancy, T.E.; Chung, D.C.; Lochhead, P.; Hold, G.L.; et al. Fusobacterium nucleatum Potentiates Intestinal Tumorigenesis and Modulates the Tumor-Immune Microenvironment. *Cell. Host. Microbe.* **2013**, *14*, 207–215. [CrossRef] [PubMed]

69. Kim, Y.; Lee, D.; Kim, D.; Cho, J.; Yang, J.; Chung, M.; Kim, K.; Ha, N. Inhibition of proliferation in colon cancer cell lines and harmful enzyme activity of colon bacteria by Bifidobacterium adolescentis SPM0212. *Arch. Pharm. Res.* **2008**, *31*, 468–473. [CrossRef] [PubMed]

70. Balamurugan, R.; Rajendiran, E.; George, S.; Samuel, G.V.; Ramakrishna, B.S. Real-time polymerase chain reaction quantification of specific butyrate-producing bacteria, Desulfovibrio and Enterococcus faecalis in the feces of patients with colorectal cancer. *J. Gastroenterol. Hepatol.* **2008**, *23*, 1298–1303. [CrossRef]

71. Ridlon, J.M.; Kang, D.J.; Hylemon, P.B.; Bajaj, J.S. Bile acids and the gut microbiome. *Curr. Opin. Gastroenterol.* **2014**, *30*, 332–338. [CrossRef]

72. Lopez-Siles, M.; Khan, T.M.; Duncan, S.H.; Harmsen, H.J.M.; Garcia-Gil, L.J.; Flint, H.J. Cultured representatives of two major phylogroups of human colonic Faecalibacteriumprausnitzii can utilize pectin, uronic acids, and host-derived substrates for growth. *Appl. Environ. Microbiol.* **2012**, *78*, 420–428. [CrossRef]

73. Li, Y.; Zhang, X.; Wang, L.; Zhou, Y.; Hassan, J.S.; Li, M. Distribution and gene mutation of enteric flora carrying β-glucuronidase among patients with colorectal cancer. *Int. J. Clin. Exp. Med.* **2015**, *8*, 5310–5316.

74. Balzola, F.; Bernstein, C.; Ho, G.T.; Lees, C. Inducible Foxp3+regulatory T-cell development by a commensal bacterium of the intestinal microbiota: Commentary. *Inflamm. Bowel Dis. Monit.* **2010**, *11*, 79–80.

75. Sokol, H.; Pigneur, B.; Watterlot, L.; Lakhdari, O.; Bermúdez-Humarán, L.G.; Gratadoux, J.-J.; Blugeon, S.; Bridonneau, C.; Furet, J.-P.; Corthier, G.; et al. Faecalibacteriumprausnitzii is an anti-inflammatory commensal

bacterium identified by gut microbiota analysis of Crohn disease patients. *Proc. Natl. Acad. Sci. USA* **2008**, *105*, 16731–16736. [CrossRef]

76. Delday, M.; Mulder, I.; Logan, E.T.; Grant, G. Bacteroides thetaiotaomicron ameliorates colon inflammation in preclinical models of Crohn's disease. *Inflamm. Bowel Dis.* **2019**, *25*, 85–96. [CrossRef] [PubMed]

77. Schultz, B.M.; Paduro, C.A.; Salazar, G.A.; Salazar-Echegarai, F.J.; Sebastián, V.P.; Riedel, C.A.; Kalergis, A.M.; Alvarez-Lobos, M.; Bueno, S.M. A potential role of Salmonella infection in the onset of inflammatory bowel diseases. *Front. Immunol.* **2017**, *8*, 191. [CrossRef] [PubMed]

78. Boshoff, A.C.; Comprehensive, H.; Boshoff, C. Adherent-invasive E coli in Crohn disease: Bacterial "agent provocateur". *J. Clin. Invest.* **2011**, *121*, 841–844.

79. Steinert, A.; Linas, I.; Kaya, B.; Ibrahim, M.; Schlitzer, A.; Hruz, P.; Radulovic, K.; Terracciano, L.; Macpherson, A.J.; Niess, J.H. The Stimulation of Macrophages with TLR Ligands Supports Increased IL-19 Expression in Inflammatory Bowel Disease Patients and in Colitis Models. *J. Immunol.* **2017**, *199*, 2570–2584. [CrossRef]

80. Islander, U.; Andersson, A.; Lindberg, E.; Adlerberth, I.; Wold, A.E.; Rudin, A. Superantigenic Staphylococcus aureus stimulates production of interleukin-17 from memory but not naive T cells. *Infect. Immun.* **2010**, *78*, 381–386. [CrossRef]

81. Sook Lee, E.; Ji Song, E.; Do Nam, Y. Dysbiosis of Gut Microbiome and Its Impact on Epigenetic Regulation. *J. Clin. Epigenetics* **2017**, *3*, 1–7. [CrossRef]

82. Neuman, H.; Forsythe, P.; Uzan, A.; Avni, O.; Koren, O.; Medicine, F.; Szold, H.; St, H.; Israel, S.; College, Z.A.; et al. Antibiotics in early life: Dysbiosis and the damage done. *FEMS Microbiol. Rev.* **2018**, *42*, 489–499. [CrossRef]

83. Kristensen, N.B.; Bryrup, T.; Allin, K.H.; Nielsen, T.; Hansen, T.H.; Pedersen, O. Alterations in fecal microbiota composition by probiotic supplementation in healthy adults: A systematic review of randomized controlled trials. *Genome Med.* **2016**, *8*, 52. [CrossRef]

84. Sáez-lara, M.J.; Robles-sanchez, C.; Ruiz-ojeda, F.J.; Plaza-diaz, J.; Gil, A. Effects of Probiotics and Synbiotics on Obesity, Insulin Resistance Syndrome, Type 2 Diabetes and Non-Alcoholic Fatty Liver Disease: A Review of Human Clinical Trials. *Int. J. Mol. Sci.* **2016**, *17*, 928. [CrossRef]

85. Villena, J.; Kitazawa, H. Modulation of intestinal TLR4-inflammatory signaling pathways by probiotic microorganisms: Lessons learned from Lactobacillus jensenii TL2937. *Front Immunol.* **2014**, *4*, 1–12. [CrossRef] [PubMed]

86. Falagas, M.E.; Betsi, G.I.; Tokas, T.; Athanasiou, S. Probiotics for Prevention of Recurrent Urinary Tract Infections in Women A Review of the Evidence from Microbiological and Clinical Studies. *Drugs* **2006**, *66*, 1253–1261. [CrossRef]

87. Ooi, L.; Ahmad, R.; Yuen, K.; Liong, M. Lactobacillus acidophilus CHO-220 and inulin reduced plasma total cholesterol and low-density lipoprotein cholesterol via alteration of lipid transporters. *J. Dairy Sci.* **2010**, *93*, 5048–5058. [CrossRef] [PubMed]

88. Brunkwall, L.; Orho-melander, M. The gut microbiome as a target for prevention and treatment of hyperglycaemia in type 2 diabetes: From current human evidence to future possibilities. *Diabetologia* **2017**, *60*, 943–951. [CrossRef] [PubMed]

89. Lumeng, C.N.; Bodzin, J.L.; Saltiel, A.R. Obesity induces a phenotypic switch in adipose tissue macrophage polarization. *J. Clin. Invest.* **2007**, *117*, 175–184. [CrossRef]

90. Chiang, J.Y.L. Bile Acid Metabolism and Signaling. In *Comprehensive Physiology*; John Wiley & Sons: Hoboken, NJ, USA, July 2013; pp. 1191–1212.

91. Wahlström, A.; Sayin, S.I.; Marschall, H.U.; Bäckhed, F. Intestinal Crosstalk between Bile Acids and Microbiota and Its Impact on Host Metabolism. *Cell Metab.* **2016**, *24*, 41–50. [CrossRef]

92. Jia, W.; Xie, G.; Jia, W. Bile acid-microbiota cross-talk in gastrointestinal inflammation and carcinogenesis. *Nat. Rev. Gastroenterol. Hepatol.* **2018**, *15*, 111–128. [CrossRef] [PubMed]

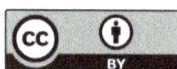

International Journal of
Molecular Sciences

MDPI

Review

Gut-Liver Axis, Gut Microbiota, and Its Modulation in the Management of Liver Diseases: A Review of the Literature

Ivana Milosevic [1,2,*], Ankica Vujovic [1,2], Aleksandra Barac [1,2], Marina Djelic [3], Milos Korac [1,2], Aleksandra Radovanovic Spurnic [1,2], Ivana Gmizic [2], Olja Stevanovic [1,2], Vladimir Djordjevic [1,4], Nebojsa Lekic [1,4], Edda Russo [5] and Amedeo Amedei [5,6]

[1] Faculty of Medicine, University of Belgrade, 11000 Belgrade, Serbia; ankica.vujovic88@gmail.com (A.V.); aleksandrabarac85@gmail.com (A.B.); milos.korac@med.bg.ac.rs (M.K.); spurnic@yahoo.com (A.R.S.); stevanovicolja74@gmail.com (O.S.); vladimir.djordjevic@kcs.ac.rs (V.D.); nesalekic67@gmail.com (N.L.)
[2] Hospital for Infectious and Tropical Diseases, Clinical Center of Serbia, 11000 Belgrade, Serbia; gmizic_ivana@yahoo.com
[3] Faculty of Medicine, Universisty of Belgrade; Institute of Medical Physiology "Rihard Burijan", 11000 Belgrade, Serbia; mdjelic011@gmail.com
[4] Clinic for Digestive Surgery, Clinical Center of Serbia, 11000 Belgrade, Serbia
[5] Department of Experimental and Clinical Medicine, University of Florence, 50134 Florence, Italy; edda.russo@unifi.it (E.R.); amedeo.amedei@unifi.it (A.A.)
[6] Department of Biomedicine, Azienda Ospedaliera Universitaria Careggi (AOUC), 50134 Florence, Italy
*   Correspondence: ivana.s.milosevic@mfub.bg.ac.rs; Tel.: +381-11-2683-366

Received: 22 December 2018; Accepted: 14 January 2019; Published: 17 January 2019

Abstract: The rapid scientific interest in gut microbiota (GM) has coincided with a global increase in the prevalence of infectious and non-infectivous liver diseases. GM, which is also called "the new virtual metabolic organ", makes axis with a number of extraintestinal organs, such as kidneys, brain, cardiovascular, and the bone system. The gut-liver axis has attracted greater attention in recent years. GM communication is bi-directional and involves endocrine and immunological mechanisms. In this way, gut-dysbiosis and composition of "ancient" microbiota could be linked to pathogenesis of numerous chronic liver diseases such as chronic hepatitis B (CHB), chronic hepatitis C (CHC), alcoholic liver disease (ALD), non-alcoholic fatty liver disease (NAFLD), non-alcoholic steatohepatitis (NASH), development of liver cirrhosis, and hepatocellular carcinoma (HCC). In this paper, we discuss the current evidence supporting a GM role in the management of different chronic liver diseases and potential new therapeutic GM targets, like fecal transplantation, antibiotics, probiotics, prebiotics, and symbiotics. We conclude that population-level shifts in GM could play a regulatory role in the gut-liver axis and, consequently, etiopathogenesis of chronic liver diseases. This could have a positive impact on future therapeutic strategies.

Keywords: gut microbiota; gut-liver axis; chronic liver diseases; fecal transplantation; probiotics

1. Gut Microbiota

The gut microbiota (GM) is a diverse ecosystem that consists of bacteria, protozoa, archaea, fungi, and viruses, which exist in a specific symbiosis between each other and the human body as well. Currently, it is well known that GM plays relevant roles in physiological and pathological conditions of human health, taking part in digestion, vitamin B synthesis, immunomodulation, and promotion of angiogenesis and nerve function. In addition, it is unavoidable that the GM has an impact on pathogenesis of gastrointestinal, hepatic, respiratory, cardiovascular, endocrine, and many other disorders, arising as "a new virtual metabolic organ" [1].

The GM colonizes human intestinal tract, which accounts for more than 100 trillion bacteria, and has a complex genome of 150-fold more genes than the human genome [2]. The majority of gut microorganisms cannot be cultured using standard techniques, so the development of culture independent molecular methods based on sequencing of the phylogenetic marker—16S/18S ribosomal RNA offer better insight in the GM structure. The GM is essentially ecomposed of the five phyla-*Firmicutes* (79.4%) (*Ruminococcus*, *Clostridium*, and *Eubacteria*), *Bacteroidetes* (16.9%) (*Porphyromonas*, *Prevotella*), *Actinobacteria* (2.5%) (*Bifidobacterium*), *Proteobacteria* (1%), and *Verrumicrobia* (0.1%) [3]. *Lactobacilli*, *Streptococci*, and *Escherichia coli* are found in small numbers in the gut. Different genetic and environmental factors influence the GM composition. For example, children born by natural childbirth inherit about 40% of the mother's intestinal flora, while GM composition is very different after the caesarean section. During the first two years of life, the diet is the most prominent factor that determines GM. Later in life, GM composition depends on age, diet, medications, and the environment.

Studies published in the last decade confirmed that the GM is implicated in the pathogenesis of various diseases, such as cancer and autism, depression, *Clostridium difficile* infection, inflammatory bowel disease, irritably bowel syndrome, colorectal carcinoma, infectious and non-infectious chronic liver diseases, obesity, diabetes mellitus type 2, atherosclerosis, and chronic kidney diseases [4–9]. In the present review, the important role of GM in the pathogenesis of most common liver diseases was discussed.

2. Gut-Liver Axis

GM as a "virtual metabolic organ" makes axis with a number of extraintestinal organs, such as kidneys, brain, cardiovascular, and the bone system, but the gut-liver axis attracts increased attention in recent years [10]. The gut-liver axis is a consequence of a close anatomical and functional, bidirectional interaction of the gastrointestinal tract and liver, primarily through a portal circulation. The symbiotic relationship between the GM and the liver is regulated and stabilized by a complex network of interactions, that encompass metabolic, immune, and neuroendocrine crosstalk between them [4]. The tight junctions (TJ) within the gut epithelium represent a natural barrier to bacteria and their metabolic products [11]. Antigens (Ag) (originating either from pathogenic micro-organisms or from food) that pass through these connections, are recognized by dendritic cells, or activate the adaptive immune system by modulating the T cell response. Minimal concentrations of pathogen-associated molecular patterns (PAMPs), such as lipopolysaccharides (LPS), peptidoglycans, and flagelin, activate the nuclear factor kappa B (NFKβ) through toll-like receptors (TLRs) and nod-like receptors (NLRs), which leads to the production of inflammatory cytokines and chemokines that enter portal circulation. In addition to hepatocyte damage, PAMPs can activate stellate cells involved in fibrosis promotion and progression, while Kupffer cells are even more responsive to LPS than hepatocytes [12]. Since the gut-liver axis affects the pathogenesis of liver diseases, it is an important focus of current clinical research (Scheme 1).

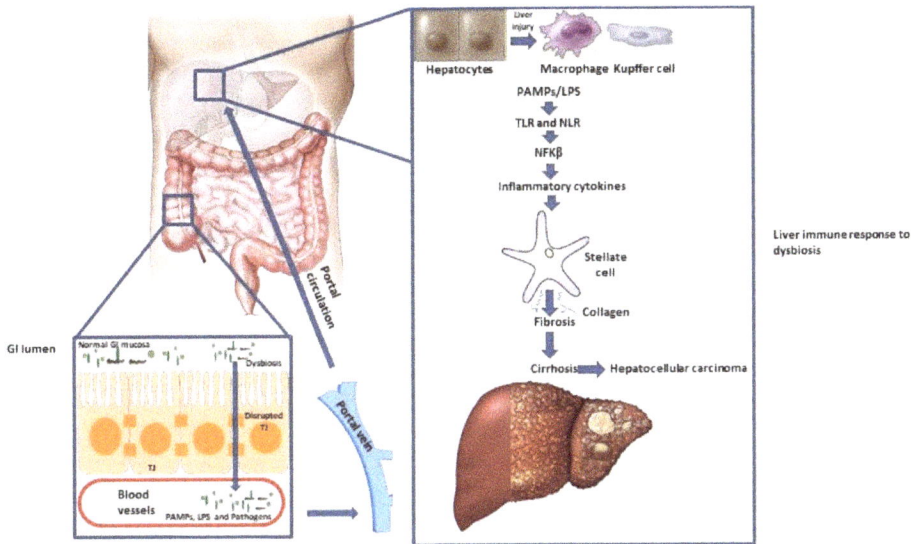

Scheme 1. Gut-liver axis pathogenesis. Abbreviations: GI, gastrointestinal, LPS, Lipopolysaccharides, NFKβ, nuclear factor kappa B, NLR, Nod-like receptors, PAMPs, Pathogen-associated molecular patterns, TJ, Tight junctions, TLR, Toll-like receptors.

3. Disbyosis and Liver Diseases

The gut-liver axis has an impact on pathogenesis of numerous chronic liver diseases such as chronic hepatitis B (CHB), chronic hepatitis C (CHC), alcoholic liver disease (ALD), non-alcoholic fatty liver disease (NAFLD), non-alcoholic steatohepatitis (NASH), development of liver cirrhosis, and hepatocellular carcinoma (HCC) (Table 1).

Table 1. Gut microbiota-associated liver diseases.

Disease	Dysbiotic Features	References
CHB	Decreased ratio of *Bifidobacteriacae/Enterobacteriaceae*: -low levels of *Bifidobacteria* and *Lactobacillus* -high levels of *Enterococcus* and *Enterobacteriaceae*	[13]
HBV related cirrhosis	Decreased *Bacteroidetes* Increased *Proteobacteria*	[14]
CHC	Decreased *Bifidobacterium* Increased *Prevotella* and *Faecalibacterium*	[15]
HCC	Decreased *Lactobacillus* spp., *Bifidobacterium* spp. and *Enterococcus* spp. Increased *Escherichia coli*	[16] [17]
HE	Production of ammonia and endotoxins by urease-producing bacteria, such as *Klebsiella* and *Proteus*	[18]
ALD	Decreased levels of butyrate-producing *Clostridiales* species Increased levels of pro-inflammatory *Enterobacteriaceae*	[19]
NAFLD/NASH	Increased *Firmicutes/Bacteroidetes* ratio	[20,21]
Cirrhosis	Decreased *Bacteroidetes* and *Firmicutes* Increased *Streptococcus* spp. and *Veillonella* spp.	[22] [16]

Abbreviations: ALD, alcoholic liver disease, CHB, chronic hepatitis B, CHC, chronic hepatitis C, HBV, hepatitis B virus, HCC, hepatocellular carcinoma, HE, hepatic encephalopathy, NAFLD, non-alcoholic fatty liver disease, and NASH, non-alcoholic steatohepatitis.

In general, an increased intestinal permeability and bacterial translocation could enable microbial metabolites to reach the liver, which would impair the bile acid (BA) metabolism and promote gut dysmotility and systemic inflammation. All these conditions could induce gut dysbiosis, which, in turn, further increases liver damage. It has been observed that the stage of liver injury correlates closely with the severity of gut dysbiosis [23]. Alterations in the fecal bacterial flora are described by changes in the composition of the dominant *Bacteroidetes* and *Firmicutes* phyla, including *Ruminococcaceae*, *Lachnospiraceae*, and *Clostridiales*, which produce short-chain fatty acids (SCFA) that are an energy source for the intestinal epithelium's cells, but can also regulate secondary BA metabolism and induce a regulatory immune process and IgA production.

3.1. Hepatitis B Virus (HBV) Infection

CHB is an important health issue worldwide. Acute HBV infection leads to CHB in just 5% of adult patients, while the proportion is quite different in children, since more than 90% of exposed neonates and 30% to 50% of children aged 1 to 5 years fail in HBV clearance. Liver injury is mediated by HBV induced immune response. TLRs play an important role in the production of interferons and proinflammatory cytokines and immune cells recruitment in order to suppress viral replication. It has been established that age-specific seroclearance depends not only on the maturity of the immune system, but on the GM stability as well [24]. Involvement of GM in HBV clearance was demonstrated in animal models. Chou et al. showed that adult mice with mature GM managed to clear HBV after six weeks of infection, which is the opposite among young mice without GM, who remained HBV positive. The fact that adult mice failed to clear HBV after gut sterilization by antibiotics (6 to 12 weeks), emphasizes the GM significance in anti-HBV immunity [25]. It also implies new therapeutic strategy for patients with HBV infection [26]. In fact, the transplantation of fecal microbiota (FMT), in addition to standard antivirals, has been shown to be effective in HBeAg clearance [27].

Compositional and structural changes of GM have been detected in patients with CHB and liver cirrhosis. These patients have a decreased ratio of *Bifidobacteriaceae*/*Enterobacteriaceae* (B/E), based on low levels of *Bifidobacteria* and *Lactobacillus*, and high levels of *Enterococcus* and *Enterobacteriacea*. In addition, gut permeability is altered when accompanied with bacterial translocation and the presence of endotoxins in the portal vein, which leads to increased TLS/NLR activation in the liver with consequential cytokine production and occurrence of liver lesions, progression of fibrosis, and development of cirrhosis and HCC [2,13]. Wei et al. have demonstrated that GM of patients with HBV-related cirrhosis contained lower levels of *Bacteroidetes* (4% vs. 53%) and increased levels of *Proteobacteria* (43% vs. 4%) compared to the heathy group [14]. In an other study, patients with alcohol-related and HBV-related cirrhosis showed decreased GM diversity, compared to healthy individuals, with a predominance of *Enterobacteriaceae* and *Streptococcaceae* [28].

3.2. Hepatitis C Virus (HCV) Infection

CHC is a global health problem that leads to progressive liver fibrosis and the cirrhosis development in 20% to 30% of untreated patients after 20 to 30 years. It has been estimated that 1% to 4% of these patients develop HCC each year [29]. GM has been rarely analyzed in patients with HCV infection. According to published data, the GM found in HCV patients shows lower microbial diversity in comparison to those in healthy controls [15,28,30]. CHC could alter microbiota composition through IgA produced by HCV infected gastric B-lymphocyte. GM found in Egyptian patients with CHC contains more *Prevotella* and *Faecalibacterium* and less *Acinetobacter*, *Veillonella*, and *Phascolarctobacterium* than healthy individuals. In the study of Aly et al., *Bifidobacterium* was detected only in GM of the healthy group, posing the possible new role of *Prevotella*/*Faecalibacterium* vs. *Bifidobacterium* ratio as a biomarker for CHC and fibrosis progression [15]. Disease progression could bring more profound changes in CHC patients' GM. Therefore, according to Heidrich et al., decreased diversity was more pronounced in HCV patients' with established cirrhosis than in those with less advanced CHC [31]. Liver cirrhosis *per se* could be an independent risk factor for dysbiosis regardless of the HCV viral load. This hypothesis is in agreement with a study performed by Bajaj et al. who found that patients with HCV cirrhosis have gut dysbiosis regardless of long-term HCV eradication. A sustained virological response (SVR) did not improve gut dysbiosis in patients with

HCV cirrhosis, due to refractory systemic inflammation and endotoxemia in these individuals [32]. Bacterial translocation was described in patients with CHC and together with increased intestinal permeability ("leaky gut"), it poses a well-established milieu with TLR/NLR activation and expression of pro-inflammatory cytokine genes, especially in those with cirrhosis [33].

3.3. Alcoholic Liver Disease

Alcohol abuse is a prominent cause of liver damage worldwide. GM is recognized as a key player in the severity of liver injury in ALD, in addition to the quantity of consumed alcohol and genetic predisposition (patatin like phospholipase domain containing 3 (PNPLA3), Transmembrane 6 superfamily 2 human gene (TM6SF2), membrane bound O-acyltransferase domain containing 7 (MBOAT7), and solute carrier family 38 member 4 (SLC38A4) etc.) [34]. Alcohol consupmtion leads to small and large intestine overgrowth and modulation of GM composition in both animals and humans [35]. Alcohol and its degradation products disrupt epithelial TJ leading to increased intestinal permeability and inflammation [34]. Gut-derived PAMPs (e.g., endotoxin) are increased after heavy alcohol intake [36]. Ethanol consumption alters the GM composition through SCFAs modulation. Intestinal levels of SCFAs are lower after alcohol consumption with the exception of increases in acetic acid levels, which is the metabolite of ethanol [37]. Alcoholic abuse was shown to be associated with decreased levels of butyrate-producing Clostridiales species order and increased levels of pro-inflammatory Enterobacteriaceae. In those with established cirrhosis, multiple members of the Bacteroidales order were depleted with a rise of taxa normally inhabiting the oral cavity [19].

3.4. Non-Alcoholic Fatty Liver Disease and Non-Alcoholic Steatohepatitis

NAFLD is one of the most important causes of liver disease worldwide, with global prevalence of 25%. NAFLD is one of the top risk factors for HCC and is predicted to become the most common indication for liver transplantation [38]. NAFLD is a consequence of triglyceride accumulation in the hepatocytes and is considered to be the hepatic manifestation of obesity and the metabolic syndrome [39]. About 20% of patients with NAFLD develop NASH, which is a chronic hepatic inflammation that can progress to cirrhosis, end stage liver disease (ESLD), and HCC. Pathogenesis of NASH is not yet fully elucidated, but it is described as a "two hit" phenomenon. The primary event is lipid accumulation with alterations of lipid homeostasis associated with obesity, insulin resistance, and adipokine abnormalities. The second "hit" is a combination of oxidative stress, lipid peroxidation, mitochondrial dysfunction, BA toxicity, cytokine-mediated recruitment, and retention of inflammatory cells [40]. Obesity is associated with dysbiotic gut microbiota, with decreased diversity and an increased *Firmicutes/Bacteroidetes* ratio [20]. A similar *Firmicutes/Bacteroidetes* ratio was found in diabetes patients as well. Endogenous ethanol is constantly produced by microbiota, regardless of oral alcohol intake, especially in those with a sugar-rich diet. Increased ethanol production by microbiota in obese humans and mice leads to the activation of TLRs in the liver, cytokine production, and alters the BA profile. Endogenous ethanol serum concentrations are significantly higher in patients with NASH compared to obese or healthy controls [41]. Gut dysbiosis in patients with NAFLD/NASH promotes insulin resistance, *de novo* lipogenesis in liver, and also increases intestinal permeability, which promotes chronic PAMPs exposure and oxidative stress caused by increased endogenous ethanol [21]. Endotoxin/TLR4 signalling contributes to the development of fibrosis and progression to cirrhosis through hepatic stellate cell activation. The GM plays a critical role in the conservation of the mainstream BA pool, which transforms BA to several metabolites by oxidation/epimerization, deconjugation, esterification, 7-dehydroxylation, and desulfatation. Changes in any of these modulations is a cause of disease. GM dysbiosis in NAFLD could affect the conversion of primary bile acids into secondary bile acids [42]. It has been observed that the bacteria able to make this transformation are decreased in the NAFLD cirrhosis fecal samples. In particular, there is a higher level of *Enterobacteriaceae* (that could be potentially pathogenic) with lower *Ruminococcaceae*, *Lachnospiraceae*, and *Blautia* (with a 7α-dehydroxylating activity) abundances.

Currently, the roles of BA and nuclear receptors are also strongly considered. The BA primarly synthesized in the liver are secreted to the gallbladder and then released into the duodenum following food ingestion. In the gut, the size and composition of the BA pool can be modified by GM via the biotransformation of primary into secondary BA. The BA contributes to the emulsification and fat solubilization but also activates the expression of a nuclear bile acid receptor FXR (farnesoid X receptor) and a membrane G protein-coupled receptor TGR5. The reduction of the secondary BA synthesis attributed to GM dysbiosis lowers the activation of nuclear receptors FXR and TGR5 in the ileum, which leads to retained bile salts, perpetuation of gut permeability, small bowel translocation, and bacterial overgrowth, which contributes to liver disease [43]. The FXR plays a key role in mediating the crosstalk between the host and GM, especially through the modulation of enterohepatic BA circulation. FXR exerts bile-acid regulatory effects via a tissue-specific mechanism. [44]. In detail, in the liver, FXR induces the expression of the small heterodimer partner (SHP), which inhibits CYP7A1 (Cholesterol 7 alpha-hydroxylase) expression, while, in the intestine, FXR increases the levels of circulating fibroblast growth factor 19 (FGF19), which decrease the expression of CYP7A1 and cytochrome P450 12a-hydroxylase B1 (CYP8B1). Therefore, this leads to the inhibition of BA synthesis [45].

FXR activation has been known to reduce triglyceride levels suppressing the synthesis and uptake of the fatty acids in the liver [46]. In addition, the FXR roles in decreasing inflammation have been emerging [47]. Lastly, related to glucide metabolism, FXR reduces insulin resistance, gluconeogenesis, increases glycogenesis, and, therefore, decreases the blood glucose amount. A more fine elucidation of FXR functions in liver and intestine needs further research. Furthermore, mice models showed that FXR activation, induced by BA products (converted by GM) might protect against bacterial overgrowth, gut permeability, and small bowel translocation [48]. The degree of FXR activation could be regulated by GM dysbiosis, inducing BA alteration and, hence, liver disease secondary to retained bile salts and a leaky gut. Bacteria, translocated from the gut, may additionally decrease FXR activation within hepatocytes, which leads to decreased BSEP (bile salt export pum) activity.

The bile acid-activated FXR and TGR5 has a protective role in liver disease progression, which means the activation of both receptors has been proposed as therapy. Many activators of FXR and TGR5 have been developed from bile acid analogues, which are able to decrease hepatic steatosis and inflammation [49]. FXR agonists such as obeticholic acid have already been recognized as a new therapeutic venue for NASH and cholestatic diseases. NASH patients exhibit increased fecal primary BAs, primary/secondary BAs fecal ratio, and plasma and hepatic BAs concentrations [50]. This cytotoxicity can lead to NASH progression and finally to liver cirrhosis.

3.5. Hepatic Encephalopathy (HE) and Spontaneous Bacterial Peritonitis (SBP)

In all patients with ESLD, regardless of its etiology, HE and SBP commonly occur. HE is considered to be a consequence of high ammonia level, but GM and bacteria's products, such as amino acid metabolites (indoles, oxindoles) and endotoxins, are also involved in HE development. The connection between HE and GM is the production of ammonia and endotoxins by urease-producing bacteria, such as Klebsiella and Proteus, which are present in GM [18]. It has been shown that microbiota of the sigmoid colon in liver cirrhosis patients differs in those with HE when compared with patients without HE [51]. Gut dysbiosis in liver cirrhosis also contributes to the development of Spontaneous Bacterial Peritonitis (SBP) through damaged intestinal barrier and a higher degree of microbial translocation [52].

3.6. Hepatocellular Carcinoma

HCC is the most common primary malignancy in adults with chronic liver disease and liver cirrhosis [53]. HBV and HCV infection, alcohol abuse, and dietary aflatoxin are major risk factors for the development of HCC. Although HBV and HCV account for 80% to 90% of overall HCC, regarding the obesity pandemic, an emergance of potent direct acting antivirals for HCV and worldwide available vaccine for HBV, it can be expected that HCC epidemiology will change in the future [54]. An alarming rise in the incidence of NAFLD and NASH was accompanied by an increased development of NASH-related HCC incidence [55].

All previously mentioned mechanisms, leaky gut, endotoxemia, TLR, dysbiosis, and immunomodulation promote the development of HCC [56]. The gastrointestinal tract contributes to homeostasis by maintaining an intact barrier against LPS and intestinal bacteria. In the case of increased intestinal permeability, bacterial translocation and LPS accumulation will lead to intestinal bacterial overgrowth and changes of GM composition. In patients with chronic liver diseases/cirrhosis, detoxification, degradation, and clearance of LPS and other bacterial products is compromised [57]. Altered microbiota is generally presented in HCC patients [58]. HCC patients have been reported to have high levels of *Escherichia coli* and other gram-negative bacteria in GM, which are associated to increased LPS serum levels [16]. *Oribacterium* and *Fusobacterium* are the most commonly isolated bacteria from tongue swab of HCC patients. On the other side, GM of HCC patients contains reduced levels of *Lactobacillus* spp., *Bifidobacterium* spp., and *Enterococcus* spp. [17]. Unlike merely microbial species, it was shown that microbial metabolism, iron transport, and energy-producing system significantly differ between GM of HCC patients and healthy control [58]. TLR4 expressed by activated stellate cells react to low LPS concentrations, which ensures the development of fibrosis and cirrhosis. The significance of GM and TLR4 activation in hepatocarcinogenesis have been studied in an animal model. It has been demonstrated that GM and TLR4 activation promote HCC development by increased cell proliferation and suppression of apoptosis [59].

4. Current Perspectives on the Therapeutic Options

Dietary modification is the focus for many studies on GM modification, but results are not encouraging due to poor compliance [11]. Different treatments options have been developed in the last decade in the attempt to modify pathogenesis factors involved in GM-liver axis, but results are still unsatisfactory [60]. Antibiotics, probiotics, prebiotics, and symbiotics are gaining increasing importance as a treatment option for GM manipulation and its impact on different liver diseases (Table 2).

Table 2. Therapeutic options for gut-microbiota alteration in liver diseases.

Disease	Therapeutic Option	References
NAFLD/NASH	-"VSL #3" (*Streptococcus thermophilus, Bifidobacterium breve, B. longum, B. infantis, Lactobacillus acidophilus, L. plantarum, L. paracasei, L. bulgaricus*) reduces liver injury	[61,62]
Cirrhosis	-Diet rich in fermented milk, vegetables, cereals, coffee, and tea is associated with a higher microbial diversity and lower risk for cirrhosis progression	[63]
HCC	-Probiotics can contribute to the inhibition of aflatoxin B-induced hepatocarcinogenesis, restore intestinal dysbiosis, reduce LPS levels and decrease tumor size	[58,99]
	-Probiotic fermented milk and chlorophyllin slow down tumor growth and volume for 40%	[64]
HE	-*Lactobacillus, Bifidobacterium*, non-pathogenetic strains of *Escherichia coli, Clostridium butyticum, Streptococcus salivarius, Saccharomyces boulardii* and VSL#3 improve HE	[65–69]

Abbreviations: NAFLD, non-alcoholic fatty liver disease, HCC, hepatocellular carcinoma, HE, hepatic encephalopathy, and NASH, non-alcoholic steatohepatitis.

4.1. Antibiotics, Probiotics, Prebiotics, and Symbiotics

Positive effects of antibiotics on small-intestinal-bacterial-overgrowth related liver damage was shown in the recent literature, which confirms the relationship between GM and liver diseases [70]. Probiotics are micro-organisms with a healthy impact to the human, while pre-biotics are food ingredients, which can not be digested and, on that way, help gut peristaltic and selectively stimulate growth of intestinal bacteria. Some prebiotic food products, like pectin, have been shown to prevent liver injury in rodent models by restoring the levels of *Bacteroides* and appears to be a promising therapeutic agent [71]. New term "symbiotics" represent combinations of a probiotic and prebiotic. From this group, the most potential for being used as potential treatment of chronic liver diseases have probiotics [11,70]. Probiotics have a significant influence on the gut-liver axis, including the immunomodulatory and anti-inflammatory role on intestinal microflora and intestinal barrier function, but also metabolic effects on non-gastrointestinal organs and systems.

Not all probiotic species have the same impact on GM modulation. For example, different strains of *Lactobacillus* spp. are associated with divergent obesity consequences, pro-obesity and anti-obesity [72]. A study on murine diet-induced obesity showed the opposite metabolic outcomes after different targeted GM manipulation with vancomycin vs. probiotic strain *Lactobacillus salivarius*, but microbiota changes were similar. On the other side, a recent human study investigating the effect of the *Lactobacillus salivarius* Ls-33 on a series of inflammatory biomarkers in obese adolescents could not detect any significant impact on the metabolic syndrome [73,74]. These results suggest that no generalization could be done. Use of probiotics and antimicrobials in chronic liver diseases should be determined in accordance to specific gut-liver axis pathology. Although there are a number of findings from animal and human studies, this topic requires more case-control prospective studies with a significant number of patients.

4.2. Fecal Microbiota Transfer (FMT)

Next to probiotics and prebiotics, fecal microbiota transfer attracts a lot of attention currently as a possible option for GM editing. FMT is the introduction of a fecal suspension derived from a healthy donor into the intestinal tract of the patient. Animal studies revealed altered GM composition after FMT in alcohol-sensitive mice and prevented alcohol-induced liver lesions [71]. Wang et al. showed potential protective effects of FMT in the improvement of motor activity in a rat model of HE. In addition, FMT had a superior impact on alteration of the intestinal mucosal barrier function, in comparison to probiotics [75]. A different study with the rat model of HE found that rectal administration of a *Lactobacillus* species suppressed bacterial cell proliferation [76]. Regarding the clinical trial, a pilot study was performed in eight male patients with severe alcoholic hepatitis (SAH) and compared outcomes with historical controls. Researchers found that one week of FMT was effective and safe in SAH patients and improved the values of liver disease severity and survival at one year [77]. In addition, an open label randomized clinical trial was performed in 20 male patients with cirrhosis and recurrent HE despite treatment with lactulose and rifaximin, comparing FMT vs. standard of care [78]. The result showed that FMT from a rationally selected donor (chosen for having the highest abundance of *Lachospiraceae* and *Ruminococcaceae* in a universal stool bank) improved cognition, reduced hospitalizations, and ameliorated the dysbiosis condition in cirrhosis with recurrent HE. However, it is not yet known what consequences FMT may excert on dysbiosis in the upper gastrointestinal tract, which may be more involved in liver disease pathogenesis. Further clinical trials benefiting FMT for management of chronic liver diseases are ongoing. It is important to highlight that FMT is a promising therapy to restore a healthy microbiota. However, its safety profile among vulnerable liver disease patients that are usually immunosuppressed and, so at risk of bacteremia, due to bacterial translocation, is unknown.

4.3. NAFLD

Several pharmacologic treatments for NAFLD exist, but a standard treatment is not yet established [79,80]. Recent animal model-studies on NAFLD and HE reported beneficial therapeutic effects of probiotics [81–83]. In mice models, probiotics had positive effects on oxidative and inflammatory liver damage mediated by c-Jun N-terminal kinase (JNK) and NF-KB correlated with TNF-α regulation and insulin resistance. The results showed improvement of histological findings including reduced fat deposits and liver damage, with decreased serum alanine aminotransferase (ALT) levels [81,83,84]. Apart from animal studies, several clinical trials of probiotics administered to patients with NAFLD have been reported. The mixture of *Streptococcus thermophilus*, *Bifidobacterium breve*, *Bifidobacterium longum*, *Bifidobacterium infantis*, *Lactobacillus acidophilus*, *Lactobacillus plantarum*, *Lactobacillus paracasei*, and *Lactobacillus bulgaricus* has joint name "VSL #3" and represent the most-studied probiotic [61]. A meta analysis of effects of probiotic on NAFLD/NASH showed that probiotic therapies can reduce liver aminotransferases, total-cholesterol, TNF-α, and improve insulin resistance in NAFLD/NASH patients [62]. Administration of non-complete VSL #3 (only *Lactobacillus bulgaricus* and *Streptococcus thermophilus*) decreased ALT and aspartate aminotransferase (AST) levels, but had no impact on cardiometabolic risk factors [85]. Ma et al. found that the probiotic therapy significantly decreased the levels of ALT, AST, total-cholesterol, high-density lipoprotein (HDL), and TNF-α in the serum, and the homeostasis model assessment of insulin resistance [62]. Comparing single strains, *Bifidobacterium longum* showed more positive effects than *Lactobacillus acidophilus* in NAFLD treatment and these beneficial effects correlated to GM modifications [61]. It was demonstrated that GM modulation by linoleic acid and *Bifidobacterium* resulted in an increase of conjugated linoleic acid (CLA) and altered fatty acid composition of liver [86]. Consequently, by producing CLA as a microbial metabolite, VSL #3 correlates with NAFLD's improvement [86]. In additional studies (of Malaguarnera et al. and Tanock et al.), probiotics were used with prebiotics in NAFLD patients, and the combination significantly reduced the AST and ALT levels and liver steatosis [87,88].

Prebiotics also hold promise for the NAFLD management. In animal models, the administration of prebiotics could lead to reduced liver inflammation in obese mice through a glucagon-like peptide-2-dependent effect on the gut barrier [89]. There is convincing evidence from short-term high quality human trials supporting the use of dietary prebiotics as a potential therapeutic intervention for NAFLD. However, further studies are needed to correlate these findings with changes in GM [90]. Although most of the conducted studies have limitations including small sample sizes and a lack of data about the patients' diets and life style, the treatments with probiotics and prebiotics for patients with NAFLD are promising [91].

Moreover, a recent meta-analysis study demonstrated that, in addition to probiotics and prebiotics, ω-3 supplementation could have effects on the gut microbiota, which improves NAFLD [92]. It has been shown that n-3polyunsaturated fatty acids (n-3 PUFAs) decrease *Akkermansia*, *Epsilon proteobacteria*, *Bacteroides*, and increase *Clostridia* [93]. Lastly, the n-3 PUFAs administration has been related to an increment of butyrate-producing bacteria [94].

4.4. Cirrhosis

Qin at el. showed reduced *Bacteroidetes* and *Firmicutes* levels and increased *Streptococcus* spp. and *Veillonella* spp. levels in GM by metagenomics analyses in cirrhotic patients, compared to a healthy population [22]. *Streptococcus* spp. and *Veillonella* spp. are bacteria regularly living in oral cavity, which implicates that an increased number of oral bacteria in GM may be related to cirrhosis development [16]. It was reported that the gut microbiome plays a role in the CHB progression to severe liver failure, including inflammation and pathogenic metabolic accumulation [75]. The connection between GM and cirrhosis was recently confirmed in the study of Bajaj et al., which showed a significant improvement of diversity and symbiosis of GM after liver transplantation in a patient with severe cirrhosis [95]. In the recent international cirrhosis cohort study, Bajaj et al. showed that diverse GM achieved by diet is associated with a lower risk for cirrhosis progression and reduced risk of hospitalization [63]. Although the functions of these bacteria in the pathogenesis and complications of liver cirrhosis is not yet clear, these findings give hope for a new therapeutic strategy against liver cirrhosis by focusing on the GM modulation.

4.5. Hepatic Encephalopathy

Probiotics inhibit the activity of bacterial ureases, modulate intestinal pH values, and reduce ammonia absorption in HE [96]. Administration of probiotics and prebiotics could improve HE by altering GM [18]. It is already shown that *Lactobacillus*, *Bifidobacterium*, non-pathogenic strains of *Escherichia coli*, *Clostridium butyricum*, *Streptococcus salivarius*, and *Saccharomyces boulardii*, and VSL #3 altered GM composition and improve HE [97]. A number of conducted clinical trials indicate that probiotics could be helpful in overt HE [65–69]. In a systematic review of McGee et al., it was found that patients treated with probiotics appeared to have reduced plasma ammonia concentrations compared to patients treated with placebo or no intervention. On the other side, treatment without probiotics and synbiotics did not significantly alter mortality and quality of life [65]. The possible explanation is that the sample of study groups was small in the reviewed control trials, as well as quantities of the probiotics were not uniform. Use of probiotics for the secondary HE prophylaxis was studied by Agrawal et al. Although not statistically significant, the occurrence rate of recurrent HE was lower in patients who received probiotics or lactulose compared to those without treatment (34% and 27%, respectively, vs. 57%) [67]. In another prospective study by Lunia et al., it was shown that probiotics could be effective in preventing overt HE. Patients with liver cirrhosis who had not experienced overt HE and who received the probiotics were less likely to develop overt HE compared to controls (1.2% vs. 19%) [67]. Among the various probiotics, the most efficacious species for HE appeared to be *Lactobacilli* and *Bifidobacteria* [97]. The most studied probiotic is the *Lactobacillus* GG AT strain 53103 (LGG). Safety and tolerability of administrated therapy is especially important for the patients with cirrhosis and HE. It is shown that LGG is safe and well tolerated in patients with cirrhosis and could cause reductions of the endotoxemia and TNF-α production [98]. However, due to a specific clinical course, randomized controlled trials are needed before probiotics can be routinely used in patients with HE.

4.6. HCC

The mouse model has shown that the obesity-induced intestinal microbial dysbiosis can lead to HCC [99]. Reports of the therapeutic prevention of HCC using probiotics are limited to aflatoxin-induced HCC. Findings of a clinical and animal model studies suggested that probiotics can contribute to the inhibition of aflatoxin B-induced hepatocarcinogenesis, restore intestinal dysbiosis, reduce LPS levels, and decrease the tumor size [59,100]. An animal study regarding the potential of Lactobacillus plantarum, isolated from Chinese traditional fermented foods, in reducing the toxicity of aflatoxin B1, showed that L. plantarum C88 treatment increased fecal aflatoxin B1 excretion and regulated defense system's deficit of antioxidant in the mice model [100]. Lastly, a study with an HCC rat model showed that probiotic fermented milk and chlorophyllin slow down tumor growth and volume for 40%, by reducing expressions of c-myc, bcl-2, cyclin D1, and rasp-21. After treatment with probiotics, mice had high levels of *Prevotella* and *Oscillibacter* in their fecal microbiota [64]. Dapito et al. also found that gut sterilization and TLR4 inactivation reduce HCC by 80% to 90% and could serve as potential HCC prevention strategies [59].

5. Conclusions

Knowledge regarding the gut-liver axis has improved in the last decade. It is confirmed that gut microbiota has a strong relationship with liver and plays a significant role in the pathogenesis of chronic liver diseases, including NAFLD, fibrosis progression, CHB, cirrhosis, HE, HCC, etc. However, the mechanism of this connection in different liver diseases is still unclear. Our knowledge about the clinical significance of probiotics' use in liver disease is starting to take shape. Although clinical and experimental studies confirmed the therapeutic potential of probiotics in chronic liver diseases, data on safety assessments, and impact on microbiota-host interactions are missing. Recently, many animal studies tried to reveal these gaps, but differences in physiology and variations in the molecular targets between mice and humans can lead to translational limitations. Large prospective controlled studies with a standardized dose of probiotics therapy and duration, liver biopsy, and patients' follow-up appointments are required to confirm these encouraging results.

Author Contributions: Conceptualization: I.M., A.V., and A.B. Writing—original draft preparation: M.Dj., M.K., A.R.S., I.G., O.S., and E.R. Writing—review and final editing: I.M., A.V., A.B., and A.A. Funding acquisition and critical reading: V.Dj. and N.L., A.A. initiated and supervised the whole work.

Funding: Marina Djelic and Ankica Vujovic received support for research from the Project of Ministry of Education, Science and Technology of the Republic of Serbia (No. III41025). Aleksandra Barac received support for research from the Project of Ministry of Education, Science and Technology of the Republic of Serbia (No. III45005).

Conflicts of Interest: The authors declare no conflicts of interest.

Abbreviations

ALD	Alcoholic liver disease
ALT	Alanine aminotransferase
AST	Aspartate aminotransferase
BA	Bile acid
CHB	Chronic hepatitis B
CHC	Chronic hepatitis C
CLA	Conjugated linoleic acid
ESLD	End-stage liver disease
FMT	Farnesoid X receptor
FXR	Fecal microbiota transfer
GM	Gut microbiota
HCC	Hepatocellular carcinoma
HDL	High-density lipoprotein
HE	Hepatic encephalopathy
JNK	c-Jun N-terminal kinase
LGG	Lactobacillus GG AT strain 53103
LPS	Lipopolysaccharides
MBOAT7	Membrane bound O-acyltransferase domain containing 7
NAFLD	Non-alcoholic fatty liver disease
NASH	Non-alcoholic steatohepatitis
NFKβ	Nuclear factor kappa B
NLRs	Nod-like receptors
PAMPs	Pathogen-associated molecular patterns
PNPLA3	Patatin like phospholipase domain containing 3
SLC38A4	Solute carrier family 38 member 4
SBP	Spontaneous bacterial peritonitis
SVR	Sustained virological response
TJ	Tight junctions
TLRs	Toll-like receptors
TM6SF2	Transmembrane 6 superfamily 2 human gene

References

1. O'Hara, A.M.; Shanahan, F. The gut flora as a forgotten organ. *EMBO J.* **2006**, *7*, 688–693. [CrossRef] [PubMed]
2. Chassaing, B.; Etienne-Mesmin, L.; Gewirtz, A.T. Microbiota-liver axis in hepatic disease. *Hepatology* **2014**, *59*, 328–339. [CrossRef] [PubMed]
3. Tap, J.; Mondot, S.; Levenez, F.; Pelletier, E.; Caron, C.; Furet, J.P.; Ugarte, E.; Muñoz-Tamayo, R.; Paslier, D.L.; Nalin, R.; et al. Towards the human intestinal microbiota phylogenetic core. *Environ. Microbiol.* **2009**, *11*, 2574–2584. [CrossRef] [PubMed]
4. Kho, Z.Y.; Lal, S.K. The Human Gut Microbiome—A Potential Controller of Wellness and Disease. *Front. Microbiol.* **2018**, *9*, 1835. [CrossRef]
5. Tao, Z.; Siew, C.N. The Gut Microbiota in the Pathogenesis and Therapeutics of Inflammatory Bowel Disease. *Front. Microbiol.* **2018**, *9*, 2247. [CrossRef]
6. Russo, E.; Amedei, A. The Role of the Microbiota in the Genesis of Gastrointestinal Cancers. In *Frontiers in Anti-Infective Drug Discovery*; Bentham Science Publishers: Emirate of Sharjah, UAE, 2018; Volume 7.

7. Al Khodor, S.; Shatat, F.I. Gut microbiome and kidney disease: A bidirectional relationship. *Pediatr. Nephrol.* **2017**, *32*, 921–931. [CrossRef] [PubMed]
8. Baothman, O.A.; Zamzami, M.A.; Taher, I.; Abubaker, J.; Abu-Farha, M. The role of Gut Microbiota in the development of obesity and Diabetes. *Lipids Health Dis.* **2016**, *15*, 108. [CrossRef]
9. Russo, E.; Bacci, G.; Chiellini, C.; Fagorzi, C.; Niccolai, E.; Taddei, A.; Ricci, F.; Ringressi, M.N.; Borrelli, R.; Melli, F.; et al. Preliminary Comparison of Oral and Intestinal Human Microbiota in Patients with Colorectal Cancer: A Pilot Study. *Front. Microbiol.* **2018**, *8*, 2699. [CrossRef]
10. Konturek, P.C.; Harsch, I.A.; Konturek, K.; Schink, M.; Konturek, T.; Neurath, M.F.; Zopf, Y. Gut–Liver Axis: How Do Gut Bacteria Influence the Liver? *Med. Sci. (Basel)* **2018**, *6*, 79. [CrossRef]
11. Vajro, P.; Paolella, G.; Fasano, A. Microbiota and gut-liver axis: A mini-review on their influences on obesity and obesity-related liver disease. *J. Pediatr. Gastroenterol. Nutr.* **2013**, *56*, 461–468. [CrossRef]
12. Yiu, J.H.; Dorweiler, B.; Woo, C.W. Interaction between gut microbiota and toll-like receptor: From immunity to metabolism. *J. Mol. Med.* **2017**, *95*, 13–20. [CrossRef]
13. Wang, J.; Wang, Y.; Zhang, X.; Liu, J.; Zhang, Q.; Zhao, Y.; Peng, J.; Feng, Q.; Dai, J.; Sun, S.; et al. Gut Microbial Dysbiosis Is Associated with Altered Hepatic Functions and Serum Metabolites in Chronic Hepatitis B Patients. *Front. Microbiol.* **2017**, *8*, 2222. [CrossRef]
14. Wei, X.; Yan, X.; Zou, D.; Yang, Z.; Wang, X.; Liu, W.; Wang, S.; Li, X.; Han, J.; Huang, L.; et al. Abnormal fecal microbiota community and functions in patients with hepatitis B liver cirrhosis as revealed by a metagenomic approach. *BMC Gastroenterol.* **2013**, *13*, 175. [CrossRef] [PubMed]
15. Aly, A.M.; Adel, A.; El-Gendy, A.O.; Essam, T.M.; Aziz, R.K. Gut microbiome alterations in patients with stage 4 hepatitis C. *Gut Pathog.* **2016**, *8*, 42. [CrossRef]
16. Grat, M.; Wronka, K.M.; Krasnodebski, M.; Masior, L.; Lewandowski, Z.; Kosinska, I.; Grat, K.; Stypulkowski, J.; Rejowski, S.; Wasilewicz, M.; et al. Profile of gut microbiota associated with the presence of hepatocel- lular cancer in patients with liver cirrhosis. *Transplant Proc.* **2016**, *48*, 1687–1691. [CrossRef]
17. Zhang, H.L.; Yu, L.X.; Yang, W.; Tang, L.; Lin, Y.; Wu, H.; Zhai, B.; Tan, Y.X.; Shan, L.; Liu, Q.; et al. Profound impact of gut homeostasis on chemically induced pro-tumorigenic inflammation and hepatocarcinogenesis in rats. *J. Hepatol.* **2012**, *57*, 803–812. [CrossRef] [PubMed]
18. Häussinger, D.; Schliess, F. Pathogenetic mechanisms of hepatic encephalopathy. *Gut* **2008**, *57*, 1156–1165. [CrossRef] [PubMed]
19. Dubinkina, V.B.; Tyakht, A.V.; Odintsova, V.Y.; Yarygin, K.S.; Kovarsky, B.A.; Pavlenko, A.V.; Ischenko, D.S.; Popenko, A.S.; Alexeev, D.G.; Taraskina, A.Y.; et al. Links of gut microbiota composition with alcohol dependence syndrome and alcoholic liver disease. *Microbiome* **2017**, *5*, 141. [CrossRef]
20. Chakraborti, C.K. New-found link between microbiota and obesity. *World J. Gastrointest. Pathophysiol.* **2015**, *6*, 110–119. [CrossRef]
21. Poeta, M.; Pierri, L.; Vajro, P. Gut-Liver Axis Derangement in Non-Alcoholic Fatty Liver Disease. *Children* **2017**, *4*, 66. [CrossRef]
22. Qin, N.; Yang, F.; Li, A.; Prifti, E.; Chen, Y.; Shao, L.; Guo, J.; Le Chatelier, E.; Yao, J.; Wu, L.; et al. Alterations of the human gut microbiome in liver cirrhosis. *Nature* **2014**, *513*, 59–64. [CrossRef] [PubMed]
23. Bajaj, J.S.; Heuman, D.M.; Hylemon, P.B.; Sanyal, A.J.; White, M.B.; Monteith, P.; Noble, N.A.; Unser, A.B.; Daita, K.; Fisher, A.R.; et al. Altered profile of human gut microbiome is associated with cirrhosis and its complications. *J. Hepatol.* **2014**, *60*, 940–947. [CrossRef] [PubMed]
24. Yang, R.; Xu, Y.; Dai, Z.; Lin, X.; Wang, H. The Immunologic Role of Gut Microbiota in Patients with Chronic HBV Infection. *J. Immunol. Res.* **2018**, *2018*, 2361963. [CrossRef] [PubMed]
25. Chou, H.H.; Chien, W.H.; Wu, L.L.; Cheng, C.H.; Chung, C.H.; Horng, J.H.; Ni, Y.H.; Tseng, H.T.; Wu, D.; Lu, X.; et al. Age-related immune clearance of hepatitis B virus infection requires the establishment of gut microbiota. *Proc. Natl. Acad. Sci. USA* **2015**, *112*, 2175–2180. [CrossRef] [PubMed]
26. Kang, Y.; Cai, Y. Gut microbiota and hepatitis-B-virus-induced chronic liver disease: Implications for faecal microbiota transplantation therapy. *J. Hosp. Infect.* **2017**, *96*, 342–348. [CrossRef]
27. Ren, Y.D.; Ye, Z.S.; Yang, L.Z.; Jin, L.X.; Wei, W.J.; Deng, Y.Y.; Chen, X.X.; Xiao, C.X.; Yu, X.F.; Xu, H.Z.; et al. Fecal microbiota transplantation induces hepatitis B virus e-antigen (HBeAg)clearance in patients with positive HBeAg after long-term antiviral therapy. *Hepatology* **2017**, *65*, 1765–1768. [CrossRef] [PubMed]
28. Chen, Y.; Yang, F.; Lu, H.; Wang, B.; Chen, Y.; Lei, D.; Wang, Y.; Zhu, B.; Li, L. Characterization of fecal microbial communities in patients with liver cirrhosis. *Hepatology* **2011**, *54*, 562–572. [CrossRef]

29. Lee, M.H.; Yang, H.I.; Yuan, Y.; L'Italien, G.; Chen, C.J. Epidemiology and natural history of hepatitis C virus infection. *World J. Gastroenterol.* **2017**, *20*, 9270–9280. [CrossRef]

30. Preveden, T.; Scarpellini, E.; Milić, N.; Luzza, F.; Abenavoli, L. Gut microbiota changes and chronic hepatitis C virus infection. *Expert Rev. Gastroenterol. Hepatol.* **2017**, *11*, 813–819. [CrossRef]

31. Heidrich, B.; Vital, M.; Plumeier, I.; Döscher, N.; Kahl, S.; Kirschner, J.; Ziegert, S.; Solbach, P.; Lenzen, H.; Potthoff, A.; et al. Intestinal microbiota in patients with chronic hepatitis C with and without cirrhosis compared with healthy controls. *Liver Int.* **2018**, *38*, 50–58. [CrossRef]

32. Bajaj, J.S.; Sterling, R.K.; Betrapally, N.S.; Nixon, D.E.; Fuchs, M.; Daita, K.; Heuman, D.M.; Sikaroodi, M.; Hylemon, P.B.; White, M.B.; et al. HCV eradication does not impact gut dysbiosis or systemic inflammation in cirrhotic patients. *Aliment. Pharmacol. Ther.* **2016**, *44*, 638–643. [CrossRef] [PubMed]

33. Munteanu, D.; Negru, A.; Radulescu, M.; Mihailescu, R.; Arama, S.S.; Arama, V. Evaluation of bacterial translocation in patients with chronic HCV infection. *Rom. J. Intern. Med.* **2014**, *52*, 91–96.

34. Cassard, A.M.; Ciocan, D. Microbiota, a key player in alcoholic liver disease. *Clin. Mol. Hepatol.* **2017**, *24*, 100–107. [CrossRef] [PubMed]

35. Hartmann, P.; Seebauer, C.T.; Schnabl, B. Alcoholic liver disease: The gut microbiome and liver cross talk. *Alcohol Clin. Exp. Res.* **2015**, *39*, 763–775. [CrossRef] [PubMed]

36. Szabo, G. Gut-liver axis in alcoholic liver disease. *Gastroenterology* **2014**, *148*, 30–36. [CrossRef] [PubMed]

37. Xie, G.; Zhong, W.; Zheng, X.; Li, Q.; Qiu, Y.; Li, H.; Chen, H.; Zhou, Z.; Jia, W. Chronic ethanol consumption alters mammalian gastrointestinal content metabolites. *J. Proteome Res.* **2013**, *12*, 3297–3306. [CrossRef] [PubMed]

38. Younossi, Z.M.; Marchesini, G.; Pinto-Cortez, H.; Petta, S. Epidemiology of Nonalcoholic Fatty Liver Disease and Nonalcoholic Steatohepatitis: Implications for Liver Transplantation. *Transplantation* **2018**, 30335697. [CrossRef] [PubMed]

39. Boppidi, H.; Daram, S.R. Nonalcoholic fatty liver disease: Hepatic manifestation of obesity and the metabolic syndrome. *Postgrad. Med.* **2008**, *120*, 1–7. [CrossRef] [PubMed]

40. Gentric, G.; Maillet, V.; Paradis, V.; Couton, D.; L'Hermitte, A.; Panasyuk, G.; Fromenty, B.; Celton-Morizur, S.; Desdouets, C. Oxidative stress promotes pathologic polyploidization in nonalcoholic fatty liver disease. *J. Clin. Investig.* **2015**, *125*, 981–992. [CrossRef]

41. Zhu, L.; Baker, S.S.; Gill, C.; Liu, W.; Alkhouri, R.; Baker, R.D.; Gill, S.R. Characterization of gut microbiomes in nonalcoholic steatohepatitis (NASH) patients: A connection between endogenous alcohol and NASH. *Hepatology* **2013**, *57*, 601–609. [CrossRef]

42. Kakiyama, G.; Pandak, W.M.; Gillevet, P.M.; Hylemon, P.B.; Heuman, D.M.; Daita, K.; Takei, H.; Muto, A.; Nittono, H.; Ridlon, J.M.; et al. Modulation of the fecal bile acid profile by gut microbiota in cirrhosis. *J. Hepatol.* **2013**, *58*, 949–955. [CrossRef] [PubMed]

43. Sinal, C.J.; Tohkin, M.; Miyata, M.; Ward, J.M.; Lambert, G.; Gonzalez, F.J. Targeted disruption of the nuclear receptor FXR/BAR impairs bile acid and lipid homeostasis. *Cell* **2000**, *102*, 731–744. [CrossRef]

44. Goodwin, B.; Jones, S.A.; Price, R.R.; Watson, M.A.; McKee, D.D.; Moore, L.B.; Galardi, C.; Wilson, J.G.; Lewis, M.C.; Roth, M.E.; et al. A regulatory cascade of the nuclear receptors FXR, SHP-1, and LRH-1 represses bile acid biosynthesis. *Mol. Cell.* **2000**, *6*, 517–526. [CrossRef]

45. Leung, D.H.; Yimlamai, D. The intestinal microbiome and paediatric liver disease. *Lancet Gastroenterol. Hepatol.* **2017**, *2*, 446–455. [CrossRef]

46. Zhu, Y.; Li, F.; Guo, G.L. Tissue-specific function of farnesoid X receptor in liver and intestine. *Pharmacol. Res.* **2011**, *63*, 259–265. [CrossRef] [PubMed]

47. Shaik, F.B.; Prasad, D.V.; Narala, V.R. Role of farnesoid X receptor in inflammation and resolution. *Inflamm. Res.* **2015**, *64*, 9–20. [CrossRef] [PubMed]

48. Inagaki, T.; Moschetta, A.; Lee, Y.K.; Peng, L.; Zhao, G.; Downes, M.; Yu, R.T.; Shelton, J.M.; Richardson, J.A.; Repa, J.J.; et al. Regulation of antibacterial defense in the small intestine by the nuclear bile acid receptor. *Proc. Natl. Acad. Sci. USA* **2006**, *103*, 3920–3925. [CrossRef]

49. Oliveira, M.C.; Gilglioni, E.H.; Boer, B.A.; Waart, D.R.; Salgueiro, C.L.; Ishii-Iwamoto, E.L.; Oude Elferink, R.P.J.; Gaemers, I.C. Bile acid receptor agonists INT747 and INT777 decrease oestrogen deficiency-related postmenopausal obesity and hepatic steatosis in mice. *Biochim. Biophys. Acta* **2016**, *1862*, 2054–2062. [CrossRef]

50. Chávez-Talavera, O.; Tailleux, A.; Lefebvre, P.; Staels, B. Bile acid control of metabolism and iInflammation in obesity, type 2 diabetes, dyslipidemia, and nonalcoholic fatty liver disease. *Gastroenterology* **2017**, *152*, 1679–1694. [CrossRef]

51. Rai, R.; Saraswat, V.A.; Dhiman, R.K. Gut microbiota: Its role in hepatic encephalopathy. *J. Clin. Exp. Hepatol.* **2015**, *5*, 29–36. [CrossRef]

52. Oikonomou, T.; Papatheodoridis, G.V.; Samarkos, M.; Goulis, I.; Cholongitas, E. Clinical impact of microbiome in patients with decompensated cirrhosis. *World J. Gastroenterol.* **2018**, *24*, 3813–3820. [CrossRef] [PubMed]

53. Kulik, L.; El-Serag, H.B. Epidemiology and Management of Hepatocellular Carcinoma. *Gastroenterology* **2018**. S0016-5085(18)35165-5. [CrossRef] [PubMed]

54. Nordenstedt, H.; White, D.L.; El-Serag, H.B. The changing pattern of epidemiology in hepatocellular carcinoma. *Dig. Liver Dis.* **2010**, *42*, 206–214. [CrossRef]

55. Cholankeril, G.; Patel, R.; Khurana, S.; Satapathy, S.K. Hepatocellular carcinoma in non-alcoholic steatohepatitis: Current knowledge and implications for management. *World J. Hepatol.* **2017**, *9*, 533–543. [CrossRef]

56. Wan, M.L.Y.; El-Nezami, H. Targeting gut microbiota in hepatocellular carcinoma: Probiotics as a novel therapy. *Hepatobiliary Surg. Nutr.* **2018**, *7*, 11–20. [CrossRef] [PubMed]

57. Tao, X.; Wang, N.; Qin, W. Gut Microbiota and Hepatocellular Carcinoma. *Gastrointest. Tumors* **2015**, *2*, 33–40. [CrossRef]

58. Lu, H.; Ren, Z.; Li, A.; Zhang, H.; Jiang, J.; Xu, S.; Luo, Q.; Zhou, K.; Sun, X.; Zheng, S.; et al. Deep sequencing reveals microbiota dysbiosis of tongue coat in patients with liver carcinoma. *Sci. Rep.* **2016**, *6*, 33142. [CrossRef]

59. Dapito, D.H.; Mencin, A.; Gwak, G.Y.; Pradere, J.P.; Jang, M.K.; Mederacke, I.; Caviglia, J.M.; Khiabanian, H.; Adeyemi, A.; Bataller, R.; et al. Promotion of hepatocellular carcinoma by the intestinal microbiota and TLR4. *Cancer Cell.* **2012**, *21*, 504–516. [CrossRef]

60. Chalasani, N.; Younossi, Z.; Lavine, J.E.; Diehl, A.M.; Brunt, E.M.; Cusi, K.; Charlton, M.; Sanyal, A.J. The diagnosis and management of non-alcoholic fatty liver disease: Practice guideline by the American Gastroenterological Association, American Association for the Study of Liver Diseases, and American College of Gastroenterology. *Gastroenterology* **2012**, *142*, 1592–1609. [CrossRef]

61. Chang, B.; Sang, L.; Wang, Y.; Tong, J.; Zhang, D.; Wang, B. The protective effect of VSL#3 on intestinal permeability in a rat model of alcoholic intestinal injury. *BMC Gastroenterol.* **2013**, *13*, 151. [CrossRef]

62. Ma, Y.Y.; Li, L.; Yu, C.H.; Shen, Z.; Chen, L.H.; Li, Y.M. Effects of probiotics on nonalcoholic fatty liver disease: A meta-analysis. *World J. Gastroenterol.* **2013**, *19*, 6911–6918. [CrossRef] [PubMed]

63. Bajaj, J.S.; Idilman, R.; Mabudian, L.; Hood, M.; Fagan, A.; Turan, D.; White, M.B.; Karakaya, F.; Wang, J.; Atalay, R.; et al. Diet Affects Gut Microbiota Modulates Hospitalization Risk Differentially In an International Cirrhosis Cohort. *Hepatology* **2018**, *68*, 234–247. [CrossRef] [PubMed]

64. Kumar, M.; Verma, V.; Nagpal, R.; Kumar, A.; Gautam, S.K.; Behare, P.V.; Grover, C.R.; Aggarwal, P.K. Effect of probiotic fermented milk and chlorophyllin on gene expressions and genotoxicity during AFB1-induced hepatocellular carcinoma. *Gene* **2011**, *490*, 54–59. [CrossRef] [PubMed]

65. McGee, R.G.; Bakens, A.; Wiley, K.; Riordan, S.M.; Webster, A.C. Probiotics for patients with hepatic encephalopathy. *Cochrane Database Syst. Rev.* **2011**, *11*, CD008716. [CrossRef]

66. Holte, K.; Krag, A.; Gluud, L.L. Systematic review and meta-analysis of randomized trials on probiotics for hepatic encephalopathy. *Hepatol. Res.* **2012**, *42*, 1008–1015. [CrossRef] [PubMed]

67. Agrawal, A.; Sharma, B.C.; Sharma, P.; Sarin, S.K. Secondary prophylaxis of hepatic encephalopathy in cirrhosis: An open-label, randomized controlled trial of lactulose, probiotics, and no therapy. *Am. J. Gastroenterol.* **2012**, *107*, 1043–1050. [CrossRef]

68. Lunia, M.K.; Sharma, B.C.; Sharma, P.; Sachdeva, S.; Srivastava, S. Probiotics prevent hepatic encephalopathy in patients with cirrhosis: A randomized controlled trial. *Clin. Gastroenterol. Hepatol.* **2014**, *12*, 1003–1008. [CrossRef]

69. Shukla, S.; Shukla, A.; Mehboob, S.; Guha, S. Meta-analysis: The effects of gut flora modulation using prebiotics, probiotics and synbiotics on minimal hepatic encephalopathy. *Aliment. Pharmacol. Ther.* **2011**, *33*, 662–671. [CrossRef] [PubMed]

70. Sajjad, A.; Mottershead, M.; Syn, W.K.; Jones, R.; Smith, S.; Nwokolo, C.U. Ciprofloxacin suppresses bacterial overgrowth, increases fasting insulin but does not correct low acylated ghrelin concentration in non-alcoholic steatohepatitis. *Aliment. Pharmacol. Ther.* **2005**, *22*, 291–299. [CrossRef]

71. Ferrere, G.; Wrzosek, L.; Cailleux, F.; Turpin, W.; Puchois, V.; Spatz, M.; Ciocan, D.; Rainteau, D.; Humbert, L.; Hugot, C.; et al. Fecal microbiota manipulation prevents dysbiosis and alcohol- induced liver injury in mice. *J. Hepatol.* **2017**, *66*, 806–815. [CrossRef]

72. Million, M.; Angelakis, E.; Paul, M.; Armougom, F.; Leibovici, L.; Raoult, D. Comparative meta-analysis of the effect of Lactobacillus species on weight gain in humans and animals. *Microb Pathog.* **2012**, *53*, 100–108. [CrossRef] [PubMed]

73. Gøbel, R.J.; Larsen, N.; Jakobsen, M.; Mølgaard, C.; Michaelsen, K.F. Probiotics to adolescents with obesity: Effects on inflammation and metabolic syndrome. *J. Pediatr. Gastroenterol. Nutr.* **2012**, *55*, 673–678. [CrossRef] [PubMed]

74. Larsen, N.; Vogensen, F.K.; Gøbel, R.J.; Michaelsen, K.F.; Forssten, S.D.; Lahtinen, S.J.; Jakobsen, M. Effect of Lactobacillus salivarius Ls-33 on fecal microbiota in obese adolescents. *Clin. Nutr.* **2013**, *32*, 935–940. [CrossRef] [PubMed]

75. Wang, W.W.; Zhang, Y.; Huang, X.B.; You, N.; Zheng, L.; Li, J. Fecal microbiota transplantation prevents hepatic encephalopathy in rats with carbon tetrachloride-induced acute hepatic dysfunction. *World J. Gastroenterol.* **2017**, *23*, 6983–6994. [CrossRef] [PubMed]

76. Adawi, D.; Kasravi, F.B.; Molin, G.; Jeppsson, B. Effect of Lactobacillus supplementation with and without arginine on liver damage and bacterial translocation in an acute liver injury model in the rat. *Hepatology* **1997**, *25*, 642–647. [CrossRef] [PubMed]

77. Philips, C.A.; Pande, A.; Shasthry, S.M.; Jamwal, K.M.; Khillan, V.; Chandel, S.S.; Kumar, G.; Sharma, M.K.; Maiwall, R.; Jindal, A.; et al. Healthy donor fecal microbiota transplantation in steroid-ineligible severe alcoholic hepatitis: A pilot study. *Clin. Gastroenterol. Hepatol.* **2017**, *15*, 600–602. [CrossRef] [PubMed]

78. Bajaj, J.S.; Kassam, Z.; Fagan, A.; Gavis, E.A.; Liu, E.; Cox, I.J.; Kheradman, R.; Heuman, D.; Wang, J.; Gurry, T.; et al. Fecal microbiota transplant from a rational stool donor improves hepatic encephalopathy: A randomized clinical trial. *Hepatology* **2017**, *66*, 1727–1738. [CrossRef]

79. Socha, P.; Horvath, A.; Vajro, P.; Dziechciarz, P.; Dhawan, A.; Szajewska, H. Pharmacological interventions for nonalcoholic fatty liver disease in adults and in children: A systematic review. *J. Pediatr. Gastroenterol. Nutr.* **2009**, *48*, 587–596. [CrossRef]

80. Minemura, M.; Shimizu, Y. Gut microbiota and liver diseases. *World J. Gastroenterol.* **2015**, *21*, 1691–1702. [CrossRef]

81. Li, Z.; Yang, S.; Lin, H. Probiotics and antibodies to TNF inhibit inflammatory activity and improve nonalcoholic fatty liver disease. *Hepatology* **2003**, *37*, 343–350. [CrossRef]

82. Chen, L.; Pan, D.D.; Zhou, J. Protective effect of selenium-enriched Lactobacillus on CCl4-induced liver injury in mice and its possible mechanisms. *World J. Gastroenterol.* **2005**, *11*, 795–800. [CrossRef]

83. Velayudham, A.; Dolganiuc, A.; Ellis, M. VSL#3 probiotic treatment attenuates fibrosis without changes in steatohepatitis in a diet-induced non-alcoholic steatohepatitis model in mice. *Hepatology* **2009**, *49*, 989–997. [CrossRef] [PubMed]

84. Ma, X.; Hua, J.; Li, Z. Probiotics improve high fat diet-induced hepatic steatosis and insulin resistance by increasing hepatic NKT cells. *J. Hepatol.* **2008**, *49*, 821–830. [CrossRef] [PubMed]

85. Aller, R.; De Luis, D.A.; Izaola, O.; Conde, R.; Gonzalez, S.M.; Primo, D.; De La Fuente, B.; Gonzalez, J. Effect of a probiotic on liver aminotransferases in nonalcoholic fatty liver disease patients: A double blind randomized clinical trial. *Eur. Rev. Med. Pharmacol. Sci.* **2011**, *15*, 1090–1095. [PubMed]

86. Wall, R.; Marques, T.M.; O'Sullivan, O.; Ross, R.P.; Shanahan, F.; Quigley, E.M.; Dinan, T.G.; Kiely, B.; Fitzgerald, G.F.; Cotter, P.D.; et al. Contrasting effects of Bifidobacterium breve NCIMB 702258 and Bifidobacterium breve DPC 6330 on the composition of murine brain fatty acids and gut microbiota. *Am. J. Clin. Nutr.* **2012**, *95*, 1278–1287. [CrossRef] [PubMed]

87. Malaguarnera, M.; Vacante, M.; Antic, T.; Giordano, M.; Chisari, G.; Acquaviva, R.; Mastrojeni, S.; Malaguarnera, G.; Mistretta, A.; Li Volti, G.; et al. Bifidobacterium longum with fructo-oligosaccharides in patients with non alcoholic steatohepatitis. *Dig. Dis. Sci.* **2012**, *57*, 545–553. [CrossRef]

88. Tannock, G.W.; Wilson, C.M.; Loach, D.; Cook, G.M.; Eason, J.; O'Toole, P.W.; Holtrop, G.; Lawley, B. Resource partitioning in relation to cohabitation of Lactobacillus species in the mouse forestomach. *ISME J.* **2012**, *6*, 927–938. [CrossRef]

89. Cani, P.D.; Possemiers, S.; Van de Wiele, T.; Guiot, Y.; Everard, A.; Rottier, O.; Geurts, L.; Naslain, D.; Neyrinck, A.; Lambert, D.M.; et al. Changes in gut microbiota control inflammation in obese mice through a mechanism involving GLP-2-driven improvement of gut permeability. *Gut* **2009**, *58*, 1091–1103. [CrossRef]

90. Gunnarsdottir, S.A.; Sadik, R.; Shev, S.; Simrén, M.; Sjövall, H.; Stotzer, P.O.; Abrahamsson, H.; Olsson, R.; Björnsson, E.S. Small intestinal motility disturbances and bacterial overgrowth in patients with liver cirrhosis and portal hypertension. *Am. J. Gastroenterol.* **2003**, *98*, 1362–1370. [CrossRef]

91. Tarantino, G.; Finelli, C. Systematic review on intervention with prebiotics/probiotics in patients with obesity-related nonalcoholic fatty liver disease. *Future Microbiol.* **2015**, *10*, 889–902. [CrossRef]

92. Musa-Veloso, K.; Venditti, C.; Lee, H.Y.; Darch, M.; Floyd, S.; West, S.; Simon, R. Systematic review and meta-analysis of controlled intervention studies on the effectiveness of long-chain Ω-3 fatty acids in patients with nonalcoholic fatty liver disease. *Nutr. Rev.* **2018**, *76*, 581–602. [CrossRef] [PubMed]

93. Robertson, R.C.; Kaliannan, K.; Strain, R.; Ross, R.P.; Stanton, C.; Kang, J.X. Maternal Ω-3 fatty acids regulate offspring obesity through persistent modulation of gut microbiota. *Microbiome* **2018**, *6*, 95. [CrossRef] [PubMed]

94. Costantini, L.; Molinari, R.; Farinon, B.; Merendino, N. Impact of omega-3 fatty acids on the gut microbiota. *Int. J. Mol. Sci.* **2017**, *18*, 2645. [CrossRef] [PubMed]

95. Bajaj, J.S.; Fagan, A.; Sikaroodi, M.; White, M.B.; Sterling, R.K.; Gilles, H.; Heuman, D.; Stravitz, R.T.; Matherly, S.C.; Siddiqui, M.S.; et al. Liver transplant modulates gut microbial dysbiosis and cognitive function in cirrhosis. *Liver Transpl.* **2017**, *23*, 907–914. [CrossRef] [PubMed]

96. Stadlbauer, V.; Mookerjee, R.P.; Hodges, S.; Wright, G.A.K.; Davies, N.A.; Jalan, R. Effect of probiotic treatment on deranged neutrophil function and cytokine responses in patients with compensated alcoholic cirrhosis. *J. Hepatol.* **2008**, *48*, 945–951. [CrossRef] [PubMed]

97. LoGuercio, C.; Federico, A.; Tuccillo, C.; Terracciano, F.; D'Auria, M.V.; De Simone, C.; Del Vecchio Blanco, C. Beneficial effects of a probiotic VSL#3 on parameters of liver dysfunction in chronic liver diseases. *J. Clin. Gastroenterol.* **2005**, *39*, 540–543. [PubMed]

98. Bajaj, J.S.; Heuman, D.M.; Hylemon, P.B.; Sanyal, A.J.; Puri, P.; Sterling, R.K.; Luketic, V.; Stravitz, R.T.; Siddiqui, M.S.; Fuchs, M.; et al. Randomised clinical trial: Lactobacillus GG modulates gut microbiome, metabolome and endotoxemia in patients with cirrhosis. *Aliment. Pharmacol. Ther.* **2014**, *39*, 1113–1125. [CrossRef]

99. Yoshimoto, S.; Loo, T.M.; Atarashi, K.; Kanda, H.; Sato, S.; Oyadomari, S.; Iwakura, Y.; Oshima, K.; Morita, H.; Hattori, M.; et al. Obesity-induced gut microbial metabolite promotes liver cancer through senescence secretome. *Nature* **2013**, *52*, 97–101. [CrossRef]

100. Huang, L.; Duan, C.; Zhao, Y.; Gao, L.; Niu, C.; Xu, J.; Li, S. Reduction of Aflatoxin B1 Toxicity by *Lactobacillus plantarum* C88: A Potential Probiotic Strain Isolated from Chinese Traditional Fermented Food "Tofu". *PLoS ONE* **2017**, *12*, e0170109. [CrossRef]

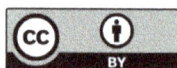

International Journal of
Molecular Sciences

MDPI

Review

Recent Advances on Microbiota Involvement in the Pathogenesis of Autoimmunity

Elena Gianchecchi [1,2] and Alessandra Fierabracci [1,*]

[1]   Infectivology and Clinical Trials Research Department, Children's Hospital Bambino Gesù, Viale San Paolo 15, 00146 Rome, Italy; elegianche@yahoo.it
[2]   VisMederi s.r.l., Strada del Petriccio e Belriguardo, 35, 53100 Siena, Italy
*   Correspondence: alessandra.fierabracci@opbg.net; Tel.: +39-06-6859-2656

Received: 23 November 2018; Accepted: 7 January 2019; Published: 11 January 2019

Abstract: Autoimmune disorders derive from genetic, stochastic, and environmental factors that all together interact in genetically predisposed individuals. The impact of an imbalanced gut microbiome in the pathogenesis of autoimmunity has been suggested by an increasing amount of experimental evidence, both in animal models and humans. Several physiological mechanisms, including the establishment of immune homeostasis, are influenced by commensal microbiota in the gut. An altered microbiota composition produces effects in the gut immune system, including defective tolerance to food antigens, intestinal inflammation, and enhanced gut permeability. In particular, early findings reported differences in the intestinal microbiome of subjects affected by several autoimmune conditions, including prediabetes or overt disease compared to healthy individuals. The present review focuses on microbiota-host homeostasis, its alterations, factors that influence its composition, and putative involvement in the development of autoimmune disorders. In the light of the existing literature, future studies are necessary to clarify the role played by microbiota modifications in the processes that cause enhanced gut permeability and molecular mechanisms responsible for autoimmunity onset.

Keywords: microbiota; autoimmunity; etiopathogenesis

---

1. Introduction

The pathogenesis of autoimmune disorders is often multifactorial; in fact, in addition to a genetic predisposition [1–3], stochastic [4] and environmental [5,6] factors also play an important role in susceptible individuals. Among the environmental factors that have gained attention during the last decade, there is the intestinal microbiota community, which is involved in performing critical tasks for the normal development and maintenance of healthy human physiology.

A growing number of investigations have highlighted that humans are not born sterile, as we thought until some time ago; instead, intracellular bacteria have been identified even in the placenta, amniotic fluid, umbilical cord, and meconium [7]. The gastrointestinal lumen, representing the widest surface area in the human body exposed to environmental factors and in contact with a high number of different antigens and microbes [8], becomes inhabited by bacteria, viruses [9], *Archaea* [10], and fungi immediately after birth [11]. *Actinobacteria, Bacteroidetes, Proteobacteria*, and *Firmicutes* are the most abundant bacterial phyla in the mouse and human intestine during homeostasis. The colonization of the gut does not represent a random event, but is the result of the evolutionary process as demonstrated by the fact that microbiome composition of humans and other mammals presents an elevated level of conservation with respect to the same phylum level [12]. The colonization of the gut by microbiota represents a dynamic, complex, and gradual process, which is also in continuous development in the early years of life in parallel with the development of the immune system of the newborn.

Distinct composition and diversity of the gut microbiome occurs even during pregnancy, along with physiologic, metabolic, and immune variations of the woman [13]. The recent study of Gomez de Agüero [14] suggests that early postnatal innate immune development could be critically influenced by maternal microbiota transfer, as well as that of its metabolites. In addition, birth delivery mode, breastfeeding, and food introduction constitute some of the factors able to influence the microbiome in the newborn. More in detail, the birth delivery mode seems to be able to drive the diversity of the infant gut microbiome, although conflicting results are reported about the putative correlation between birth delivery mode and the risk of developing non-communicable diseases later in life [15].

Indeed, when natural delivery occurs, contact with vaginal and fecal microbiota of the mother is favored, while during the caesarian section (CS), contact with commensal bacteria on other surfaces, such as the skin is promoted, avoiding or dramatically reducing contact with maternal vaginal and fecal microbiota [16]. CS was not only associated with a reduced microbiome diversity, with respect to natural delivery [17], which persisted until 7 years of age [18], but was also correlated with diminished Th1 chemokines in the blood [18] and with an increased risk to develop childhood T1D [17,19].

The crosstalk between the microbiome and the host is fundamental since it induces the proper gut epithelial construction and activity, as well as metabolism and nutrition. The gut epithelial barrier, constituted by a single cell layer, represents the interface between the host and microbiota, allowing metabolites to access and interact with host cells. On the other hand, maintenance of gut integrity is fundamental since impairment of the gut and mucosal barrier could allow microbes to enter the *lamina propria* and systemic blood circulation inducing an imbalance in the host immune homeostasis and leading to systemic immune hyperactivation.

Several functions can be exploited only upon bacterial activity. More in detail, these include the metabolism of complex glycans, amino acids, and xenobiotic, and the synthesis of short-chain fatty acids (SCFAs) and vitamins [16]. Moreover, the microbiome is able to impede pathogens, such as *Shigella flexneri* and *Salmonella*, that could enter host cells, preventing development of inflammation promoted by dysbiosis. An inflammatory condition can be elicited by microbes identified as pathobionts in host harboring an aberrant microbiota caused by the use of antibiotics or in genetically predisposed individuals [11].

If, on one side, the host immune system controls microbial ecology, on the other side, microbiota produces a wide variety of biochemically active compounds, such as neurotransmitters and tryptophan-derived metabolites [20,21] influencing both the maturation and activity of the immune system. Given the importance of a proper regulation of host immune response, increasing interest in the wide microbial metabolite repertoire has emerged. These metabolites represent compounds produced by the host or by the microbiome itself (such as polyamines), or are derived from the bacterial metabolism of substances introduced with the diet. Among the latter are found ligands of the aryl hydrocarbon receptor (AHR), polyamines, and SCFAs, which encompasses butyric acid, acetic acid, and propionic acid, and that originate from undigested complex carbohydrates [22].

AHR signaling is fundamental for the maintenance of host immune homeostasis. Indeed, the protective role of AHR ligands has been demonstrated against the fungal pathogen *Candida* (*C.*) *albicans* and against mucosal inflammation through the IL-22 synthesis [23].

Polyamines reinforce the intestinal epithelial cell barrier by inducing the synthesis of intercellular junction proteins, such as E-cadherin, *zonula occludens* 1, and occludin [24]. Furthermore, they play a role in host immunity through the inhibition of macrophage activation and pro-inflammatory cytokine synthesis. In addition, they can modulate mucosal and systemic adaptive immunity [22].

SCFAs exert several functions affecting host physiology: they represent a considerable source of energy for intestinal epithelial cells, induce mucin gene transcription [25], and influence the permeability of tight junctions. As a consequence, the epithelial barrier is strengthened, thus preventing toxic compounds from entering the blood stream. In addition, as AHR activation, SCFAs also have an effect on host immunity. Indeed, the tolerogenic phenotype and thus immune homeostasis, as well as T regulatory cell (Treg) development, are promoted by SCFAs through the inhibition of histone deacetylases [26].

The majority of intercellular signals is mediated by bioactive molecules, such as lipopolysaccharide (LPS), proteins, toxic and immunomodulatory mediators, RNA or DNA, and ATP [27] contained into secreted extracellular vesicles (EVs) [28]. EVs are spherical particles that are membrane-bounded and characterized by a diameter of 50–250 nm. This protects their content from nucleases and proteases, and properly delivers it to neighboring or distant cells [29]. EVs can be secreted by eukaryotic cells, and Gram-negative [28] and Gram-positive bacteria [29].

The symbiotic interaction between the human host and microbiome is so strict that the microbiome has also been defined as a prokaryotic organ with complex endocrine functions [26]. Increasing evidence has reported that alterations in the composition and/or abundance of the gut microbiome and subsequent alterations in its metabolic network correlated with the onset and even the progression of various intestinal and systemic autoimmune conditions. Nevertheless, the mechanisms underlying the dysregulation of gut microbiota and autoimmunity remain to be elucidated.

2. Microbiome Composition and Autoimmune Conditions

Recently, increasing interest has been directed towards the identification of the gut microbiome, the principal source of microbes, and the understanding of its positive or negative effects on health of human beings, in particular in the light of the recent evidence that the inflammatory process could be elicited by the microbiome.

A growing number of studies have supported the striking linking of altered microbiota composition with the onset of several different autoimmune disorders (Table 1). These include Type I diabetes (T1D) [16,30–53]; rheumatoid arthritis (RA) [54–62]; systemic lupus erythematosus (SLE) [63–67]; inflammatory bowel disease (IBD) encompassing Crohn's disease (CD) and ulcerative colitis (UC) [68–78]; Behcet's disease (BD) [79–82]; autoimmune skin conditions including vitiligo [83], psoriasis vulgaris [84–88], and atopic dermatitis [89–97]; and autoimmune neurological diseases [98–106]. Several alterations involving microbiome have been identified in autoimmune patients and thus hypothesized to have a role in the onset of the different autoimmune conditions (Table 2).

Table 1. Microbiome alterations in different autoimmune conditions respect to healthy subjects.

Autoimmune Conditions	Microbiome Alterations in Autoimmunity Respect to Healthy Subjects	References
Type I diabetes	↓ bacterial diversity in high-risk children	[35,42,43]
	↑ *Bacteroidetes/Firmicutes* ratio	[36,44,51]
	↑ *Bacteroidetes, Clostridium*, and *Veillonella*; ↓ *Bifidobacterium, Lactobacillus, Blautia coccoides/Eubacterium rectale* group, and *Prevotella*	[37]
	↑ *Bacteroides dorei* in high-risk children	[39]
	↑ *Bacteroides* and ↓ *Prevotella* in newly diagnosed T1D patients	[40]
	↓ *Bifidobacterium*	[36,41]
	↑ *Bacteroides* and *Clostridium* cluster XVa and cluster IV; ↓ *Bifidobacterium*	[47]
	↑ *Candida albicans* and *Enterobacteriaceae*	[41]
Rheumatoid arthritis	↑ of the pathobiont *Prevotella (Prevotella copri)* in new-onset RA subjects	[107]
	Gut and oral microbiome dysbiosis; ↓ *Haemophilus spp.* and ↑ *Lactobacillus salivarius*	[56]
	↓ gut bacterial diversity and expansion of rare lineage intestinal microbes	[57]
	Association between periodontal infection due to *Porphyromonas gingivalis* and RA	[54,108]
	↑ *Fretibacterium, Selenomonas* and *Prevotella nigrescens*	[55]
	↑ *Bacilli* and *Lactobacillales*; ↓ genus *Faecalibacterium* and the specie *Faecalibacterium prausnitzii*; Absence of the genus *Flavobacterium* and the species *Blautia coccoides* in RA patients present instead in controls	[62]
	↑ *Prevotella copri* and ↓ *Bacteroides* in new-onset untreated RA patients	[107]

Table 1. *Cont.*

Autoimmune Conditions	Microbiome Alterations in Autoimmunity Respect to Healthy Subjects	References
Systemic lupus erythematosus	↑ *Bacteroidetes/Firmicutes* ratio	[65]
	Association between SLE and periodontal disease; Dysbiosis of the subgingival microbiota; ↑ subgingival bacterial load; ↓ subgingival microbial diversity at diseased sites	[67]
	↑ *Fretibacterium*, *Selenomonas*, and *Prevotella nigrescens*;	[109]
	Association with periodontal pathogens (*Treponema denticola*, *Porphyromonas gingivalis*, *Fretibacterium fastidiosum* and *Tannerella forsythia*	[109,110]
Behcet's disease	↓ *Roseburia* and *Subdoligranulum* genera	[79]
	↑ *Bifidobacterium* and *Eggerthella* genera and ↓ *Megamonas* and *Prevotella* genera	[81]
	↑ *Bilophila spp.* and several opportunistic pathogens (e.g., *Parabacteroides spp.* and *Paraprevotella spp.*); ↓ butyrate-producing bacteria *Clostridium spp.* and methanogens (*Methanoculleus spp.* and *Methanomethylophilus spp.*).	[82]
Inflammatory bowel disease	↓ gut bacterial diversity	[68]
	↓ diversity in the bacterial phylum *Firmicutes faecal*; ↓ *Clostridium leptum* phylogenetic group	[70]
	↑ *Proteobacteria* phylum including Escherichia *coli*; ↓ *Firmicutes* phylum was reduced	[69,70,73, 111]
	↓ *Faecalibacterium prausnitzii* is associated with an ↑ risk of postoperative recurrence of ileal CD	[72]
	↓ in several butyrate-producing bacteria species	[74,76]
	↓ of the genera *Bacteroides*, *Eubacterium*, *Faecalibacterium* and *Ruminococcus*; ↑ genera *Actinomyces* and *Bifidobacterium*; ↓ butyrate-producing bacterial species, as *Blautia faecis*, *Roseburia inulinivorans*, *Ruminococcus torques*, *Clostridium lavalense*, *Bacteroides uniformis*, and *Faecalibacterium prausnitzii*	[76]
	Dysbiosis	[112]
	↑ *Caudovirales* bacteriophages and fungal composition	[113]
Vitiligo	↑ *Actinobacteria*, *Proteobacteria*, *Firmicutes*, and *Bacteroidetes*	[83,114]
	↓ bacterial diversity	[83]
Psoriasis vulgaris	↑ *Proteobacteria*; ↓ *Staphylococci* and *Propionibacteria*	[85]
	↓ bacterial diversity; ↑ *Corynebacterium*, *Propionibacterium*, *Staphylococcus*, and *Streptococcus*; ↓ *Cupriavidus*, *Flavisolibacter*, *Methylobacterium*, and *Schlegelella* genera. Association between lesion samples with *Firmicutes*-associated microbiota	[86]
	↓ diversity and ↑ *Staphylococcus* in psoriatic ear sites	[87]
	↑ diversity and ↑ heterogeneity ↑ *Staphylococcus aureus*; ↓ *Staphylococcus epidermidis* and *Propionibacterium acnes*	[88]
Atopic dermatitis	↑ *Faecalibacterium prausnitzii* subspecies	[93]
	↑ *Staphylococcus aureus*	[94]
	↓ *Propionibacterium acnes* and *Lawsonella clevelandensis*; ↑ *Staphylococcus aureus* in non-lesional relative to lesional AD patients	[95]
Autoimmune neurological diseases	↓ species belonging to *Clostridia XIVa* and *IV Clusters*	[101]
	↑ *Pseudomonas*, *Mycoplana*, *Haemophilus*, *Blautia*, and *Dorea* in relapsing remitting MS patients; ↓ *Parabacteroides*, *Adlercreutzia*, and *Prevotella* genera	[102]
	↑ *Methanobrevibacter* and *Akkermansia*; ↓ *Butyricimonas*	[103]
	↑ *Akkermansia muciniphila* and *Acinetobacter calcoaceticus*; ↓ *Parabacteroides distasonis*	[106]

Table 2. Bacterial associated mechanisms promoting autoimmunity.

Autoimmune Disorders	Bacterial Associated Mechanisms Promoting Autoimmunity	References
Type I diabetes	Perturbation in the integrity of epithelial barrier	[49,115–119]
	Changes in gut microbiota following antibiotic treatment	[120–122]
	Functional enrichment in core energy metabolism proteins, in particular on sugar transport and processing	[47]
	Perturbations in the integrity of epithelial tight junctions	[44]
	Blockage of Treg differentiation via products generated with the anaerobic respiration, such as acetate and succinate	[44]
	Increased intestinal inflammation and reduced barrier activity due to depletion in microbiota taxa related with host proteins implicated in the maintenance of mucous barrier functionality, microvilli adhesion, and exocrine pancreas	[48]
	Reduced presence of beneficial anaerobic gut bacteria *Lactobacillus*, *Bifidobacterium*, and *Bacteroides* species exerting an inhibitory function by synthetizing short-chain fatty acids and antimicrobial compounds	[36,41]
Lung autoimmunity in rheumatoid arthritis	Bacterial metabolites can affect host immune system leading to pro- or anti-inflammatory reactions	[53]
	Modulation of host immune response by gut-residing segmented filamentous bacteria via increased Th17cells percentages induced by the strong Th17 chemoattractant CCL20	[123–125]
Rheumatoid arthritis	Promotion of autoantibodies by gut residing segmented filamentous bacteria during the pre-arthritic phase	[126]
	Molecular mimicry between several gut microbe epitopes and two autoantigens *N*-acetylglucosamine-6-sulfatase and filamin A greatly expressed in inflamed synovial tissue	[58]
	Citrullinated proteins via the peptidylarginine deiminase (PAD) enzyme derived from bacteria	[127–129]
Systemic lupus erythematosus	Correlation between dysbiotic periodontal inflammation and more severe SLE scores	[67]
Behcet's disease	Altered Th1, Th17, and Treg functions	[130,131]
	Reduction in butyrate-producing bacteria and methanogens, with enhanced oxidation-reduction process, capsular polysaccharide transport system, and type III and IV secretion systems	[82]
	Strong intraocular inflammatory reaction	[82]
Inflammatory bowel disease	Impaired epithelial barrier and increased intestinal permeability	[111]
	Cellular stress responses interacting with microbiome in the gastrointestinal tract. Interaction between bacteria and endoplasmic reticulum	[78]
	Reduction of several butyrate-producing bacteria	[74,76]
	Reduced AHR agonists in the inflamed intestinal tissue samples that modulate T cell responses AHR agonists exert an anti-inflammatory effect inducing IL-22	[132–134]
Vitiligo	Aberrant intra-community network in the lesional skin areas respect to those of non-lesional sites. Dysbiosis of diverse microbial community in vitiligo lesional skin	[135]
Psoriasis vulgaris	Increased Th17 response which could have a role in IL-17-driven inflammation	[88]
Atopic dermatitis	Increase of IgE response, inflammatory and Th2/Th22 transcripts, promotion of Th2 activation, and suppression of resident Treg cells by secretomes of skin microbiota	[91]
	Induction of an imbalanced Th1/Th2 skin immunity	[94]
	Decrease of butyrate and propionate producers (molecules with an anti-inflammatory activity)	[93]
	EVs derived from the microbiome and increase of inflammation	[89,136]
Multiple sclerosis	Reduced levels of circulating AHR agonists and reduced AHR agonistic activity	[104]
	Modulation by fecal microbiota abundance of expression of host immune genes involved in dendritic cell maturation, and interferon and NF-kB signaling pathways in circulating T lymphocytes and monocytes	[103]
	Reduced Treg compartment associated with increased percentages of effector CD4$^+$ lymphocytes that differentiated into IFNγ-producing Th1 cells Reduced IL-10$^+$ Treg subset in mice transplanted with microbiota from MS patients	[106]
	Diet skewed gut microbial and metabolic profiles	[105,137,138]

2.1. Type 1 Diabetes

Type 1 diabetes (T1D) is an organ-specific autoimmune condition characterized by the specific destruction of pancreatic β cells of the islet of Langerhans deputed to insulin release. This destructive process is operated by cytotoxic T lymphocytes (Tc) [139]. As a consequence, glucose cannot be absorbed by cells. The insulitis lesion is characterized by several infiltrating cells, such as B and T lymphocytes. T-helper 1 (Th1) lymphocytes are responsible for the pancreatic infiltration and for the sustenance of cytotoxic T (Tc) lymphocyte activity by secreting cytokines [140]. Millions of people are affected by T1D worldwide, whose etiology is multifactorial [141]. In more detail, it has been suggested that a combination of environmental, genetic, and stochastic factors are responsible for its pathogenesis [142,143]. T1D incidence has been steadily rising during the last 50 years, probably due to modifications in the gut microbiota associated with modern lifestyles, which may be responsible for a defective development of the immune system.

Recent investigations conducted on animal models [30–34,38,45] and humans [36,37,39,40,42,43,47] have implicated a causal role for the alterations in the normal flora in T1D development [41] through an upsurge in gut permeability [115–118]. The shifts in the intestinal microbial populations before T1D clinical onset support the role played by gut bacteria in T1D etiopathogenesis. The identification of these changes is fundamental to understand the events implicated in the progression of the disease, even though limited knowledge regarding bacterial functions involved in T1D is available yet.

Bosi et al. [119] observed that T1D onset was preceded by enhanced intestinal permeability.

Non-obese diabetic (NOD) mice carried a "diabetes-permissive" microbiota different from that harbored by T1D-protected inbred strains. Furthermore, important imbalances affecting microbiota can both reduce and accelerate T1D onset [144].

T1D incidence was increased when NOD mice were grown in a specific-pathogen-free (SPF) environment or clean housing facilities compared to conventional conditions [33] and changes perturbing gut microbiome, like diet modifications, can prevent disease [145]. Also, antibiotic treatment accelerated T1D onset in mice by substantially shifting the gut microbiota [120–122], and this was particularly important in the case of early life antibiotics exposure [121]. Roesch et al. [146] found a higher *Bifidobacter/Lactobacilli* ratio in the diabetic-resistant rat group with respect to the diabetic sensitive rat group. Sun et al. [45] demonstrated that changes in gut microbiome limited autoimmune diabetes in NOD mice by synthetizing an immunoregulatory cathelicidin-related antimicrobial peptide in islets.

High-risk children presenting islet-autoantibodies had distinct bacterial diversity with respect to low-risk autoantibody-negative children [35,36]. Kostic et al. [43] reported a reduced bacterial diversity prior to the onset of clinical disease in an investigation conducted on high-risk Finnish children; these data were in accordance with those reported by Alkanani [42] demonstrating the correlation between T1D susceptibility and intestinal microbiome perturbations in a U.S.-based cohort.

Most of the studies assessing impairment of the gut microbiome balance and T1D have been conducted on Caucasians; however, the incidence of the disorder was quickly rising during the past decade in China, allowing us to speculate the role of non-genetic factors. Therefore, Huang et al. [51] have evaluated gut microbiota profiling in 12 T1D Han Chinese and 10 healthy controls by using 16S rRNA sequencing followed by analyses of the gut microbiota composition. The study proved important differences in 28 bacterial taxa (13 increased and 15 decreased) in T1D patients as compared to controls. In T1D subjects and controls, *Bacteroidetes* and *Firmicutes* constituted the dominant phyla, respectively. The raised *Bacteroidetes/Firmicutes* ratio was in accordance with a previous study conducted on Caucasians T1D and high-risk cohorts [44]. Also, Murri [37] reported an increase in *Bacteroides* in Spanish T1D children respect to controls along with a higher abundance of *Clostridium* and *Veillonella* and a reduction in the populations of *Bifidobacterium*, *Lactobacillus*, the *Blautia coccoides/Eubacterium rectale* group, and *Prevotella*.

Likewise, the Pinto [47] group reported the rise in *Bacteroides* and *Clostridium* cluster XVa and cluster IV concurrently with a reduction in *Bifidobacterium*. The proteome analysis distributed the most representative bacterial proteins in functional groups thus revealing marked differences between Portuguese T1D children and controls. In fact, whereas in the latter most of the proteins correlated with metabolism and transport of carbohydrates, in the former group, among the most abundant proteins some were specific for T1D, such as those involved in transport and metabolism of amino acids and coenzymes, meaning that a functional enrichment in core energy metabolism proteins, in particular on sugar transport and processing is involved.

It has been speculated that a *Bacteroides* expansion could affect the integrity of epithelial tight junctions and halt Treg differentiation by the products, such as acetate and succinate, generated with the anaerobic respiration [44]. The recent intestinal metaproteomics study conducted by Gavin [48] on 33 subjects with recent-onset T1D, 17 islet autoantibody-positive subjects, 29 low-risk autoantibody-negative subjects, and 22 healthy individuals revealed the presence of specific host-microbiota interactions in T1D patients presenting considerable alterations in the prevalence of host proteins correlated with exocrine pancreas output, inflammation, and mucosal function. In addition, T1D subjects showed a higher intestinal inflammation and reduced barrier activity due to a depletion in microbiota taxa related with host proteins implicated in the maintenance of microvilli adhesion, mucous barrier, and exocrine pancreas functionality.

The evaluation of the possible correlation between autoantibodies and bacterial abundances revealed a positive association between anti-islet cell autoantibodies with *Bacteriodes* and *Bilophila*, while a negative association was found with *Streptococcus* and *Ruminococcaceae*. In addition, *Faecalibacterium* abundance was negatively correlated with levels of glycated hemoglobin A1c (HbA1c) [51], in contrast with the study of Hornef [147] reporting similarity in the phylum level between T1D Han Chinese children and healthy controls.

Recently, Gursoy et al. [49] have investigated the potential role played by the intestinal colonization of the opportunistic fungus *C. albicans*, which is part of the normal intestinal microflora, on T1D onset and gut integrity. Intestinal *C. albicans* colonization was found in 50% of T1D patients and 23.8% of controls at the time of diagnosis in a total of 42 newly-diagnosed T1D patients and 42 healthy controls. These findings support the hypothesis that the autoimmune response, like that responsible for T1D onset, could be due to alterations in the normal gut microbiome composition by enhancing intestinal permeability. Soyucen et al. [41] analyzed the fecal flora of 35 newly diagnosed Turkish T1D patients and 35 healthy subjects reporting a significant decrease in *Bifidobacterium* colonization, in accordance with de Goffau et al. [36], and a considerable increase in *C. albicans* and *Enterobacteriaceae* in T1D patients was found with respect to controls. Regarding *Escherichia (E.) coli*, no differences between the two groups were observed. Although a reduction in *Bacteroides* spp. and *Lactobacillus* colonization characterized T1D subjects with respect to controls, these differences did not reach significance. However, it has been supposed that the higher *C. albicans* colonization could be due to the reduction of *Lactobacillus*, *Bifidobacterium*, and *Bacteroides* species. Indeed, they constitute beneficial anaerobic bacteria within the gut since they exert an inhibitory function by synthetizing short-chain fatty acids and antimicrobial compounds. These alterations, besides *Enterobacteriaceae* and the slight and non-significative *E. coli* increase observed in the T1D group, could lead to islet destruction as a final step of the autoimmune process.

Although more data are necessary to fully understand the correlation between β islet destruction and the potential causal role of microbiome and diet, their interaction is critical, as demonstrated by the correlation between early probiotic supplementation and diminished risk of islet autoimmunity in children with a high genetic risk for T1D [46].

Recently, Henschel [50] reported that the peripheral inflammatory state correlated with autoimmune diabetes susceptibility was kept under control following modulation of the diet and gastrointestinal microbiota. More specific, spontaneous diabetic BB DR*lyp*/*lyp* and diabetes inducible BB DR⁺/⁺ weanings fed with a standard cereal diet presented a considerable pro-inflammatory transcriptional expression consistent with microbial antigen exposure. This inherent inflammatory state (i.e., the presence of the pro-inflammatory islet transcriptome as well as β-cell chemokine expression) was reverted when DR⁺/⁺ weanings were fed with a gluten-free hydrolyzed casein diet (HCD) or treated with antibiotics and reduced T1D incidence was proven in lymphopenic DR*lyp*/*lyp* rats. Moreover, the introduction of gluten to HCD reverted these effects. The sequencing of bacterial 16S rRNA gene highlighted that diet changes or antibiotic treatments disrupt ileal and cecal microbiota, with an enhancement in *Firmicutes/Bacteriodetes* ratio and in the relative abundances of lactobacilli and butyrate producing taxa [50]. A recent study of Mullaney et al. [52] found that specific gut microbial imbalance were linked to T1D susceptibility alleles in mice. Accordingly, immune tolerance towards islet antigens was re-established upon disease protective allele introduction which induced a restoration of the gut immune regulatory system and microbiome modifications. Additional studies demonstrate bacterial metabolites can affect host immune system and induce beta cell autoimmunity and T1D [53].

2.2. Rheumatoid Arthritis

Rheumatoid arthritis (RA) constitutes a systemic inflammatory chronic disorder wherein joints, representing the target of the inflammatory process, undergo destruction. In addition to joints, other organs can also be affected by the autoimmune process, such as the lungs and the gastrointestinal tract. The etiopathogenesis is multifactorial: environmental, genetic, hormonal, and immunological factors have been hypothesized to have a role in RA onset [148,149].

The involvement of gut microbiome in RA pathogenesis is supported by the observation that germ-free mice were protected against experimental arthritis [123].

Although segmented filamentous bacteria (SFB) constitute a smaller though important component of the commensal flora, its ability to shape the immune response of the host by inducing intestinal T helper 17 (Th17) lymphocytes [124] has been demonstrated. It was shown that autoimmune arthritis was caused by gut-residing SFB via Th17 cells [123,125], which, in association with a T follicular helper (Tfh), promoted autoantibodies in young K/BxN mice [125].

In accordance with these observations, interleukin-17 (IL-17) neutralization inhibited AR onset [150] and a substantial amelioration in the production of autoantibodies, as well as in autoimmune arthritis development that occurred when Tfh and Th17 cells were lost [125]. It has been thought that Th17 compartment carrying dual T cell receptors (TCRs) recognizing both microbial and self-antigens may be specifically expanded by SFB causing lung autoimmunity onset, an important extra-articular RA manifestation and the principal cause of RA-related mortality. In detail, whereas during the pre-arthritic phase SFB promoted autoantibodies, the RA-related lung pathological changes were due to Th17 recruitment as a consequence of the strong chemokine (C-C motif) ligand 20 (CCL20) expression, representing a chemoattractant for Th17 in this organ [126].

A perturbation of the gut microbiome in RA patients has been reported [56,107] with a higher abundance of the pathobiont *Prevotella* (*P. copri*) in new-onset RA subjects, while the reduction observed in established RA subjects could be due to the treatment [107]. The role of this bacterium is also sustained by the study of Pianta [58], who found molecular mimicry between its epitopes and two autoantigens, *N*-acetylglucosamine-6-sulfatase (GNS) and filamin A (FLNA). In addition to gut dysbiosis, the microbiome of the dental region and saliva were also altered [56]. In particular, an association between periodontal infections due to *Porphyromonas* (*P.*) *gingivalis* and RA have been envisaged [54,108]. This hypothesis is supported by both the correlation between oral and gut flora and the higher incidence of periodontitis in RA subjects [108] and by a recent investigation conducted on animal model of RA demonstrating worsening of collagen-induced arthritis (CIA) upon the oral administration of *P. gingivalis* [59] through the enhanced synthesis of IL-17 [55].

The research conducted by Teng [60] using young and middle-aged K/BxN T cells aimed to investigate the impact exerted by age and microbiome on autoimmune arthritis, since this pathology usually develops in middle age, whereas most of the studies conducted until now were performed on young adult mice. When compared with younger mice, the old counterparts with the same TCR specificity presented a higher number of Tfh, representing a reminiscence of those differentiated during the early age that have survived during the aging process. Tfh had an effector memory phenotype (CD62L^{lo}CD44^{hi}) in the majority of the cases. Tfh presented a low response when antigen was newly introduced in middle age, but they recognized the self-antigen from youth as occurring in RA during the latent phase [151]. This alteration was associated with a significantly impaired Th17 response not due to a defective Th17 proliferation but to an inefficiency of middle-aged autoimmune CD4+ T cells to differentiate into Th17. In addition, a reduced IL-23 expression level was found, which is fundamental for the maintenance of Th17. Likewise, a lower differentiation of IL-17-producing cells from naive CD4+ T cells in older mice with respect to the younger group was observed, resembling the observation obtained in humans [152,153]. The discrepancies concerning Th17 number were probably due to the age of mice used in the two studies [60]. The investigation of the contribution of age on AR is particularly important since it represents a risk factor for AR.

A correlation between dysbiosis of the oral microbiome, periodontitis, and the production of citrullinated proteins was also observed in RA patients. Indeed, among the autoantibody profile characterizing RA patients, there are antibodies recognizing anti-citrullinated products that could represent novel epitopes upon being targeted by the post-transcriptional modification of citrullination. According to this hypothesis, a recent study of Pianta [58] reported the identification of two self-antigens FLNA and GNS recognized by B and T lymphocytes in RA subjects. More in detail, GNS was citrullinated, and GNS antibody values correlated with anti–citrullinated protein antibody (ACPA) levels. Not only were FLNA and GNS both greatly expressed in inflamed synovial tissue, but their T cell epitopes presented also homology with *Prevotella, Parabacteroides sp., Butyricimonas sp.,* and other gut microbes [58]. This evidence has allowed us to speculate the putative role of citrullinated products as a self-antigen in subjects with a genetic predisposition for RA [154]. Along with citrullinated proteins, proinflammatory cytokines have also been hypothesized to be implicated in the linkage of RA with periodontal disease as witnessed by the rapid RA development in the adjuvant arthritis model in case of pre-existing extra-synovial inflammation due to *P. gingivalis* [155].

Recent studies have in fact highlighted the role played by the peptidylarginine deiminase (PAD) enzyme derived from *P. gingivalis* and *Aggregatibacter* (*A.*) *actinomycetemcomitans*, which citrullinates human fibrinogen, alpha-enolase [127], and peptides from critical RA autoantigens [128] and causes hypercitrullination in the rheumatoid joint in host neutrophils [129].

As reported for other autoimmune conditions, in RA subjects, several alterations in gut microbiome with respect to healthy individuals have also been reported [57,61,62]. A stronger reduction in gut microbial diversity was proven in RA patients with respect to controls, and it was related to disease duration and autoantibodies levels. Furthermore, Chen et al. observed a decrease in abundant taxa accompanied by an expansion of rare lineage intestinal microbes in RA patients respect to controls [57].

Picchianti et al. [62] noted substantial changes involving mainly lower taxonomic levels, while the relative abundance of the microbial phyla was not modified. More specifically, *Bacilli* and *Lactobacillales* were enhanced, while the genus *Faecalibacterium* and the species *Faecalibacterium* (*F.*) *prausnitzii* were importantly decreased in RA patients with respect to controls. Moreover, the latter presented the genus *Flavobacterium* and the species *Blautia* (*B.*) *coccoides*, which have not been observed in RA subjects [62].

2.3. Systemic Lupus Erythematosus

Systemic lupus erythematosus (SLE) is a systemic autoimmune disease characterized by B cell hyperactivity and the presence of several circulating autoantibodies [156,157], with a higher incidence in women. Several factors, such as genetic and environmental factors, drugs, infections, and immune system defects (reviewed in Reference [157]), seem to contribute to SLE etiology. In addition to the investigation of the putative correlation between SLE and the human microbiota [65,158], the role of periodontal disease in SLE condition [63,64,66,159] has been furthered since, as demonstrated in RA (*vide supra*), periodontal pathology may aggravate SLE severity by increasing systemic inflammation. Furthermore, a limited number of studies with opposite results, partially attributed to small sample size, are available so far.

Recently, Corrêa and colleagues [67] investigated for the first time the influence of SLE on the oral microbiota on 52 SLE patients and 52 healthy subjects finding a positive correlation between SLE and periodontal disease that affected 67% of SLE patients. Moreover, SLE patients showed a dysbiotic subgingival microbiota, with a more elevated subgingival bacterial load and a reduced microbial diversity at the diseased sites than controls. A dysbiotic condition correlated with an increased inflammation, as revealed by higher levels of inflammatory cytokines (IL-6, IL-17, and IL-33) in SLE subjects with periodontitis, is in accordance with the finding of Mendonça [109]. Independently from periodontal status, SLE patients presented an expansion of bacterial species frequently characterizing periodontitis, including *Fretibacterium*, *Selenomonas*, and *Prevotella* (*P.*) *nigrescens*; the latter has also been found to be increased in RA [55]. In addition, the analysis of the subgingival microbiota collected from SLE patients and healthy subjects revealed that the microbiome was influenced by SLE since they were characterized by a shift toward greater proportions of pathogenic bacteria. This was in accordance with previous data [110] reporting a positive association among periodontal pathogens (*Treponema denticola*, *P. gingivalis*, *Fretibacterium fastidiosum*, and *Tannerella forsythia*). A higher periodontal damage or inflammatory response favoring periodontitis could be promoted via dysbiosis of the subgingival microbiota; on the other hand, severity of SLE could be worsened by the presence of a periodontal condition as demonstrated by the fact that periodontal inflammation correlated with more severe SLE scores [67]. In light of these observations, the importance of a strict monitoring of dental health status of SLE patients is evident, and eventually treating periodontal inflammation during the starting phase becomes urgent.

2.4. Behcet's Disease

Behcet's disease (BD) represents a chronic multisystemic inflammatory condition characterized by the presence of uveitis, skin lesions, recurrent oral aphthous, and genital ulcers [160,161], and can involve the gastrointestinal tract (intestinal BD) [160–162] and the central nervous system (CNS) [150,161]. Importantly, it represents one of the principal causes of blindness. IBD etiology is caused by environmental and genetic factors [150,161,163], including microbial factors in genetically susceptible individuals [150,160,164]. BD patients show defects in Th1, Th17, and Treg cell functions [165,166], which have been demonstrated to be regulated by the gut microbiome [130,131]. The possible association between BD and specific changes in the gut microbial community has been showed [79–81].

The presence of marked modifications in BD conditions has been recently confirmed by the metagenomic study conducted by Ye et al. [82] analyzing fecal and saliva samples collected from 32 active BD patients and 74 healthy controls. *Bilophila* spp. and several opportunistic pathogens (e.g., *Parabacteroides* spp. and *Paraprevotella* spp.) resulted in an increase in fecal samples from active BD patients, whereas a reduction was observed in butyrate-producing bacteria (BPB) *Clostridium* spp. and methanogens (*Methanoculleus* spp. and *Methanomethylophilus* spp.). These changes were associated with altered biological microbial functions with an enhanced oxidation–reduction process, capsular polysaccharide transport system, and type III and IV secretion systems. Accordingly, the fecal microbiota transplant from active BD patients in B10RIII mice strongly exacerbated experimental autoimmune uveitis (EAU) activity with strong inflammatory cell infiltration within the retina, the choroid, and the vitreous cavity. Conversely, healthy control-recipient mice and PBS-treated group showed merely a weak intraocular inflammatory reaction. Moreover BD-recipient mice had an enhanced inflammatory cytokine synthesis of IL-17 and interferon gamma (IFN-γ) with respect to the two control groups [82].

2.5. Inflammatory Bowel Disease

IBD encompasses Crohn's disease (CD) and ulcerative colitis (UC). IBD is a complex disorder in which a chronic inflammation affects the gastrointestinal tract with frequent extra-intestinal manifestations [167]. A combination of non-genetic and genetic factors could be responsible for IBD pathogenesis, although its etiology remains to be elucidated [168]. The disease is supposed to be due to altered innate and adaptive immune responses directed towards pathogen associated molecular patterns (PAMPs) derived from microorganisms constituting the intestinal flora in genetically susceptible individuals. A role for the intestinal microbial community in the onset and chronicity of

CD is strongly suspected. However, investigation of such a complex ecosystem is difficult, even with culture-independent molecular approaches.

An impaired epithelial barrier and increased intestinal permeability observed in UC and CD patients sustain this hypothesis [167]. A correlation between IBD and a decrease in gut bacterial diversity upon an imbalance from commensal in favor of potentially pathogenic species (identified as "dysbiosis") has been reported [68,70,71,77]. In particular, recent data are supporting the critical role of cellular stress signaling involving the gut microbiome in the mucosa of the gastrointestinal tract. The microbiome fosters intestinal health and at the same time could have a role in IBD onset through complex interactions with the stress signaling pathways in host cells [78].

In the metagenomic study performed by Manichanh et al. [70], a full range of intestinal microbes were investigated by using two libraries of genomic DNA isolated from fecal samples obtained from six CD patients and six healthy donors. The study revealed a diminished diversity in the bacterial phylum *Firmicutes* (*F.*) *faecal* in the microbiota of CD subjects. In more detail, a significant reduction of the *Clostridium leptum* phylogenetic group was reported in CD patients compared to healthy subjects. In addition, novel bacterial species were observed [70].

Frequently, an enhancement in the *Proteobacteria* phylum including *E. coli* has been observed in patients with UC or CD, whereas *Firmicutes* phylum was reduced in the fecal samples of CD patients respect to healthy individuals [69,70,73].

Takahashi [76] found a decline in several butyrate-producing bacteria species in the fecal microbiome of CD patients in accordance with a previous study performed by Wang [74]. More specifically, a meaningful reduced abundance of the genera *Bacteroides*, *Eubacterium*, *Faecalibacterium*, and *Ruminococcus*, and increased proportion of the genera *Actinomyces* and *Bifidobacterium* were reported in CD patients respect to healthy controls. At the species level, a considerable reduction of butyrate-producing bacterial species, as *Blautia faecis*, *Roseburia inulinivorans*, *Ruminococcus torques*, *Clostridium lavalense*, *Bacteroides uniformis*, and *F. prausnitzii* characterized CD patients respect to healthy subjects. Similar results were observed in further CD patients ($n = 68$) and healthy controls ($n = 46$) [76].

The presence of important differences in mucosa-associated gut microbiota have also been observed in children affected by IBD [112,169,170]. Dysbiosis could be present before CD onset, as demonstrated by the group of Gevers, who found disturbances in the microbiota composition of the stool and mucosal in newly diagnosed, treatment-naive children affected by CD [171]. IBD subjects also showed alterations in the composition of bacteriophages with an increase in *Caudovirales bacteriophages* [113], as well as in fungal composition. Alterations in the diversity of the latter characterized mucosa and fecal samples. Even though the exact role of fungi in IBD development has not been clarified, host metabolism and mucosal immune response, as well as the microbiome composition, and thus the homeostasis of the gut more in general, could be influenced by fungi as supported by animal studies [172]. Indeed, even fungi and viruses constitutes the microbiome of the gut, with the predominance of bacteriophages as demonstrated by metagenomic analyses executed on viral particles from human stool samples [173,174]. Recently, Van Belleghem [175] observed that *Staphylococcus* (*S.*) *aureus* and *Pseudomonas aeruginosa* phages exert immunomodulatory activities on human peripheral mononuclear cells, whereas a limited number of studies have investigated the role of bacteriophages in IBD pathogenesis [176]. Concerning the contribution of diet and metabolism to IBD pathogenesis, aryl hydrocarbon receptor (AHR) agonists seem to play a role in several autoimmune conditions, including IBD by modulating T cell responses. Intriguingly, reduced levels of AhR expression agonists characterized the inflamed intestinal tissue samples collected from CD respect to uninvolved areas of the same patients, and UC and control subjects. The anti-inflammatory effect exerted by the Ahr agonist on the gastrointestinal tract was mediated by the induction of IL-22 [177], accordingly with previous studies reporting the anti-inflammatory [178] and protective [132] role of this cytokine. On the light of these results, AhR-related molecules could represent a promising treatment for CD.

2.6. Autoimmune Skin Conditions

2.6.1. Vitiligo

Vitiligo is a chronic pigmentary disorder affecting 1% of the population. It represents an acquired depigmentary skin disorder leading to the development of white macules that are caused by a reduction of the number and function of melanocytes in the skin and/or hair [133]. The pathology presents a systemic involvement since melanocytes are located not only in the skin but also on various parts of the body [134]. Its origin remains to be elucidated and among the various hypothesis [179,180], the main one is an autoimmune attack of melanocytes. Furthermore, it is frequently associated with other autoimmune diseases [181]. The available treatment aims to reduce the exaggerated immune reaction, although with limited positive results.

The group of Ganju [83] investigated the differences in bacterial community of lesional and non-lesional skin of vitiligo subjects. The analysis of community composition revealed that four phyla (*Actinobacteria, Proteobacteria, Firmicutes,* and *Bacteroidetes*) dominated in both skin types, in accordance with previous data of microbiota composition of healthy skin [114]. However, they highlighted the presence of dysbiosis in the diversity of the microbial community structure in the lesional skin of vitiligo subjects with a reduction in taxonomic richness. Furthermore, they evaluated the presence of networks between individual microbiota members through intra-community network analysis investigating various network properties (which includes nodes, edges, density, diameter, etc.), and centrality measures (degree and betweenness). The study allowed for the reveal of a specific pattern of interactions between resident bacterial populations of the two sites (lesional and non-lesional). Lesional skin areas present an aberrant intra-community network since bacteria had a reduced number of interactions respect to those of non-lesional sites. In more detail, *Actinobacterial* sp. and *Firmicutes* prevailed in the central regulatory nodes of non-lesional skin and in lesional sites, respectively. Although the dynamics characterizing the bacteria constituting the cutaneous microbiome remains to be elucidated, the alterations observed in the microbiome composition of vitiligo lesions allowed researchers to envisage their implication in the persistence and the severity of vitiligo. If such a hypothesis will be confirmed, skin bacterial populations could represent a valuable target for vitiligo treatment.

2.6.2. Psoriasis Vulgaris

Psoriasis vulgaris represents a common chronic inflammatory skin disease caused by iper-activated immune pathways of both the innate and adaptive immunity that in normal conditions are constitutive or inducible [182]. The common type of psoriasis is also denominated by large plaque psoriasis or psoriasis vulgaris and is characterized by red colored plaques with well-defined borders and silvery-white dry scale, involving elbows, knees, scalp, and the lumbosacral area. However, psoriasis lesions can also be more extensive. Besides this form of psoriasis, there are also further variants of the disease: guttate, inverse, pustular, erythrodermic, palmo-plantar, and drug-associated psoriasis [135,183,184]. The possible correlation between the disease and the skin microbiome has been investigated by a small number of studies. The existing contrasting results can be caused by the absence of standardized sampling and protocols, or to an intrinsic variability of microbes among humans [84–87,185].

The study performed by the group of Alekseyenko [86] focused on the characterization of skin microbiota of psoriatic lesions, unaffected contralateral skin from 75 chronic plaque psoriatic patients, and similar skin loci in 124 matched healthy subjects through high-throughput 16S rRNA gene sequencing. Psoriasis was characterized by physiological alterations, both at the lesion site and at the systemic level, which were able to modulate microbiome composition among the clinical skin types evaluated. More specifically, a reduction in the taxonomic diversity as well as in the evenness in both lesion and unaffected microbiota communities from psoriatic patients with respect to the control was observed. The analysis of the relative abundance of the taxa constituting the skin microbiota revealed that three phyla *Proteobacteria, Firmicutes,* and *Actinobacteria* prevailed in the skin microbial communities in all three subgroups, according to previous studies [85]. Furthermore, psoriasis correlated with relative abundance and presence of specific taxa. More in detail, even though the three subgroups evaluated (lesion, unaffected, and control) did not present significant differences in the genera usually present on skin, i.e., *Propionibacterium, Corynebacterium, Streptococcus,* and *Staphylococcus;* they were characterized by considerable differences in the combined relative abundance of the four taxa. *Corynebacterium, Propionibacterium, Staphylococcus,* and *Streptococcus* showed a higher abundance, whereas a marked reduction in relative abundances of *Cupriavidus, Flavisolibacter, Methylobacterium,* and *Schlegelella* genera were observed in psoriatic patients with respect to controls. The study highlighted the association between lesion samples with *Firmicutes*-associated microbiota. A recent investigation conducted by Chang [88] confirmed alterations affecting skin microbiome in psoriasis, and further analysis conducted on mice colonized with *S. aureus* demonstrated a marked upregulation of Th17 response, which could have a role in IL-17-driven inflammation in psoriasis. Accordingly, mice colonized with *Staphylococcus epidermidis* or un-colonized mice (controls) did not present this response.

2.6.3. Atopic Dermatitis

Atopic dermatitis (AD) represents a chronic recurrent inflammatory cutaneous disease whose patients present itching and xerosis [186]. AD is also associated with other allergic diseases. An enhancement of its prevalence has been observed in developed countries, affecting from 15% to 30% and 2% to 10% of children and adults, respectively [187]. The pathology is in fact the skin manifestation of a systemic disorder in which both local and systemic factors are implicated in its etiology. AD skin is characterized by dysbiosis with marked *S. aureus* colonization [94], which has also been positively associated with disease severity.

The investigation conducted by Laborel-Préneron [91] revealed the correlation between *S. aureus* in inflamed skin of AD subjects and elevated IgE response and up-regulation of inflammatory and Th2/Th22 transcripts. Furthermore, secretomes from *S. aureus* and *S. epidermidis* from the skin microbiota of AD children induced monocyte-derived dendritic cells to produce pro-inflammatory IFN-γ and anti-inflammatory IL-10, respectively. *S. aureus* and *S. epidermidis* secretomes also exerted the opposite effect on CD4$^+$ T cell activation, which was induced by the former, whereas CD4$^+$ proliferation was inhibited by the concurrent presence of *S. epidermidis* secretome. The two secretomes also have effects on Treg function. More specific, the secretome of *S. epidermidis* elicited Treg activity favoring the suppression of CD4$^+$ T cell activation, whereas when the *S. aureus* secretome was present, Treg did not show this effect. This study supports the involvement of *S. aureus* in the onset and promotion of cutaneous inflammation by inducing Th2 activation and suppressing the resident Treg cells.

Iwamoto et al. [94] reported that *S. aureus* from AD skin was able to change the synthesis of cytokines via monocyte-derived Langerhans cells inducing an imbalanced Th1/Th2 skin immunity. In addition to *S. aureus,* the other microbes constituting the cutaneous microbiome could have an important role in the onset and progression of AD [92].

Song et al. [93] observed a significant correlation between the high abundance of *F. prausnitzii* subspecies in the gut microbiome and AD. This enrichment could lead to a reduction of butyrate and propionate producers and thus a diminishment in these two molecules with anti-inflammatory activity. In particular, among the species producing butyrate and propionate, those related to the strain A2-165 are also affected by the change in composition, and their deficiency has been related to CD.

The Suzuki [97] group has investigated whether an abnormal immune response toward microbial stimuli derived via the colonization of beneficial bacteria could be implicated in AD onset. They reported that the stimulation with heat-killed Gram-positive bacteria (*Bifidobacterium bifidum* and *Lactobacillus rhamnosus GG*) and *Lactobacillus*-derived peptidoglycan of cord-blood mononuclear cells (CBMCs) derived from AD infants produced a lower synthesis of IL-10 with respect to infants without AD. This finding has suggested a putative correlation between these bacteria and a higher risk of infantile AD.

AD pathogenesis is not only due to microbiome, but also to extracellular vesicles (EVs) released from bacteria and containing pathogenic proteins from *S. aureus*. These have been correlated with AD onset as demonstrated by in vitro and in vivo studies performed by Hong et al. [89]. More in detail, *S. aureus* EVs were able to promote inflammatory responses via dermal fibroblasts and the thickening of the epidermis associated with the infiltration of mast cells and eosinophils when EVs were applied to tape-stripped mouse skin [89]. EVs derived from the microbiome have been identified in the blood [89], as well as in other organ systems to promote inflammation [187]. AD subjects presented meaningfully elevated serum levels of *S. aureus* EV-specific IgE respect to healthy subjects [89].

As demonstrated recently by Kim et al. [96] on 27 AD patients and 6 healthy controls, the bacterial EV composition differs significantly between the two groups evaluated, with a marked reduction of *Lactococcus*, *Leuconostoc*, and *Lactobacillus* EV proportions and an increase of those from *Alicyclobacillus* and *Propionibacterium* in AD patients with respect to controls. In addition, EVs produced from lactic acid bacteria exerted a protective function against the *S. aureus* EV-induced AD mouse model. Also, Francuzik et al. [95] recently observed differences between lesional and non-lesional skin in AD patients, where the latter showed a diminished abundance of *Propionibacterium* (*P.*) *acnes* and *Lawsonella clevelandensis* and an increase of *S. aureus*. The observation that the products of fermentation of *P. acnes* blocked *S. aureus* and *S. epidermidis* growth, as well as serum collected from AD patients halted *S. aureus* growth more efficiently than serum from healthy individuals, allowed the researchers to hypothesize that specific changes in the cutaneous microbiota could represent a possible strategy for AD treatment.

2.7. Autoimmune Neurological Diseases

The incidence of autoimmune neurological diseases, including multiple sclerosis (MS), as well as other autoimmune disorders, has dramatically increased in industrialized Western countries [136,188]. It has been supposed that the diet present in these societies, with rich fat content and reduced intake of fibers, as opposite to societies characterized by a traditional lifestyle [53,189], could induce changes in the composition of the gut microbiome and its activities promoting the onset of autoimmune conditions [190,191].

The intake of fiber through the diet are important for the health of humans since they exert several physiological effects, as modulation of the gut immunological microenvironment of the gut and the protection against autoimmune and allergic diseases induced by short chain fatty acids (SCFAs) representing the final-products of the fiber fermentation [53,189–193]. The role of insoluble fibers, including cellulose, in the etiology of autoimmune conditions remains to be elucidated, though they are able to shape the diversity of the microbiome [192,193]. MS onset has been linked to dietary exposure [98,194,195]. Berer et al. [105] observed that autoimmune demyelination was promoted by auto-reactive B lymphocytes induced after the stimulation of the commensal microbiome with the autoantigen myelin oligodendrocyte glycoprotein (MOG). Conversely, CNS inflammation in mice was contrasted with the expansion of CD4$^+$ Foxp3$^+$ Tregs via TLR2-mediated CD39 signaling upon the administration of polysaccharide A (PSA), an intestinal commensal product derived from *B. fragilis* [99,100]. Other microbial metabolites able to reduce neuroinflammation are those derived from dietary tryptophan (Trp), which is introduced with the diet and metabolized by the commensal gut microbiome [196] into several AHR agonists and exerts its activity on astrocytes [104]. In association with Trp-derived metabolites, type I interferon (IFN-I) is also synthesized in the CNS function and the axis IFN-I/AhR is involved in the regulation of astrocyte functions and the inflammatory process affecting the CNS [104]. However, MS patients presented lower levels of circulating AHR agonists and a reduced AhR agonistic activity than controls in order to hypothesize the involvement of the commensal microbiome metabolism, diet, or the environment in MS pathogenesis [104].

Furthermore, recent studies have highlighted the presence of dysbiosis in the gut microbiome of patients with MS [101–103]. Miyake et al. [101] observed a considerable reduction of species belonging to *Clostridia XIVa* and *IV Clusters*. The study conducted by Jangi et al. [103] on 60 MS patients and 43 healthy controls revealed gut microbiome alterations which included an increased abundance of *Methanobrevibacter* and *Akkermansia* and a reduction in *Butyricimonas*. These defects were associated with an altered expression of genes playing a role in dendritic cell maturation, interferon signaling and nuclear factor-κB (NF-κB) signaling pathways in circulating T lymphocytes and monocytes. In addition, a decrease in *Sarcina* and a rise in *Prevotella* and *Sutterella* occurred in patients on disease-modifying treatment respect to untreated patients [103]. The presence of dysbiosis involving *Akkermansia* (*A.*) *muciniphila* has also been confirmed recently by Cekanaviciute et al. [106] who reported an enhancement in *A. muciniphila* and *Acinetobacter* (*A.*) *calcoaceticus* in MS patients associated with a reduction in *Parabacteroides* (*P.*) *distasonis*. The exposure of human peripheral blood mononuclear cells and monocolonized mice to *A. muciniphila* and *A. calcoaceticus* individual bacterial cultures shifted T lymphocytes towards a pro-inflammatory phenotype. A reduction in Treg compartment associated with a higher number of effector CD4$^+$ lymphocytes that differentiated into IFNγ-producing Th1 cells were induced by *A. calcoaceticus*. Th1 lymphocyte differentiation was even more marked upon exposure to *A. muciniphila*. Conversely, *P. distasonis* induced anti-inflammatory IL-10-expressing human CD4$^+$ CD25$^+$ T cells and IL-10$^+$ FoxP3$^+$ Tregs in mice [106].

The group of Chen [102] reported an enhancement of *Pseudomonas*, *Mycoplana*, *Haemophilus*, *Blautia*, and *Dorea* in relapsing remitting MS (RRMS) (*n* = 31) patients, while *Parabacteroides*, *Adlercreutzia* and *Prevotella* genera were increased in healthy controls (*n* = 36).

Recently, the groups of Berer [105] and Cekanaviciute [106] demonstrated that microbiome transplantation from MS patients into germ-free mice enables spontaneous experimental autoimmune encephalomyelitis (EAE) in mice [105,106] and a IL-10$^+$ Treg subset was lowered with respect to mice transplanted with microbiota from healthy controls [106].

The recent study conducted by Berer et al. [105] found that spontaneous CNS-directed autoimmunity onset is suppressed by a diet with a crude high non-fermentable fiber content (26% of cellulose content, cellulose rich (CR)) during early adult life. In detail, they use genetically engineered spontaneous experimental opticospinal encephalomyelitis (OSE) mice as a spontaneous model for EAE [197] with respect to classic active EAE models such that microbiota composition and immune responses could not be exogenously biased by the use of adjuvants [197]. In the control diet-fed mice (standard rodent diet), spontaneous EAE (sEAE) incidence was about 55%, whereas EAE incidence was strongly decreased (23%) when a CR diet was used, and moreover, OSE mice showed delayed neurological symptom onset. Disease severity, as well as inflammatory marker expression in the spinal cord in EAE mice, did not show any differences. The investigation of the cytokine expression profile revealed that CR diet was correlated with a reduction in the pathogenic T cell response with respect to control diet-fed animals, and in addition, T lymphocytes from mice fed with a CR diet had higher transcript levels of the Th2 cell-associated cytokines than T cells from control mice. The characterization of the cecal microbiota of CR diet and control diet-fed revealed that dietary regimens skewed gut microbial and metabolic profiles. More specifically, OSE mice fed with a CR diet presented an increase of the genera *Helicobacter*, *Enterococcus*, *Desulfovibrio*, *Parabacteroides*, *Pseudoflavonifractor*, and *Oscillibacter*, whereas *Lactobacillus*, *Parasutterella*, *Coprobacillus*, and *TM7 genera Incertae Sedis* were considerably diminished with respect to the control group. It has been hypothesized that the increased Th2 cell response was promoted in CR diet-fed mice and thus the protective effect against EAE onset could have been a consequence of the modified gut microbiota and/or the altered metabolic profile [198].

3. Conclusions

In the last few years, autoimmune and inflammatory disorder incidence has considerably increased worldwide, and increasing observations have reported a correlation between the presence of microbiome dysbiosis and the development of different autoimmune conditions, although the precise mechanism remains to be elucidated. Furthermore, limited knowledge is currently available on whether these modifications in microbiome composition could be causally related to the pathogenesis of autoimmunity or these alterations could be a consequence of an abnormal immune response. However, since the gut microbiome is able to shape the host adaptive immune responses through mediator and nutrient release, and moreover dysbiosis of specific human gut bacteria has been found in several different autoimmune conditions, the manipulation of the microbiome could represent a potential therapeutic strategy for the improvement and potentially complete restoration of the normal immune response in different autoimmune diseases.

As emphasized above, diet has the strongest influence on gut microbiota [137]. Nevertheless, to date, few clinical studies of dietary interventions on human gut microbiota have been reported [137]. Definitively, a healthy status is associated with a low energy and high fiber and vegetables intake. In the future, perspectives of human health can certainly be derived from diet regimen control together with synbiotic administration of microbial taxa in order to equilibrate gut microbiota composition [189,192,193,199–202]. Regarding in particular the focus of the present review, several studies pointed to the selection of microbial species that could improve the treatment of chronic inflammatory disorders in addition to other conditions, including atherosclerosis, behavior abnormalities, cancer, *Clostridium difficile* infection, and obesity. Indeed, Treg expansion was promoted by certain gut bacterial species [137,138]. In mouse models of colitis and allergic inflammation, *Lactococcus lactis*-expressing IL-10 treated inflammation [203] and was safe when administered in a human phase I trial [204]. *E. coli*-secreted proteins were shown to activate anorexigenic pathways to control satiety for obesity treatment [205]. Further in diabetic rats, metabolism control was ameliorated using glucagon-like peptide 1-releasing bacterial strains with the effect of inducing insulin secretion [206].

A future avenue for treatment is fecal microbiota transplantation (FMT). Studies have already documented FMT as a medically actionable tool, for example, in treating recurrent diarrhea using *Clostridium difficile* or insulin-resistance in obese patients [207]. This evidence could foster future application studies aimed to control inflammation in patients affected by autoimmunity.

Author Contributions: Writing—original draft preparation: E.G. Writing—review and editing, supervision, and funding acquisition: A.F.

Funding: This study was supported by the Italian Ministry of Health Ricerca Corrente 201802P004265.

Conflicts of Interest: The authors declare no conflict of interest.

Abbreviations

ACPA	anti–citrullinated protein antibody
AD	atopic dermatitis
AHR	aryl hydrocarbon receptor
BD	Behcet's disease
BPB	butyrate-producing bacteria
CBMCs	cord-blood mononuclear cells
CCL20	chemokine (C-C motif) ligand 20
CD	Crohn's disease
CIA	collagen-induced arthritis
CNS	central nervous system
CR	cellulose rich
CS	caesarian section
EAE	autoimmune encephalomyelitis
EVs	extracellular vesicles
FLNA	filamin A
FMT	fecal microbiota transplantation
GNS	*N*-acetylglucosamine-6-sulfatase
HbA1c	hemoglobin A1c
HCD	hydrolyzed casein diet

IBD	inflammatory bowel disease
IFN-I	type I interferon
IFN-γ	interferon gamma
IL	Interleukin
LPS	lipopolysaccharide
MOG	myelin oligodendrocyte glycoprotein
MS	multiple sclerosis
NF-κB	nuclear factor-κB
NOD	non-obese diabetic mice
OSE	opticospinal encephalomyelitis
PAD	peptidylarginine deiminase
PAMPs	pathogen associated molecular patterns
PSA	polysaccharide A
RA	rheumatoid arthritis
RRMS	relapsing remitting MS
SCFAs	short-chain fatty acids
SCFAs	short chain fatty acids
sEAE	spontaneous EAE
SFB	segmented filamentous bacteria
SLE	systemic lupus erythematosus
SPF	specific-pathogen-free
T1D	type I diabetes
Tc	cytotoxic T lymphocytes
TCRs	T cell receptors
Tfh	T follicular helper
Th	T lymphocytes. T-helper
Treg	regulatory T
Trp	tryptophan
UCs	ulcerative colitis

References

1. Ajayi, T.; Innes, C.L.; Grimm, S.A.; Rai, P.; Finethy, R.; Coers, J.; Wang, X.; Bell, D.A.; McGrath, J.A.; Schurman, S.H.; et al. Crohn's disease IRGM risk alleles are associated with altered gene expression in human tissues. *Am. J. Physiol. Gastrointest. Liver Physiol.* **2019**, *316*, G95–G105. [CrossRef] [PubMed]

2. Batura, V.; Muise, A.M. Very early onset IBD: Novel genetic aetiologies. *Curr. Opin. Allergy Clin. Immunol.* **2018**, *18*, 470–480. [CrossRef]

3. Zhang, J.; Meng, Y.; Wu, H.; Wu, Y.; Yang, B.; Wang, L. Association between PPP2CA polymorphisms and clinical features in southwest Chinese systemic lupus erythematosus patients. *Medicine* **2018**, *97*, e11451. [CrossRef] [PubMed]

4. Wu, Y.L.; Ding, Y.P.; Gao, J.; Tanaka, Y.; Zhang, W. Risk factors and primary prevention trials for type 1 diabetes. *Int. J. Biol. Sci.* **2013**, *9*, 666–679. [CrossRef] [PubMed]

5. Barbeau, W.E. What is the key environmental trigger in type 1 diabetes—Is it viruses, or wheat gluten, or both? *Autoimmun. Rev.* **2012**, *12*, 295–299. [CrossRef]

6. Lindoso, L.; Mondal, K.; Venkateswaran, S.; Somineni, H.K.; Ballengee, C.; Walters, T.D.; Griffiths, A.; Noe, J.D.; Crandall, W.; Snapper, S.; et al. The Effect of Early-Life Environmental Exposures on Disease Phenotype and Clinical Course of Crohn's Disease in Children. *Am. J. Gastroenterol.* **2018**, *113*, 1524–1529. [CrossRef] [PubMed]

7. Jimenez, E.; Marin, M.L.; Martin, R.; Odriozola, J.M.; Olivares, M.; Xaus, J.; Fernández, L.; Rodríguez, J.M. Is meconium from healthy newborns actually sterile? *Res. Microbiol.* **2008**, *159*, 187–193. [CrossRef]

8. Vereecke, L.; Beyaert, R.; van Loo, G. Enterocyte death and intestinal barrier maintenance in homeostasis and disease. *Trends Mol. Med.* **2011**, *17*, 584–593. [CrossRef] [PubMed]

9. Ogilvie, L.A.; Jones, B.V. The human gut virome: A multifaceted majority. *Front. Microbiol.* **2015**, *6*, 918. [CrossRef]

10. Gough, E.K.; Prendergast, A.J.; Mutasa, K.E.; Stoltzfus, R.J.; Manges, A.R. Sanitation Hygiene Infant Nutrition Efficacy (SHINE) Trial Team. Assessing the Intestinal Microbiota in the SHINE Trial. *Clin. Infect. Dis.* **2015**, *61*, S738–S744. [CrossRef]

11. Kaiko, G.E.; Stappenbeck, T.S. Host-microbe interactions shaping the gastrointestinal environment. *Trends Immunol.* **2014**, *35*, 538–548. [CrossRef]

12. Consortium, H.M.P. Structure, function and diversity of the healthy human microbiome. *Nature* **2012**, *486*, 207–214.

13. DiGiulio, D.B.; Callahan, B.J.; McMurdie, P.J.; Costello, E.K.; Lyell, D.J.; Robaczewska, A.; Sun, C.L.; Goltsman, D.S.; Wong, R.J.; Shaw, G.; et al. Temporal and spatial variation of the human microbiota during pregnancy. *Proc. Natl. Acad. Sci. USA* **2015**, *112*, 11060–11065. [CrossRef] [PubMed]

14. Gomez de Agüero, M.; Ganal-Vonarburg, S.C.; Fuhrer, T.; Rupp, S.; Uchimura, Y.; Li, H.; Steinert, A.; Heikenwalder, M.; Hapfelmeier, S.; Sauer, U.; et al. The maternal microbiota drives early postnatal innate immune development. *Science* **2016**, *351*, 1296–1302. [CrossRef] [PubMed]

15. Clausen, T.D.; Bergholt, T.; Eriksson, F.; Rasmussen, S.; Keiding, N.; Løkkegaard, E.C. Prelabor Cesarean Section and Risk of Childhood Type 1 Diabetes: A Nationwide Register-based Cohort Study. *Epidemiology* **2016**, *27*, 547–555. [CrossRef] [PubMed]

16. Gianchecchi, E.; Fierabracci, A. On the pathogenesis of insulin-dependent diabetes mellitus: The role of microbiota. *Immunol. Res.* **2017**, *65*, 242–256. [CrossRef] [PubMed]

17. Cardwell, C.R.; Stene, L.C.; Joner, G.; Cinek, O.; Svensson, J.; Goldacre, M.J.; Parslow, R.C.; Pozzilli, P.; Brigis, G.; Stoyanov, D.; et al. Caesarean section is associated with an increased risk of childhood-onset type 1 diabetes mellitus: A meta-analysis of observational studies. *Diabetologia* **2008**, *51*, 726–735. [CrossRef] [PubMed]

18. Salminen, S.; Gibson, G.R.; McCartney, A.L.; Isolauri, E. Influence of mode of delivery on gut microbiota composition in seven year old children. *Gut* **2004**, *53*, 1388–1389. [CrossRef] [PubMed]

19. Magne, F.; Puchi Silva, A.; Carvajal, B.; Gotteland, M. The Elevated Rate of Cesarean Section and Its Contribution to Non-Communicable Chronic Diseases in Latin America: The Growing Involvement of the Microbiota. *Front. Pediatr.* **2017**, *5*, 192. [CrossRef]

20. Wikoff, W.R.; Anfora, A.T.; Liu, J.; Schultz, P.G.; Lesley, S.A.; Peters, E.C.; Siuzdak, G. Metabolomics analysis reveals large effects of gut microflora on mammalian blood metabolites. *Proc. Natl. Acad. Sci. USA* **2009**, *106*, 3698–3703. [CrossRef] [PubMed]

21. Clarke, G.; Stilling, R.M.; Kennedy, P.J.; Stanton, C.; Cryan, J.F.; Dinan, T.G. Minireview: Gut microbiota: The neglected endocrine organ. *Mol. Endocrinol.* **2014**, *28*, 1221–1238. [CrossRef] [PubMed]

22. Rooks, M.G.; Garrett, W.S. Gut microbiota, metabolites and host immunity. *Nat. Rev. Immunol.* **2016**, *16*, 341–352. [CrossRef] [PubMed]

23. Zelante, T.; Iannitti, R.G.; Cunha, C.; De Luca, A.; Giovannini, G.; Pieraccini, G.; Zecchi, R.; D'Angelo, C.; Massi-Benedetti, C.; Fallarino, F.; et al. Tryptophan catabolites from microbiota engage aryl hydrocarbon receptor and balance mucosal reactivity via interleukin-22. *Immunity* **2013**, *39*, 372–385. [CrossRef]

24. Chen, J.; Rao, J.N.; Zou, T.; Liu, L.; Marasa, B.S.; Xiao, L.; Zeng, X.; Turner, D.J.; Wang, J.Y. Polyamines are required for expression of Toll-like receptor 2 modulating intestinal epithelial barrier integrity. *Am. J. Physiol. Gastrointest. Liver Physiol.* **2007**, *293*, G568–G576. [CrossRef]

25. Willemsen, L.E.M.; Koetsier, M.A.; van Deventer, S.J.H.; van Tol, E.A.F. Short chain fatty acids stimulate epithelial mucin 2 expression through differential effects on prostaglandin E1 and E2 production by intestinal myofibroblasts. *Gut* **2003**, *52*, 1442–1447. [CrossRef] [PubMed]

26. Tao, R.; de Zoeten, E.F.; Ozkaynak, E.; Chen, C.; Wang, L.; Porrett, P.M.; Li, B.; Turka, L.A.; Olson, E.N.; Greene, M.I.; et al. Deacetylase inhibition promotes the generation and function of regulatory T cells. *Nat. Med.* **2007**, *13*, 1299–1307. [CrossRef] [PubMed]

27. Renelli, M.; Matias, V.; Lo, R.Y.; Beveridge, T.J. DNA-containing membrane vesicles of Pseudomonas aeruginosa PAO1 and their genetic transformation potential. *Microbiology* **2004**, *50*, 2161–2169. [CrossRef]

28. Muraca, M.; Putignani, L.; Fierabracci, A.; Teti, A.; Perilongo, G. Gut microbiota-derived outer membrane vesicles: Under-recognized major players in health and disease? *Discov. Med.* **2015**, *19*, 343–348.

29. Avila-Calderón, E.D.; Araiza-Villanueva, M.G.; Cancino-Diaz, J.C.; López-Villegas, E.O.; Sriranganathan, N.; Boyle, S.M.; et al. Roles of bacterial membrane vesicles. *Arch. Microbiol.* **2015**, *197*, 1–10. [CrossRef]

30. Graham, S.; Courtois, P.; Malaisse, W.J.; Rozing, J.; Scott, F.W.; Mowat, A.M. Enteropathy precedes type 1 diabetes in the BB rat. *Gut* **2004**, *53*, 1437–1444. [CrossRef]
31. Neu, J.; Reverte, C.M.; Mackey, A.D.; Liboni, K.; Tuhacek-Tenace, L.M.; Hatch, M.; Li, N.; Caicedo, R.A.; Schatz, D.A.; Atkinson, M. Changes in intestinal morphology and permeability in the biobreeding rat before the onset of type 1 diabetes. *J. Pediatr. Gastroenterol. Nutr.* **2005**, *40*, 589–595. [CrossRef] [PubMed]
32. Brugman, S.; Klatter, F.A.; Visser, J.T.; Wildeboer-Veloo, A.C.; Harmsen, H.J.; Rozing, J.; Bos, N.A. Antibiotic treatment partially protects against type 1 diabetes in the Bio-Breeding diabetes-prone rat. Is the gut flora involved in the development of type 1 diabetes? *Diabetologia* **2006**, *49*, 2105–2108. [CrossRef] [PubMed]
33. Wen, L.; Ley, R.E.; Volchkov, P.Y.; Stranges, P.B.; Avanesyan, L.; Stonebraker, A.C.; Hu, C.; Wong, F.S.; Szot, G.L.; Bluestone, J.A.; et al. Innate immunity and intestinal microbiota in the development of Type 1 diabetes. *Nature* **2008**, *455*, 1109–1113. [CrossRef] [PubMed]
34. Valladares, R.; Sankar, D.; Li, N.; Williams, E.; Lai, K.K.; Abdelgeliel, A.S.; Gonzalez, C.F.; Wasserfall, C.H.; Larkin, J.; Schatz, D.; et al. Lactobacillus johnsonii N6.2 mitigates the development of type 1 diabetes in BB-DP rats. *PLoS ONE* **2010**, *5*, e10507. [CrossRef]
35. Giongo, A.; Gano, K.A.; Crabb, D.B.; Mukherjee, N.; Novelo, L.L.; Casella, G.; Drew, J.C.; Ilonen, J.; Knip, M.; Hyöty, H.; et al. Toward defining the autoimmune microbiome for type 1 diabetes. *ISME J.* **2011**, *5*, 82–91. [CrossRef] [PubMed]
36. de Goffau, M.C.; Luopajärvi, K.; Knip, M.; Ilonen, J.; Ruohtula, T.; Härkönen, T.; Orivuori, L.; Hakala, S.; Welling, G.W.; Harmsen, H.J.; et al. Fecal microbiota composition differs between children with β-cell autoimmunity and those without. *Diabetes* **2013**, *62*, 1238–1244. [CrossRef]
37. Murri, M.; Leiva, I.; Gomez-Zumaquero, J.M.; Tinahones, F.J.; Cardona, F.; Soriguer, F.; Queipo-Ortuño, M.I. Gut microbiota in children with type 1 diabetes differs from that in healthy children: A case-control study. *BMC Med.* **2013**, *11*, 46. [CrossRef]
38. Patrick, C.; Wang, G.S.; Lefebvre, D.E.; Crookshank, J.A.; Sonier, B.; Eberhard, C.; Mojibian, M.; Kennedy, C.R.; Brooks, S.P.; Kalmokoff, M.L.; et al. Promotion of autoimmune diabetes by cereal diet in the presence or absence of microbes associated with gut immune activation.; regulatory imbalance; and altered cathelicidin antimicrobial Peptide. *Diabetes* **2013**, *62*, 2036–2047. [CrossRef]
39. Davis-Richardson, A.G.; Ardissone, A.N.; Dias, R.; Simell, V.; Leonard, M.T.; Kemppainen, K.M.; Drew, J.C.; Schatz, D.; Atkinson, M.A.; Kolaczkowski, B.; et al. Bacteroides dorei dominates gut microbiome prior to autoimmunity in Finnish children at high risk for type 1 diabetes. *Front. Microbiol.* **2014**, *5*, 678. [CrossRef]
40. Mejía-León, M.E.; Petrosino, J.F.; Ajami, N.J.; Domínguez-Bello, M.G.; de la Barca, A.M. Fecal microbiota imbalance in Mexican children with type 1 diabetes. *Sci. Rep.* **2014**, *4*, 3814. [CrossRef]
41. Soyucen, E.; Gulcan, A.; Aktuglu-Zeybek, A.C.; Onal, H.; Kiykim, E.; Aydin, A. Differences in the gut microbiota of healthy children and those with type 1 diabetes. *Pediatr. Int.* **2014**, *56*, 336–343. [CrossRef] [PubMed]
42. Alkanani, A.K.; Hara, N.; Gottlieb, P.A.; Ir, D.; Robertson, C.E.; Wagner, B.D.; Frank, D.N.; Zipris, D. Alterations in intestinal microbiota correlate with susceptibility to type 1 diabetes. *Diabetes* **2015**, *64*, 3510–3520. [CrossRef] [PubMed]
43. Kostic, A.D.; Gevers, D.; Siljander, H.; Vatanen, T.; Hyötyläinen, T.; Hämäläinen, A.M.; Peet, A.; Tillmann, V.; Pöhö, P.; Mattila, I.; et al. The dynamics of the human infant gut microbiome in development and in progression toward type 1 diabetes. *Cell Host Microbe* **2015**, *17*, 260–273. [CrossRef] [PubMed]
44. Mejia-Leon, M.E.; Barca, A.M. Diet, microbiota and immune system in type 1 diabetes development and evolution. *Nutrients* **2015**, *7*, 9171–9184. [CrossRef] [PubMed]
45. Sun, J.; Furio, L.; Mecheri, R.; van der Does, A.M.; Lundeberg, E.; Saveanu, L.; Chen, Y.; van Endert, P.; Agerberth, B.; Diana, J. Pancreatic β-Cells Limit Autoimmune Diabetes via an Immunoregulatory Antimicrobial Peptide Expressed under the Influence of the Gut Microbiota. *Immunity* **2015**, *43*, 304–317. [CrossRef]
46. Uusitalo, U.; Liu, X.; Yang, J.; Aronsson, C.A.; Hummel, S.; Butterworth, M.; Lernmark, Å.; Rewers, M.; Hagopian, W.; She, J.X.; et al. Association of Early Exposure of Probiotics and Islet Autoimmunity in the TEDDY Study. *JAMA Pediatr.* **2016**, *170*, 20–28. [CrossRef] [PubMed]
47. Pinto, E.; Anselmo, M.; Calha, M.; Bottrill, A.; Duarte, I.; Andrew, P.W.; Faleiro, M.L. The intestinal proteome of diabetic and control children is enriched with different microbial and host proteins. *Microbiology* **2017**, *163*, 161–174. [CrossRef] [PubMed]

48. Gavin, P.G.; Mullaney, J.A.; Loo, D.; Cao, K.L.; Gottlieb, P.A.; Hill, M.M.; Zipris, D.; Hamilton-Williams, E.E. Intestinal Metaproteomics Reveals Host-Microbiota Interactions in Subjects at Risk for Type 1 Diabetes. *Diabetes Care* **2018**, *41*, 2178–2186. [CrossRef]

49. Gürsoy, S.; Koçkar, T.; Atik, S.U.; Önal, Z.; Önal, H.; Adal, E. Autoimmunity and intestinal colonization by Candida albicans in patients with type 1 diabetes at the time of the diagnosis. *Korean J. Pediatr.* **2018**, *61*, 217–220. [CrossRef]

50. Henschel, A.M.; Cabrera, S.M.; Kaldunski, M.L.; Jia, S.; Geoffrey, R.; Roethle, M.F.; Lam, V.; Chen, Y.G.; Wang, X.; Salzman, N.H.; et al. Modulation of the diet and gastrointestinal microbiota normalizes systemic inflammation and β-cell chemokine expression associated with autoimmune diabetes susceptibility. *PLoS ONE* **2018**, *13*, e0190351. [CrossRef] [PubMed]

51. Huang, Y.; Li, S.C.; Hu, J.; Ruan, H.B.; Guo, H.M.; Zhang, H.H.; Wang, X.; Pei, Y.F.; Pan, Y.; Fang, C. Gut microbiota profiling in Han Chinese with type 1 diabetes. *Diabetes Res. Clin. Pract.* **2018**, *141*, 256–263. [CrossRef]

52. Mullaney, J.A.; Stephens, J.E.; Costello, M.E.; Fong, C.; Geeling, B.E.; Gavin, P.G.; Wright, C.M.; Spector, T.D.; Brown, M.A.; Hamilton-Williams, E.E. Correction to: Type 1 diabetes susceptibility alleles are associated with distinct alterations in the gut microbiota. *Microbiome* **2018**, *6*, 51. [CrossRef] [PubMed]

53. Arpaia, N.; Campbell, C.; Fan, X.; Dikiy, S.; van der Veeken, J.; deRoos, P.; Liu, H.; Cross, J.R.; Pfeffer, K.; Coffer, P.J.; et al. Metabolites produced by commensal bacteria promote peripheral regulatory T-cell generation. *Nature* **2013**, *504*, 451–455. [CrossRef] [PubMed]

54. Liao, F.; Li, Z.; Wang, Y.; Shi, B.; Gong, Z.; Cheng, X. Porphyromonas gingivalis may play an important role in the pathogenesis of periodontitis-associated rheumatoid arthritis. *Med. Hypotheses* **2009**, *72*, 732–735. [CrossRef] [PubMed]

55. de Aquino, S.G.; Abdollahi-Roodsaz, S.; Koenders, M.I.; van de Loo, F.A.; Pruijn, G.J.; Marijnissen, R.J.; Walgreen, B.; Helsen, M.M.; van den Bersselaar, L.A.; de Molon, R.S.; et al. Periodontal pathogens directly promote autoimmune experimental arthritis by inducing a TLR2- and IL-1-driven Th17 response. *J. Immunol.* **2014**, *192*, 4103–4111. [CrossRef] [PubMed]

56. Zhang, X.; Zhang, D.; Jia, H.; Feng, Q.; Wang, D.; Liang, D.; Wu, X.; Li, J.; Tang, L.; Li, Y.; et al. The oral and gut microbiomes are perturbed in rheumatoid arthritis and partly normalized after treatment. *Nat. Med.* **2015**, *21*, 895–905. [CrossRef]

57. Chen, J.; Wright, K.; Davis, J.M.; Jeraldo, P.; Marietta, E.V.; Murray, J.; Nelson, H.; Matteson, E.L.; Taneja, V. An expansion of rare lineage intestinal microbes characterizes rheumatoid arthritis. *Genome Med.* **2016**, *8*, 43. [CrossRef]

58. Pianta, A.; Arvikar, S.L.; Strle, K.; Drouin, E.E.; Wang, Q.; Costello, C.E.; Steere, A.C. Two rheumatoid arthritis-specific autoantigens correlate microbial immunity with autoimmune responses in joints. *J. Clin. Investig.* **2017**, *127*, 2946–2956. [CrossRef] [PubMed]

59. Sato, K.; Takahashi, N.; Kato, T.; Matsuda, Y.; Yokoji, M.; Yamada, M.; Nakajima, T.; Kondo, N.; Endo, N.; Yamamoto, R.; et al. Aggravation of collagen-induced arthritis by orally *administered Porphyromonas gingivalis* through modulation of the gut microbiota and gut immune system. *Sci. Rep.* **2017**, *7*, 6955. [CrossRef]

60. Teng, F.; Felix, K.M.; Bradley, C.P.; Naskar, D.; Ma, H.; Raslan, W.A.; Wu, H.J. The impact of age and gut microbiota on Th17 and Tfh cells in K/BxN autoimmune arthritis. *Arthritis Res. Ther.* **2017**, *19*, 188. [CrossRef]

61. Jubair, W.K.; Hendrickson, J.D.; Severs, E.L.; Schulz, H.M.; Adhikari, S.; Ir, D.; Pagan, J.D.; Anthony, R.M.; Robertson, C.E.; Frank, D.N.; et al. Modulation of Inflammatory Arthritis in Mice by Gut Microbiota Through Mucosal Inflammation and Autoantibody Generation. *Arthritis Rheumatol.* **2018**, *70*, 1220–1233. [CrossRef]

62. Picchianti-Diamanti, A.; Panebianco, C.; Salemi, S.; Sorgi, M.L.; Di Rosa, R.; Tropea, A.; Sgrulletti, M.; Salerno, G.; Terracciano, F.; D'Amelio, R.; et al. Analysis of Gut Microbiota in Rheumatoid Arthritis Patients: Disease-Related Dysbiosis and Modifications Induced by Etanercept. *Int. J. Mol. Sci.* **2018**, *19*, 2938. [CrossRef] [PubMed]

63. Mutlu, S.; Richards, A.; Maddison, P.; Scully, C. Gingival and periodontal health in systemic lupus erythematosus. *Community Dent. Oral Epidemiol.* **1993**, *21*, 158–161. [CrossRef] [PubMed]

64. de Araújo Navas, E.A.F.; Sato, E.I.; Pereira, D.F.A.; Back-Brito, G.N.; Ishikawa, J.A.; Jorge, A.O.C.; Brighenti, F.L.; Koga-Ito, C.Y. Oral microbial colonization in patients with systemic lupus erythematous: Correlation with treatment and disease activity. *Lupus* **2012**, *21*, 969–977. [CrossRef]

65. Hevia, A.; Milani, C.; López, P.; Cuervo, A.; Arboleya, S.; Duranti, S.; Turroni, F.; González, S.; Suárez, A.; Gueimonde, M.; et al. Intestinal dysbiosis associated with systemic lupus erythematosus. *mBio* **2014**, *5*, 1–10. [CrossRef]

66. Calderaro, D.C.; Ferreira, G.A.; de Mendonça, S.M.S.; Corrêa, J.D.; Santos, F.X.; Sanção, J.G.C.; da Silva, T.A.; Teixeira, A.L. Há associação entre o lúpus eritematoso sistêmico e a doença periodontal? *Rev. Bras. Reumatol.* **2016**, *56*, 280–284. [CrossRef]

67. Corrêa, J.D.; Calderaro, D.C.; Ferreira, G.A.; Mendonça, S.M.; Fernandes, G.R.; Xiao, E.; Teixeira, A.L.; Leys, E.J.; Graves, D.T.; Silva, T.A. Subgingival microbiota dysbiosis in systemic lupus erythematosus: Association with periodontal status. *Microbiome* **2017**, *5*, 34. [CrossRef] [PubMed]

68. Ott, S.J.; Musfeldt, M.; Wenderoth, D.F.; Hampe, J.; Brant, O.; Fölsch, U.R.; Timmis, K.N.; Schreiber, S. Reduction in diversity of the colonic mucosa associated bacterial microflora in patients with active inflammatory bowel disease. *Gut* **2004**, *53*, 685–693. [CrossRef]

69. Gophna, U.; Sommerfeld, K.; Gophna, S.; Doolittle, W.F.; Veldhuyzen van Zanten, S.J. Differences between tissue-associated intestinal microfloras of patients with Crohn's disease and ulcerative colitis. *J. Clin. Microbiol.* **2006**, *44*, 4136–4141. [CrossRef]

70. Manichanh, C.; Rigottier-Gois, L.; Bonnaud, E.; Gloux, K.; Pelletier, E.; Frangeul, L.; Nalin, R.; Jarrin, C.; Chardon, P.; Marteau, P.; et al. Reduced diversity of faecal microbiota in Crohn's disease revealed by a metagenomic approach. *Gut* **2006**, *55*, 205–211. [CrossRef] [PubMed]

71. Frank, D.N.; St Amand, A.L.; Feldman, R.A.; Boedeker, E.C.; Harpaz, N.; Pace, N.R. Molecular-phylogenetic characterization of microbial community imbalances in human inflammatory bowel diseases. *Proc. Natl. Acad. Sci. USA* **2007**, *104*, 13780–13785. [CrossRef] [PubMed]

72. Sokol, H.; Pigneur, B.; Watterlot, L.; Lakhdari, O.; Bermúdez-Humarán, L.G.; Gratadoux, J.J.; Blugeon, S.; Bridonneau, C.; Furet, J.P.; Corthier, G.; et al. Faecalibacterium prausnitzii is an anti-inflammatory commensal bacterium identified by gut microbiota analysis of Crohn disease patients. *Proc. Natl. Acad. Sci. USA* **2008**, *105*, 16731–16736. [CrossRef] [PubMed]

73. Walker, A.W.; Sanderson, J.D.; Churcher, C.; Parkes, G.C.; Hudspith, B.N.; Rayment, N.; Brostoff, J.; Parkhill, J.; Dougan, G.; Petrovska, L. High-throughput clone library analysis of the mucosa-associated microbiota reveals dysbiosis and differences between inflamed and non-inflamed regions of the intestine in inflammatory bowel disease. *BMC Microbiol.* **2011**, *11*, 7. [CrossRef] [PubMed]

74. Wang, W.; Chen, L.; Zhou, R.; Wang, X.; Song, L.; Huang, S.; Wang, G.; Xia, B. Increased proportions of Bifidobacterium and the Lactobacillus group and loss of butyrate-producing bacteria in inflammatory bowel disease. *J. Clin. Microbiol.* **2014**, *52*, 398–406. [CrossRef]

75. Norman, J.M.; Handley, S.A.; Baldridge, M.T.; Droit, L.; Liu, C.Y.; Keller, B.C.; Kambal, A.; Monaco, C.L.; Zhao, G.; Fleshner, P.; et al. Disease specific alterations in the enteric virome in inflammatory bowel disease. *Cell* **2015**, *160*, 447–460. [CrossRef] [PubMed]

76. Takahashi, K.; Nishida, A.; Fujimoto, T.; Fujii, M.; Shioya, M.; Imaeda, H.; Inatomi, O.; Bamba, S.; Sugimoto, M.; Andoh, A. Reduced Abundance of Butyrate-Producing Bacteria Species in the Fecal Microbial Community in Crohn's Disease. *Digestion* **2016**, *93*, 59–65. [CrossRef] [PubMed]

77. Ni, J.; Wu, G.D.; Albenberg, L.; Tomov, V.T. Gut microbiota and IBD: Causation or correlation? *Nat. Rev. Gastroenterol. Hepatol.* **2017**, *14*, 573–584. [CrossRef]

78. Cao, S.S. Cellular Stress Responses and Gut Microbiota in Inflammatory Bowel Disease. *Gastroenterol. Res. Pract.* **2018**, *2018*, 7192646. [CrossRef]

79. Consolandi, C.; Turroni, S.; Emmi, G.; Severgnini, M.; Fiori, J.; Peano, C.; Biagi, E.; Grassi, A.; Rampelli, S.; Silvestri, E.; et al. Behcet's syndrome patients exhibit specific microbiome signature. *Autoimmun. Rev.* **2015**, *14*, 269–276. [CrossRef]

80. Seoudi, N.; Bergmeier, L.A.; Drobniewski, F.; Paster, B.; Fortune, F. The oral mucosal and salivary microbial community of Behcet's syndrome and recurrent aphthous stomatitis. *J. Oral Microbiol.* **2015**, *7*, 27150. [CrossRef]

81. Shimizu, J.; Kubota, T.; Takada, E.; Takai, K.; Fujiwara, N.; Arimitsu, N.; Ueda, Y.; Wakisaka, S.; Suzuki, T.; Suzuki, N. Bifidobacteria abundance-featured gut microbiota compositional change in patients with Behcet's disease. *PLoS ONE* **2016**, *11*, e0153746. [CrossRef] [PubMed]

82. Ye, Z.; Zhang, N.; Wu, C.; Zhang, X.; Wang, Q.; Huang, X.; Du, L.; Cao, Q.; Tang, J.; Zhou, C.; et al. A metagenomic study of the gut microbiome in Behcet's disease. *Microbiome* **2018**, *6*, 135. [CrossRef] [PubMed]

83. Ganju, P.; Nagpal, S.; Mohammed, M.H.; Nishal Kumar, P.; Pandey, R.; Natarajan, V.T.; Mande, S.S.; Gokhale, R.S. Microbial community profiling shows dysbiosis in the lesional skin of Vitiligo subjects. *Sci. Rep.* **2016**, *6*, 18761. [CrossRef]

84. Gao, Z.; Tseng, C.; Strober, B.E.; Pei, Z.; Blaser, M.J. Substantial alterations of the cutaneous bacterial biota in psoriatic lesions. *PLoS ONE* **2008**, *3*, e2719. [CrossRef] [PubMed]

85. Fahlen, A.; Engstrand, L.; Baker, B.S.; Powles, A.; Fry, L. Comparison of bacterial microbiota in skin biopsies from normal and psoriatic skin. *Arch. Dermatol. Res.* **2012**, *304*, 15–22. [CrossRef] [PubMed]

86. Alekseyenko, A.V.; Perez-Perez, G.I.; De Souza, A.; Strober, B.; Gao, Z.; Bihan, M.; Li, K.; Methé, B.A.; Blaser, M.J. Community differentiation of the cutaneous microbiota in psoriasis. *Microbiome* **2013**, *1*, 31. [CrossRef] [PubMed]

87. Tett, A.; Pasolli, E.; Farina, S.; Truong, D.T.; Asnicar, F.; Zolfo, M.; Beghini, F.; Armanini, F.; Jousson, O.; De Sanctis, V.; et al. Unexplored diversity and strain-level structure of the skin microbiome associated with psoriasis. *NPJ Biofilms Microbiomes* **2017**, *3*, 14. [CrossRef]

88. Chang, H.W.; Yan, D.; Singh, R.; Liu, J.; Lu, X.; Ucmak, D.; Lee, K.; Afifi, L.; Fadrosh, D.; Leech, J.; et al. Alteration of the cutaneous microbiome in psoriasis and potential role in Th17 polarization. *Microbiome* **2018**, *6*, 154. [CrossRef]

89. Hong, S.W.; Kim, M.R.; Lee, E.Y.; Kim, J.H.; Kim, Y.S.; Jeon, S.G.; Yang, J.M.; Lee, B.J.; Pyun, B.Y.; Gho, Y.S. Extracellular vesicles derived from Staphylococcus aureus induce atopic dermatitis-like skin inflammation. *Allergy* **2011**, *66*, 351–359. [CrossRef]

90. Kong, H.H.; Oh, J.; Deming, C.; Conlan, S.; Grice, E.A.; Beatson, M.A.; Nomicos, E.; Polley, E.C.; Komarow, H.D.; NISC Comparative Sequence Program; et al. Temporal shifts in the skin microbiome associated with disease flares and treatment in children with atopic dermatitis. *Genome Res.* **2012**, *22*, 850–859. [CrossRef]

91. Laborel-Préneron, E.; Bianchi, P.; Boralevi, F.; Lehours, P.; Fraysse, F.; Morice-Picard, F.; Sugai, M.; Sato'o, Y.; Badiou, C.; Lina, G.; et al. Effects of the Staphylococcus aureus and Staphylococcus epidermidis Secretomes Isolated from the Skin Microbiota of Atopic Children on CD4+ T Cell Activation. *PLoS ONE* **2015**, *10*, e0141067. [CrossRef]

92. Williams, M.R.; Gallo, R.L. The role of the skin microbiome in atopic dermatitis. *Curr. Allergy Asthma Rep.* **2015**, *15*, 65. [CrossRef] [PubMed]

93. Song, H.; Yoo, Y.; Hwang, J.; Na, Y.C.; Kim, H.S. Faecalibacterium prausnitzii subspecies-level dysbiosis in the human gut microbiome underlying atopic dermatitis. *J. Allergy Clin. Immunol.* **2016**, *137*, 852–860. [CrossRef] [PubMed]

94. Iwamoto, K.; Moriwaki, M.; Niitsu, Y.; Saino, M.; Takahagi, S.; Hisatsune, J.; Sugai, M.; Hide, M. Staphylococcus aureus from atopic dermatitis skin alters cytokine production triggered by monocyte-derived Langerhans cell. *J. Dermatol. Sci.* **2017**, *88*, 271–279. [CrossRef] [PubMed]

95. Francuzik, W.; Franke, K.; Schumann, R.R.; Heine, G.; Worm, M. Propionibacterium acnes Abundance Correlates Inversely with Staphylococcus aureus: Data from Atopic Dermatitis Skin Microbiome. *Acta Derm. Venereol.* **2018**, *98*, 490–495. [CrossRef] [PubMed]

96. Kim, M.H.; Choi, S.J.; Choi, H.I.; Choi, J.P.; Park, H.K.; Kim, E.K.; Kim, M.J.; Moon, B.S.; Min, T.K.; Rho, M.; et al. Lactobacillus plantarum-derived Extracellular Vesicles Protect Atopic Dermatitis Induced by Staphylococcus aureus-derived Extracellular Vesicles. *Allergy Asthma Immunol. Res.* **2018**, *10*, 516–532. [CrossRef] [PubMed]

97. Suzuki, S.; Campos-Alberto, E.; Morita, Y.; Yamaguchi, M.; Toshimitsu, T.; Kimura, K.; Ikegami, S.; Katsuki, T.; Kohno, Y.; Shimojo, N. Low Interleukin 10 Production at Birth Is a Risk Factor for Atopic Dermatitis in Neonates with Bifidobacterium Colonization. *Int. Arch. Allergy Immunol.* **2018**, *11*, 1–8. [CrossRef]

98. Berer, K.; Mues, M.; Koutrolos, M.; Rasbi, Z.A.; Boziki, M.; Johner, C.; Wekerle, H.; Krishnamoorthy, G. Commensal microbiota and myelin autoantigen cooperate to trigger autoimmune demyelination. *Nature* **2011**, *479*, 538–541. [CrossRef]

99. Wang, Y.; Begum-Haque, S.; Telesford, K.M.; Ochoa-Reparaz, J.; Christy, M.; Kasper, E.J.; Robson, S.C.; Kasper, L.H. A commensal bacterial product elicits and modulates migratory capacity of CD39(+) CD4 T regulatory subsets in the suppression of neuroinflammation. *Gut Microbes* **2014**, *5*, 552–561. [CrossRef]

100. Wang, Y.; Telesford, K.M.; Ochoa-Reparaz, J.; Haque-Begum, S.; Christy, M.; Kasper, E.J.; Wang, L.; Wu, Y.; Robson, S.C.; Kasper, D.L.; et al. An intestinal commensal symbiosis factor controls neuroinflammation via TLR2-mediated CD39 signalling. *Nat. Commun.* **2014**, *5*, 4432. [CrossRef]

101. Miyake, S.; Kim, S.; Suda, W.; Oshima, K.; Nakamura, M.; Matsuoka, T.; Chihara, N.; Tomita, A.; Sato, W.; Kim, S.W.; et al. Dysbiosis in the Gut Microbiota of Patients with Multiple Sclerosis, with a Striking Depletion of Species Belonging to Clostridia XIVa and IV Clusters. *PLoS ONE* **2015**, *10*, e0137429. [CrossRef] [PubMed]

102. Chen, J.; Chen, J.; Chia, N.; Kalari, K.R.; Yao, J.Z.; Novotna, M.; Paz Soldan, M.M.; Luckey, D.H.; Marietta, E.V.; Jeraldo, P.R.; et al. Multiple sclerosis patients have a distinct gut microbiota compared to healthy controls. *Sci. Rep.* **2016**, *6*, 28484. [CrossRef] [PubMed]

103. Jangi, S.; Gandhi, R.; Cox, L.M.; Li, N.; von Glehn, F.; Yan, R.; Patel, B.; Mazzola, M.A.; Liu, S.; Glanz, B.L.; et al. Alterations of the human gut microbiome in multiple sclerosis. *Nat. Commun.* **2016**, *7*, 12015. [CrossRef] [PubMed]

104. Rothhammer, V.; Mascanfroni, I.D.; Bunse, L.; Takenaka, M.C.; Kenison, J.E.; Mayo, L.; Chao, C.C.; Patel, B.; Yan, R.; Blain, M.; et al. Type I interferons and microbial metabolites of tryptophan modulate astrocyte activity and central nervous system inflammation via the aryl hydrocarbon receptor. *Nat. Med.* **2016**, *22*, 586–597. [CrossRef] [PubMed]

105. Berer, K.; Gerdes, L.A.; Cekanaviciute, E.; Jia, X.; Xiao, L.; Xia, Z.; Liu, C.; Klotz, L.; Stauffer, U.; Baranzini, S.E.; et al. Gut microbiota from multiple sclerosis patients enables spontaneous autoimmune encephalomyelitis in mice. *Proc. Natl. Acad. Sci. USA* **2017**, *114*, 10719–10724. [CrossRef] [PubMed]

106. Cekanaviciute, E.; Yoo, B.B.; Runia, T.F.; Debelius, J.W.; Singh, S.; Nelson, C.A.; Kanner, R.; Bencosme, Y.; Lee, Y.K.; Hauser, S.L.; et al. Gut bacteria from multiple sclerosis patients modulate human T cells and exacerbate symptoms in mouse models. *Proc. Natl. Acad. Sci. USA* **2017**, *114*, 10713–10718. [CrossRef] [PubMed]

107. Scher, J.U.; Sczesnak, A.; Longman, R.S.; Segata, N.; Ubeda, C.; Bielski, C.; Rostron, T.; Cerundolo, V.; Pamer, E.G.; Abramson, S.B.; et al. Expansion of intestinal Prevotella copri correlates with enhanced susceptibility to arthritis. *Elife* **2013**, *2*, e01202. [CrossRef] [PubMed]

108. Terao, C.; Asai, K.; Hashimoto, M.; Yamazaki, T.; Ohmura, K.; Yamaguchi, A.; Takahashi, K.; Takei, N.; Ishii, T.; Kawaguchi, T.; et al. Significant association of periodontal disease with anticitrullinated peptide antibody in a Japanese healthy population—The Nagahama study. *J. Autoimmun.* **2015**, *59*, 85–90.

109. Mendonça, S.M.S.; Corrêa, J.D.; Souza, A.F.; Travassos, D.V.; Calderaro, D.C.; Rocha, N.P.; Vieira, É.L.M.; Teixeira, A.L.; Ferreira, G.A.; Silva, T.A. Immunological signatures in saliva of systemic lupus erythematosus patients: Influence of periodontal condition. *Clin. Exp. Rheumatol.* **2018**.

110. Socransky, S.S.; Haffajee, A.D.; Cugini, M.A.; Smith, C.; Kent, R.L., Jr. Microbial complexes in subgingival plaque. *J. Clin. Periodontol.* **1998**, *25*, 134–144. [CrossRef] [PubMed]

111. Rehman, A.; Rausch, P.; Wang, J.; Skieceviciene, J.; Kiudelis, G.; Bhagalia, K.; Amarapurkar, D.; Kupcinskas, L.; Schreiber, S.; Rosenstiel, P.; et al. Geographical patterns of the standing and active human gut microbiome in health and IBD. *Gut* **2016**, *65*, 238–248. [CrossRef] [PubMed]

112. Assa, A.; Butcher, J.; Li, J.; Elkadri, A.; Sherman, P.M.; Muise, A.M.; Stintzi, A.; Mack, D. Mucosa-Associated Ileal Microbiota in New-Onset Pediatric Crohn's Disease. *Inflamm. Bowel Dis.* **2016**, *22*, 1533–1539. [CrossRef]

113. Wagner, J.; Maksimovic, J.; Farries, G.; Sim, W.H.; Bishop, R.F.; Cameron, D.J.; Catto-Smith, A.G.; Kirkwood, C.D. Bacteriophages in gut samples from pediatric Crohn's disease patients: Metagenomic analysis using 454 pyrosequencing. *Inflamm. Bowel Dis.* **2013**, *19*, 1598–1608. [CrossRef] [PubMed]

114. Grice, E.A.; Kong, H.H.; Conlan, S.; Deming, C.B.; Davis, J.; Young, A.C.; NISC Comparative Sequencing Program; Bouffard, G.G.; Blakesley, R.W.; Murray, P.R.; et al. Topographical and temporal diversity of the human skin microbiome. *Science* **2009**, *324*, 1190–1192. [CrossRef] [PubMed]

115. Carratù, R.; Secondulfo, M.; de Magistris, L.; Iafusco, D.; Urio, A.; Carbone, M.G.; Pontoni, G.; Cartenì, M.; Prisco, F. Altered intestinal permeability to mannitol in diabetes mellitus type I. *J. Pediatr. Gastroenterol. Nutr.* **1999**, *28*, 264–269. [CrossRef] [PubMed]

116. Westerholm-Ormio, M.; Vaarala, O.; Pihkala, P.; Ilonen, J.; Savilahti, E. Immunologic activity in the small intestinal mucosa of pediatric patients with type 1 diabetes. *Diabetes* **2003**, *52*, 2287–2295. [CrossRef]

117. Secondulfo, M.; Iafusco, D.; Carratù, R.; deMagistris, L.; Sapone, A.; Generoso, M.; Mezzogiomo, A.; Sasso, F.C.; Cartenì, M.; De Rosa, R.; et al. Ultrastructural mucosal alterations and increased intestinal permeability in non-celiac.; type I diabetic patients. *Dig. Liver Dis.* **2004**, *36*, 35–45. [CrossRef]

118. Sapone, A.; de Magistris, L.; Pietzak, M.; Clemente, M.G.; Tripathi, A.; Cucca, F.; Lampis, R.; Kryszak, D.; Cartenì, M.; Generoso, M.; et al. Zonulin upregulation is associated with increased gut permeability in subjects with type 1 diabetes and their relatives. *Diabetes* **2006**, *55*, 1443–1449. [CrossRef]

119. Bosi, E.; Molteni, L.; Radaelli, M.G.; Folini, L.; Fermo, I.; Bazzigaluppi, E.; Piemonti, L.; Pastore, M.R.; Paroni, R. Increased intestinal permeability precedes clinical onset of type 1 diabetes. *Diabetologia* **2006**, *49*, 2824–2827. [CrossRef]

120. Brown, K.; Godovannyi, A.; Ma, C.; Zhang, Y.; Ahmadi-Vand, Z.; Dai, C.; Gorzelak, M.A.; Chan, Y.; Chan, J.M.; Lochner, A.; et al. Prolonged antibiotic treatment induces a diabetogenic intestinal microbiome that accelerates diabetes in NOD mice. *ISME J.* **2016**, *10*, 321–332. [CrossRef]

121. Candon, S.; Perez-Arroyo, A.; Marquet, C.; Valette, F.; Foray, A.P.; Pelletier, B.; Milani, C.; Ventura, M.; Bach, J.F.; Chatenoud, L. Antibiotics in Early Life Alter the Gut Microbiome and Increase Disease Incidence in a Spontaneous Mouse Model of Autoimmune Insulin-Dependent Diabetes. *PLoS ONE* **2016**, *11*, e0147888. [CrossRef] [PubMed]

122. Livanos, A.E.; Greiner, T.U.; Vangay, P.; Pathmasiri, W.; Stewart, D.; McRitchie, S.; Li, H.; Chung, J.; Sohn, J.; Kim, S.; et al. Antibiotic-mediated gut microbiome perturbation accelerates development of type 1 diabetes in mice. *Nat. Microbiol.* **2016**, *1*, 16140. [CrossRef] [PubMed]

123. Wu, H.J.; Ivanov, I.I.; Darce, J.; Hattori, K.; Shima, T.; Umesaki, Y.; Littman, D.R.; Benoist, C.; Mathis, D. Gut residing segmented filamentous bacteria drive autoimmune arthritis via T helper 17 cells. *Immunity* **2010**, *32*, 815–827. [CrossRef] [PubMed]

124. Ivanov, I.I.; Atarashi, K.; Manel, N.; Brodie, E.L.; Shima, T.; Karaoz, U.; Wei, D.; Goldfarb, K.C.; Santee, C.A.; Lynch, S.V.; et al. Induction of intestinal Th17 cells by segmented filamentous bacteria. *Cell* **2009**, *139*, 485–498. [CrossRef]

125. Teng, F.; Klinger, C.N.; Felix, K.M.; Bradley, C.P.; Wu, E.; Tran, N.L.; Umesaki, Y.; Wu, H.J. Gut microbiota drive autoimmune arthritis by promoting differentiation and migration of Peyer's patch T follicular helper cells. *Immunity* **2016**, *44*, 875–888. [CrossRef] [PubMed]

126. Bradley, C.P.; Teng, F.; Felix, K.M.; Sano, T.; Naskar, D.; Block, K.E.; Huang, H.; Knox, K.S.; Littman, D.R.; Wu, H.J. Segmented filamentous bacteria provoke lung autoimmunity by inducing gut–lung axis Th17 cells expressing dual TCRs. *Cell Host Microbe* **2017**, *22*, 697–704.e4. [CrossRef]

127. Wegner, N.; Wait, R.; Sroka, A.; Eick, S.; Nguyen, K.A.; Lundberg, K.; Kinloch, A.; Culshaw, S.; Potempa, J.; Venables, P.J. Peptidylarginine deiminase from *Porphyromonas gingivalis* citrullinates human fibrinogen and alpha-enolase: Implications for autoimmunity in rheumatoid arthritis. *Arthritis Rheum.* **2010**, *62*, 2662–2672. [CrossRef]

128. Montgomery, A.B.; Kopec, J.; Shrestha, L.; Thezenas, M.L.; Burgess-Brown, N.A.; Fischer, R.; Yue, W.W.; Venables, P.J. Crystal structure of *Porphyromonas gingivalis* peptidylarginine deiminase: Implications for autoimmunity in rheumatoid arthritis. *Ann. Rheum. Dis.* **2016**, *75*, 1255–1261. [CrossRef]

129. Konig, M.F.; Abusleme, L.; Reinholdt, J.; Palmer, R.J.; Teles, R.P.; Sampson, K.; Rosen, A.; Nigrovic, P.A.; Sokolove, J.; Giles, J.T.; et al. Aggregatibacter actinomycetemcomitans-induced hypercitrullination links periodontal infection to autoimmunity in rheumatoid arthritis. *Sci. Transl. Med.* **2016**, *8*, 369ra176. [CrossRef]

130. Atarashi, K.; Tanoue, T.; Shima, T.; Imaoka, A.; Kuwahara, T.; Momose, Y.; Cheng, G.; Yamasaki, S.; Saito, T.; Ohba, Y.; et al. Induction of colonic regulatory T cells by indigenous clostridium species. *Science* **2011**, *331*, 337–341. [CrossRef]

131. Tanabe, S. The effect of probiotics and gut microbiota on Th17 cells. *Int. Rev. Immunol.* **2013**, *32*, 511–525. [CrossRef] [PubMed]

132. Zenewicz, L.A.; Yancopoulos, G.D.; Valenzuela, D.M.; Murphy, A.J.; Stevens, S.; Flavell, R.A. Innate and adaptive interleukin-22 protects mice from inflammatory bowel disease. *Immunity* **2008**, *29*, 947–957. [CrossRef] [PubMed]

133. Ezzedine, K.; Eleftheriadou, V.; Whitton, M.; van Geel, N. Vitiligo. *Lancet* **2015**, *386*, 74–84. [CrossRef]

134. Lotti, T.; D'Erme, A.M. Vitiligo as a systemic disease. *Clin. Dermatol.* **2014**, *32*, 430–434. [CrossRef] [PubMed]

135. Lebwohl, M. Psoriasis. *Lancet* **2003**, *361*, 1197–1204. [CrossRef]

136. Bach, J.F. The hygiene hypothesis in autoimmunity: The role of pathogens and commensals. *Nat. Rev. Immunol.* **2017**, *18*, 105–120. [CrossRef]

137. Lynch, S.V.; Pedersen, O.P. The human intestinal microbiome in health and disease. *N. Engl. J. Med.* **2016**, *375*, 2369–2379. [CrossRef]

138. Ahern, P.P.; Faith, J.J.; Gordon, J.I. Mining the human gut microbiota for effector strains that shap the immune system. *Immunity* **2014**, *40*, 815–823. [CrossRef] [PubMed]

139. American Diabetes Association. Diagnosis and Classification of Diabetes Mellitus. *Diabetes Care* **2009**, *32*, S62–S67. [CrossRef] [PubMed]

140. Stechova, K.; Kolar, M.; Blatny, R.; Halbhuber, Z.; Vcelakova, J.; Hubackova, M.; Petruzelkova, L.; Sumnik, Z.; Obermannova, B.; Pithova, P.; et al. Healthy first degree relatives of patients with type 1 diabetes exhibit significant differences in basal gene expression pattern of immunocompetent cells compared to controls: Expression pattern as predeterminant of autoimmune diabetes. *Scand. J. Immunol.* **2011**, *75*, 210–219. [CrossRef] [PubMed]

141. La Marca, V.; Gianchecchi, E.; Fierabracci, A. Type 1 Diabetes and Its Multi-Factorial Pathogenesis: The Putative Role of NK Cells. *Int. J. Mol. Sci.* **2018**, *19*, 794. [CrossRef] [PubMed]

142. Silveira, P.A.; Grey, S.T. B cells in the spotlight: Innocent bystanders or major players in the pathogenesis of type 1 diabetes. *Trends Endocrinol. Metab.* **2006**, *17*, 128–135. [CrossRef] [PubMed]

143. Gianchecchi, E.; Palombi, M.; Fierabracci, A. The putative role of the C1858T polymorphismof protein tyrosine phosphatase PTPN22 gene in autoimmunity. *Autoimmun. Rev.* **2013**, *12*, 717–725. [CrossRef] [PubMed]

144. Hildebrand, F.; Nguyen, T.L.; Brinkman, B.; Yunta, R.G.; Cauwe, B.; Vandenabeele, P.; Liston, A.; Raes, J. Inflammation-associated enterotypes, host genotype, cage and inter-individual effects drive gut microbiota variation in common laboratory mice. *Genome Biol.* **2013**, *14*, R4. [CrossRef] [PubMed]

145. Nielsen, D.S.; Krych, Ł.; Buschard, K.; Hansen, C.H.; Hansen, A.K. Beyond genetics. Influence of dietary factors and gut microbiota on type 1 diabetes. *FEBS Lett.* **2014**, *588*, 4234–4243. [CrossRef] [PubMed]

146. Roesch, L.F.; Lorca, G.L.; Casella, G.; Giongo, A.; Naranjo, A.; Pionzio, A.M.; Li, N.; Mai, V.; Wasserfall, C.H.; Schatz, D.; et al. Culture-independent identification of gut bacteria correlated with the onset of diabetes in a rat model. *ISME J.* **2009**, *3*, 536–548. [CrossRef] [PubMed]

147. Hornef, M.W.; Pabst, O. Real friends: Faecalibacterium prausnitzii supports mucosal immune homeostasis. *Gut* **2016**, *65*, 365–367. [CrossRef] [PubMed]

148. Espinoza, L.R.; Garcia-Valladares, I. Of bugs and joints: The relationship between infection and joints. *Reumatología Clínica* **2013**, *9*, 229–238. [CrossRef]

149. Taneja, V. Cytokines pre-determined by genetic factors are involved in pathogenesis of rheumatoid arthritis. *Cytokine* **2014**, *75*, 216–221. [CrossRef]

150. Lehner, T. Immunopathogenesis of Behçet's disease. *Ann. Med. Interne* **1999**, *150*, 483–487.

151. Goodnow, C.C. Multistep pathogenesis of autoimmune disease. *Cell* **2007**, *130*, 25–35. [CrossRef] [PubMed]

152. Lee, J.S.; Lee, W.W.; Kim, S.H.; Kang, Y.; Lee, N.; Shin, M.S.; Kang, S.W.; Kang, I. Age-associated alteration in naive and memory Th17 cell response in humans. *Clin. Immunol.* **2011**, *140*, 84–91. [CrossRef] [PubMed]

153. Zhou, M.; Zou, R.; Gan, H.; Liang, Z.; Li, F.; Lin, T.; Luo, Y.; Cai, X.; He, F.; Shen, E. The effect of aging on the frequency, phenotype and cytokine production of human blood CD4 + CXCR5 + T follicular helper cells: Comparison of aged and young subjects. *Immun. Ageing* **2014**, *11*, 12. [CrossRef] [PubMed]

154. Malmstrom, V.; Catrina, A.I.; Klareskog, L. The immunopathogenesis of seropositive rheumatoid arthritis: From triggering to targeting. *Nat. Rev. Immunol.* **2017**, *17*, 60–75. [CrossRef] [PubMed]

155. Bartold, P.M.; Marino, V.; Cantley, M.; Haynes, D.R. Effect of Porphyromonas gingivalis-induced inflammation on the development of rheumatoid arthritis. *J. Clin. Periodontol.* **2010**, *37*, 405–411. [CrossRef]

156. Kotzin, B.L. Systemic lupus erythematosus. *Cell* **1996**, *85*, 303–306. [CrossRef]

157. Pacheco, G.V.; Cruz, D.C.; González Herrera, L.J.; Pérez Mendoza, G.J.; Adrián Amaro, G.I.; Nakazawa Ueji, Y.E.; Angulo Ramírez, A.V. Copy number variation of TLR-7 gene and its association with the development of systemic lupus erythematosus in female patients from Yucatan Mexico. *Genet. Epigenet.* **2014**, *6*, 31–36. [CrossRef]

158. Zhang, H.; Liao, X.; Sparks, J.B.; Luo, X.M. Dynamics of gut microbiota in autoimmune lupus. *Appl. Environ. Microbiol.* **2014**, *80*, 7551–7560. [CrossRef]

159. Al-Mutairi, K.; Al-Zahrani, M.; Bahlas, S.; Kayal, R.; Zawawi, K. Periodontal findings in systemic lupus erythematosus patients and healthy controls. *Saudi Med. J.* **2015**, *36*, 463–468. [CrossRef]

160. Sakane, T.; Takeno, M.; Suzuki, N.; Inaba, G. Behçet's disease. *N. Engl. J. Med.* **1999**, *341*, 1284–1291. [CrossRef]

161. Yurdakul, S.; Hamuryudan, V.; Yazici, H. Behçet syndrome. *Curr. Opin. Rheumatol.* **2004**, *16*, 38–42. [CrossRef] [PubMed]

162. Takada, Y.; Fujita, Y.; Igarashi, M.; Katsumata, T.; Okabe, H.; Saigenji, K.; Takahashi, T.; Atari, E. Intestinal Behçet's disease-pathognomonic changes in intramucosal lymphoid tissues and effect of a "rest cure" on intestinal lesions. *J. Gastroenterol.* **1997**, *32*, 598–604. [CrossRef] [PubMed]

163. Karasneh, J.; Gül, A.; Ollier, W.E.; Silman, A.J. Worthington, J. Whole-genome screening for susceptibility genes in multicase families with Behçet's disease. *Arthritis Rheum.* **2005**, *52*, 1836–1842. [CrossRef] [PubMed]

164. Melikoglu, M.; Uysal, S.; Krueger, J.G.; Kaplan, G.; Gogus, F.; Yazici, H.; Oliver, S. Characterization of the divergent wound-healing responses occurring in the pathergy reaction and normal healthy volunteers. *J. Immunol.* **2006**, *177*, 6415–6421. [CrossRef] [PubMed]

165. Takeuchi, M.; Kastner, D.L.; Remmers, E.F. The immunogenetics of Behcet's disease: A comprehensive review. *J. Autoimmun.* **2015**, *64*, 137–148. [CrossRef]

166. Zeidan, M.J.; Saadoun, D.; Garrido, M.; Klatzmann, D.; Six, A.; Cacoub, P. Behcet's disease physiopathology: A contemporary review. *Auto. Immun. Highlights* **2016**, *7*, 4. [CrossRef] [PubMed]

167. Geremia, A.; Biancheri, P.; Allan, P.; Corazza, G.R.; Di Sabatino, A. Innate and adaptive immunity in inflammatory bowel disease. *Autoimmun. Rev.* **2014**, *13*, 3–10. [CrossRef]

168. Ananthakrishnan, A.N.; Bernstein, C.N.; Iliopoulos, D.; Macpherson, A.; Neurath, M.F.; Ali, R.A.R.; Vavricka, S.R.; Fiocchi, C. Environmental triggers in IBD: A review of progress and evidence. *Nat. Rev. Gastroenterol. Hepatol.* **2018**, *15*, 39–49. [CrossRef]

169. Kellermayer, R.; Mir, S.A.; Nagy-Szakal, D.; Cox, S.B.; Dowd, S.E.; Kaplan, J.L.; Sun, Y.; Reddy, S.; Bronsky, J.; Winter, H.S. Microbiota separation and C-reactive protein elevation in treatment-naïve pediatric granulomatous Crohn disease. *J. Pediatr. Gastroenterol. Nutr.* **2012**, *55*, 243–250. [CrossRef]

170. Shah, R.; Cope, J.L.; Nagy-Szakal, D.; Dowd, S.; Versalovic, J.; Hollister, E.B.; Kellermayer, R. Composition and function of the pediatric colonic mucosal microbiome in untreated patients with ulcerative colitis. *Gut Microbes* **2016**, *7*, 384–396. [CrossRef]

171. Gevers, D.; Kugathasan, S.; Denson, L.A.; Vázquez-Baeza, Y.; Van Treuren, W.; Ren, B.; Schwager, E.; Knights, D.; Song, S.J.; Yassour, M.; et al. The treatment-naive microbiome in new-onset Crohn's disease. *Cell Host Microbe* **2017**, *21*, 301–304. [CrossRef]

172. Akazawa, Y.; Isomoto, H.; Matsushima, K.; Kanda, T.; Minami, H.; Yamaghchi, N.; Taura, N.; Shiozawa, K.; Ohnita, K.; Takeshima, F.; et al. Endoplasmic reticulum stress contributes to Helicobacter pylori VacA induced apoptosis. *PLoS ONE* **2013**, *8*, e82322. [CrossRef] [PubMed]

173. Reyes, A.; Haynes, M.; Hanson, N.; Angly, F.E.; Heath, A.C.; Rohwer, F.; Gordon, J.I. Viruses in the faecal microbiota of monozygotic twins and their mothers. *Nature* **2010**, *466*, 334–338. [CrossRef] [PubMed]

174. Minot, S.; Sinha, R.; Chen, J.; Li, H.; Keilbaugh, S.A.; Wu, G.D.; Lewis, J.D.; Bushman, F.D. The human gut virome: Inter-individual variation and dynamic response to diet. *Genome Res.* **2011**, *21*, 1616–1625. [CrossRef] [PubMed]

175. Van Belleghem, J.D.; Clement, F.; Merabishvili, M.; Lavigne, R.; Vaneechoutte, M. Pro- and anti-inflammatory responses of peripheral blood mononuclear cells induced by Staphylococcus aureus and Pseudomonas aeruginosa phages. *Sci. Rep.* **2017**, *7*, 8004. [CrossRef] [PubMed]

176. Magin, W.S.; Van Kruiningen, H.J.; Colombel, J.F. Immunohistochemical search for viral and bacterial antigens in Crohn's disease. *J. Crohns Colitis* **2013**, *7*, 161–166. [CrossRef]

177. Monteleone, I.; Rizzo, A.; Sarra, M.; Sica, G.; Sileri, P.; Biancone, L.; MacDonald, T.T.; Pallone, F.; Monteleone, G. Aryl hydrocarbon receptor-induced signals up-regulate IL-22 production and inhibit inflammation in the gastrointestinal tract. *Gastroenterology* **2011**, *141*, 237–248.e1. [CrossRef]

178. Sugimoto, K.; Ogawa, A.; Mizoguchi, E.; Shimomura, Y.; Andoh, A.; Bhan, A.K.; Blumberg, R.S.; Xavier, R.J.; Mizoguchi, A. IL-22 ameliorates intestinal inflammation in a mouse model of ulcerative colitis. *J. Clin. Investig.* **2008**, *118*, 534–544. [CrossRef]

179. Guerra, L.; Dellambra, E.; Brescia, S.; Raskovic, D. Vitiligo: Pathogenetic hypotheses and targets for current therapies. *Curr. Drug Metab.* **2010**, *11*, 451–467. [CrossRef]

180. Malhotra, N.; Dytoc, M. The pathogenesis of vitiligo. *J. Cutan. Med. Surg.* **2013**, *17*, 153–172. [CrossRef]

181. Amerio, P.; Tracanna, M.; De Remigis, P.; Betterle, C.; Vianale, L.; Marra, M.E.; Di Rollo, D.; Capizzi, R.; Feliciani, C.; Tulli, A. Vitiligo associated with other autoimmune diseases: Polyglandular autoimmune syndrome types 3B+C and 4. *Clin. Exp. Dermatol.* **2006**, *31*, 746–749. [CrossRef] [PubMed]

182. Lowes, M.A.; Suárez-Fariñas, M.; Krueger, J.G. Immunology of psoriasis. *Annu. Rev. Immunol.* **2014**, *32*, 227–255. [CrossRef] [PubMed]

183. Nestle, F.O.; Kaplan, D.H.; Barker, J. Psoriasis. *N. Engl. J. Med.* **2009**, *361*, 496–509. [CrossRef] [PubMed]

184. Perera, G.K.; Di Meglio, P.; Nestle, F.O. Psoriasis. *Annu. Rev. Pathol. Mech. Dis.* **2012**, *7*, 385–422. [CrossRef]

185. Loesche, M.A.; Farahi, K.; Capone, K.; Fakharzadeh, S.; Blauvelt, A.; Duffin, K.C.; DePrimo, S.E.; Muñoz-Elías, E.J.; Brodmerkel, C.; Dasgupta, B.; et al. Longitudinal study of the psoriasis-associated skin microbiome during therapy with ustekinumab in a randomized phase 3b clinical trial. *J. Investig. Dermatol.* **2018**, *138*, 1973–1981. [CrossRef] [PubMed]

186. Sabin, B.R.; Peters, N.; Peters, A.T. Chapter 20: Atopic dermatitis. *Allergy Asthma Proc.* **2012**, *33*, 67–69. [CrossRef] [PubMed]

187. Jang, S.C.; Kim, S.R.; Yoon, Y.J.; Park, K.S.; Kim, J.H.; Lee, J.; Kim, O.Y.; Choi, E.J.; Kim, D.K.; Choi, D.S.; et al. In vivo kinetic biodistribution of nano-sized outer membrane vesicles derived from bacteria. *Small* **2015**, *11*, 456–461. [CrossRef] [PubMed]

188. Koch-Henriksen, N.; Sorensen, P.S. The changing demographic pattern of multiple sclerosis epidemiology. *Lancet Neurol.* **2010**, *9*, 520–532. [CrossRef]

189. Matveeva, O.; Bogie, J.F.J.; Hendriks, J.J.A.; Linker, R.A.; Haghikia, A.; Kleinewietfeld, M. Western lifestyle and immunopathology of multiple sclerosis. *Ann. N. Y. Acad. Sci.* **2018**, *1417*, 71–86. [CrossRef]

190. Maslowski, K.M.; Mackay, C.R. Diet, gut microbiota and immune responses. *Nat. Immunol.* **2011**, *12*, 5–9. [CrossRef]

191. Levy, M.; Kolodziejczyk, A.A.; Thaiss, C.A.; Elinav, E. Dysbiosis and the immune system. *Nat. Rev. Immunol.* **2017**, *17*, 219–232. [CrossRef] [PubMed]

192. Cox, L.M.; Cho, I.; Young, S.A.; Anderson, W.H.; Waters, B.J.; Hung, S.C.; Gao, Z.; Mahana, D.; Bihan, M.; Alekseyenko, A.V.; et al. The nonfermentable dietary fiber hydroxypropyl methylcellulose modulates intestinal microbiota. *FASEB J.* **2012**, *27*, 692–702. [CrossRef] [PubMed]

193. Bindels, L.B.; Segura Munoz, R.R.; Gomes-Neto, J.C.; Mutemberezi, V.; Martínez, I.; Salazar, N.; Cody, E.A.; Quintero-Villegas, M.I.; Kittana, H.; de Los Reyes-Gavilán, C.G.; et al. Resistant starch can improve insulin sensitivity independently of the gut microbiota. *Microbiome* **2017**, *5*, 12. [CrossRef] [PubMed]

194. Farinotti, M.; Simi, S.; Di Pietrantonj, C.; McDowell, N.; Brait, L.; Lupo, D.; Filippini, G. Dietary interventions for multiple sclerosis. *Cochrane Database Syst. Rev.* **2012**, *12*, Cd004192. [CrossRef] [PubMed]

195. Yamamura, T.; Miyake, S. Diet, Gut Flora, and Multiple Sclerosis: Current Research and Future Perspectives. In *Multiple Sclerosis Immunology: A Foundation for Current and Future Treatments*; Springer: New York, NY, USA, 2013; Volume 6, pp. 115–126.

196. Quintana, F.J.; Sherr, D.H. Aryl hydrocarbon receptor control of adaptive immunity. *Pharmacol. Rev.* **2013**, *65*, 1148–1161. [CrossRef] [PubMed]

197. Krishnamoorthy, G.; Lassmann, H.; Wekerle, H.; Holz, A. Spontaneous opticospinal encephalomyelitis in a double-transgenic mouse model of autoimmune T cell/B cell cooperation. *J. Clin. Investig.* **2006**, *116*, 2385–2392. [CrossRef] [PubMed]

198. Berer, K.; Martínez, I.; Walker, A.; Kunkel, B.; Schmitt-Kopplin, P.; Walter, J.; Krishnamoorthy, G. Dietary non-fermentable fiber prevents autoimmune neurological disease by changing gut metabolic and immune status. *Sci. Rep.* **2018**, *8*, 10431. [CrossRef]

199. Smith, P.M.; Howitt, M.R.; Panikov, N.; Michaud, M.; Gallini, C.A.; Bohlooly-Y, M.; Glickman, J.N.; Garrett, W.S. The Microbial Metabolites, Short-Chain Fatty Acids, Regulate Colonic Treg Cell Homeostasis. *Science* **2013**, *341*, 569–573. [CrossRef]

200. Trompette, A.; Gollwitzer, E.S.; Yadava, K.; Sichelstiel, AK.; Sprenger, N.; Ngom-Bru, C.; Blanchard, C.; Junt, T.; Nicod, L.P.; Harris, N.L.; et al. Gut microbiota metabolism of dietary fiber influences allergic airway disease and hematopoiesis. *Nat. Med.* **2014**, *20*, 159–166. [CrossRef]

201. Haghikia, A.; Jörg, S.; Duscha, A.; Berg, J.; Manzel, A.; Waschbisch, A.; Hammer, A.; Lee, D.H.; May, C.; Wilck, N.; et al. Dietary fatty acids directly impact central nervous system autoimmunity via the small intestine. *Immunity* **2015**, *43*, 817–829. [CrossRef] [PubMed]

202. Mariño, E.; Richards, J.L.; McLeod, K.H.; Stanley, D.; Yap, Y.A.; Knight, J.; McKenzie, C.; Kranich, J.; Oliveira, A.C.; Rossello, F.J.; et al. Gut microbial metabolites limit the frequency of autoimmune T cells and protect against type 1 diabetes. *Nat. Immunol.* **2017**, *18*, 552–562. [CrossRef] [PubMed]

203. Marinho, F.A.; Pacifico, L.G.; Miyoshi, A.; Azevedo, V.; Le Loir, Y.; Guimarães, V.D.; Langella, P.; Cassali, G.D.; Fonseca, C.T.; Oliveira, S.C. An intranasal administration of Lactococcus lactis strains expressing recombinat interleukin-10 modulates acute allergic airway inflammation in a murine model. *Clin Exp Allergy* **2010**, *40*, 1541–1551. [CrossRef]

204. Braat, H.; Rottiers, P.; Hommes, D.W.; Huyghebaert, N.; Remaut, E.; Remon, J.P.; van Deventer, S.J.; Neirynck, S.; Peppelenbosch, M.P.; Steidler, L. A phase I trial with transgenic bacteria expressing interleukin-10 in Crohn's disease. *Clin. Gastroenterol. Hepatol.* **2006**, *4*, 745–749. [CrossRef] [PubMed]

205. Breton, J.; Tennoune, N.; Lucas, N.; Francois, M.; Legrand, R.; Jacquemot, J.; Goichon, A.; Guérin, C.; Peltier, J.; Pestel-Caron, M.; et al. Gut commensal E. Coli proteins activate host satiety pathways following nutrient-induced bacterial growth. *Cell Metab.* **2016**, *23*, 324–334. [CrossRef] [PubMed]

206. Duan, F.F.; Liu, J.H.; March, J.C. Engineered commensal bacteria reprogram intestinal cells into glucose-responsive insulin-secreting cells for the treatment of diabetes. *Diabetes* **2015**, *64*, 1794–1803. [CrossRef] [PubMed]

207. Vrieze, A.; Van Nood, E.; Holleman, F.; Salojärvi, J.; Kootte, R.S.; Bartelsman, J.F.; Dallinga-Thie, G.M.; Ackermans, M.T.; Serlie, M.J.; Oozeer, R.; et al. Transfer of intestinal microbiota from lean donors increases insulin sensitivity in individuals with metabolic syndrome. *Gastroenterology* **2012**, *143*, 913–916.e7. [CrossRef] [PubMed]

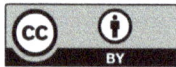

International Journal of
Molecular Sciences

MDPI

Article

Analysis of Gut Microbiota in Rheumatoid Arthritis Patients: Disease-Related Dysbiosis and Modifications Induced by Etanercept

Andrea Picchianti-Diamanti [1,*,†], Concetta Panebianco [2,†], Simonetta Salemi [1],
Maria Laura Sorgi [1], Roberta Di Rosa [1], Alessandro Tropea [1], Mayla Sgrulletti [1],
Gerardo Salerno [1], Fulvia Terracciano [2], Raffaele D'Amelio [1,‡], Bruno Laganà [1] and
Valerio Pazienza [2,*]

[1] Department of Clinical and Molecular Medicine, Sant'Andrea University Hospital, Sapienza University of
   Rome, 00185 Rome, Italy; s.salemi@gmail.com (S.S.); marialaura.sorgi@uniroma1.it (M.L.S.);
   roberta.dirosa@uniroma1.it (R.D.R.); alessandro.tropea3@gmail.com (A.T.);
   Mayla.sgrulletti@uniroma1.it (M.S.); Gerardo.salerno@uniroma1.it (G.S.);
   raffaele.damelio@uniroma1.it (R.D.); bruno.lagana@uniroma1.it (B.L.)
[2] Gastroenterology Unit, IRCCS "Casa Sollievo della Sofferenza" Hospital, Viale dei Cappuccini, 1,
   71013 San Giovanni Rotondo, Italy; panebianco.c@gmail.com (C.P.); terracciano74@hotmail.com (F.T.)
* Correspondence: andrea.picchiantidiamanti@uniroma1.it (A.P.-D.); v.pazienza@operapadrepio.it (V.P.)
† These authors contributed equally to the manuscript.
‡ Retired.

Received: 23 August 2018; Accepted: 25 September 2018; Published: 27 September 2018

Abstract: A certain number of studies were carried out to address the question of how dysbiosis could affect the onset and development of rheumatoid arthritis (RA), but little is known about the reciprocal influence between microbiota composition and immunosuppressive drugs, and how this interaction may have an impact on the clinical outcome. The aim of this study was to characterize the intestinal microbiota in a groups of RA patients treatment-naïve, under methotrexate, and/or etanercept (ETN). Correlations between the gut microbiota composition and validated immunological and clinical parameters of disease activity were also evaluated. In the current study, a 16S analysis was employed to explore the gut microbiota of 42 patients affected by RA and 10 healthy controls. Disease activity score on 28 joints (DAS-28), erythrocyte sedimentation rate, C-reactive protein, rheumatoid factor, anti-cyclic citrullinated peptides, and dietary and smoking habits were assessed. The composition of the gut microbiota in RA patients free of therapy is characterized by several abnormalities compared to healthy controls. Gut dysbiosis in RA patients is associated with different serological and clinical parameters; in particular, the phylum of Euryarchaeota was directly correlated to DAS and emerged as an independent risk factor. Patients under treatment with ETN present a partial restoration of a beneficial microbiota. The results of our study confirm that gut dysbiosis is a hallmark of the disease, and shows, for the first time, that the anti-tumor necrosis factor alpha (TNF-α) ETN is able to modify microbial communities, at least partially restoring a beneficial microbiota.

Keywords: microbiota; rheumatoid arthritis; anti-TNF-α; methotrexate; etanercept; disease activity

1. Introduction

The human intestinal microbiota is a complex microcosm composed of more than 1000 different bacterial species, archaea, fungi, and viruses [1]. There is growing knowledge that these bacteria are not only involved in the digestion and absorption of food, but they can also exert a protective function by preventing adherence of pathogenic bacteria to the mucosal layer, and they play a pivotal role in modulating the innate and acquired immunity of the host [2–4].

Recent advances in sequencing technologies led to a deep characterization of the human gut microbiota in healthy subjects. This enabled the investigation of modifications in the structure of gut commensal communities (called dysbiosis), which could be involved in the onset and maintenance of different chronic autoimmune diseases, such as inflammatory bowel diseases (IBD) and arthritis [5,6]. Dysbiosis could lead to alterations in the intestinal epithelial cell layer with an increased exposure to a variety of bacteria and bacterial products leading to a chronic antigenic stimulation, spreading of inflammatory mediators, and T cell activation [7,8].

It was recently demonstrated that different environmental factors are involved in the development of both intestinal/oral dysbiosis and arthritis onset and outcome, among which the most relevant are diet, smoking, infections, and drugs [9–12].

Rheumatoid arthritis (RA) is an inflammatory autoimmune disease of unknown etiology, potentially leading to progressive joint destruction and disability. In RA patients, an accumulating body of studies demonstrated a pathogenic role of dysbiosis of the oral microbiota, in particular, an association between *Porphyromonas gingivalis*, periodontitis, and the generation of citrullinated products was clearly demonstrated [13–15].

On the other hand, data regarding the role of intestinal microbiota in these patients are not conclusive, and no studies address the reciprocal influence between biotechnological immunosuppressants and microbiota on RA outcome.

Etanercept (ETN, a dimeric recombinant fully human fusion protein consisting of a human 75-kDa tumor necrosis factor (TNF) receptor linked to the Fc portion of human immunoglobulin G1 (IgG1)) is one of the five currently available biotechnological agents that target TNF-α. ETN proved to be safe and effective in reducing disease activity and limiting the progression of joint damage in RA patients; it can be administered as monotherapy or in combination therapy with methotrexate (MTX) [16].

The aim of this study was to characterize the intestinal microbiota in a group of RA patients treatment-naïve, under MTX, and/or ETN. Correlations between the gut microbiota composition and validated immunological and clinical parameters of disease activity were also evaluated.

2. Results

2.1. Microbiota Profile in Rheumatoid Arthritis (RA) Patients Free of Therapy versus Healthy Controls(HCs)

Lifestyle factors, as well as demographic, serologic, and clinical parameters, of the four RA treatment groups are shown in Table 1.

No significant differences were observed among the RA groups except for the disease duration, which, as expected, was shorter in the group of naïve and MTX monotherapy patients. HCs were also similar to RA patients regarding lifestyle factors, but they were significantly younger ($p < 0.05$).

After passing quality control filters, a mean of 281,218 sequences per sample were obtained. The assessment of the Shannon index in each sample revealed that α-diversity was neither changed in naïve patients compared with the HCs, nor in each treatment group (naïve, ETN, MTX, or ETN plus MTX) relative to patients free of therapy (Figure 1A). Similarly, no significant change in species richness was observed (Figure 1B).

Table 1. Main demographic, clinical, and serologic data of the 42 rheumatoid arthritis (RA) patients.

Patient Characteristics	Naïve	ETN	MTX	ETN + MTX	p-Value
Male *n* (%)	1 (9)	1 (10)	2 (18)	2 (20)	ns
Age	55.7	59.8	62.3	64.6	ns
Varied and balanced diet *n* (%)	10 (91)	9 (90)	10 (91)	9 (90)	ns
Smokers *n* (%)	1 (9)	3 (30)	1 (9)	1 (10)	ns
Disease Duration (years)	6.4	14.8	11.2	19.9	0.007 * 0.07 0.002 0.04
DAS-28	4.3	3.9	4	3.7	ns
RF pos *n* (%)	8 (73)	6 (60)	8 (73)	6 (60)	ns
ACPA pos *n* (%)	8 (73)	6 (60)	8 (73)	6 (60)	ns
ESR (mm/h)	27.4	28.3	22.4	22.6	ns
CRP (mg/L)	5.7	6.5	5.1	6.4	ns

RA = Rheumatoid arthritis; Naïve = patients naïve to immunosuppressants; ETN = etanercept; MTX = methotrexate; ACPA = anti-citrullinated peptide antibodies; RF = rheumatoid factor; ESR = erythrocyte sedimentation rate; CRP = C-reactive protein; DAS-28 = disease activity score on 28 joints. Data are expressed as means. * Naïve vs. ETN; naïve vs. MTX; naïve vs. ETN + MTX; MTX vs. ETN + MTX. ns = not significant.

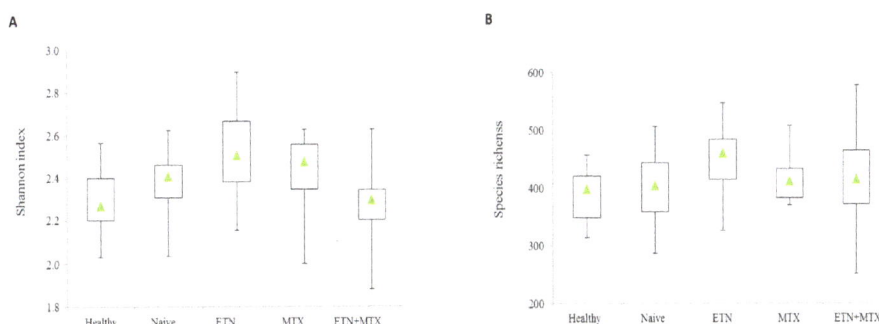

Figure 1. Box plots of Shannon diversity index (**A**) and species richness (**B**) of microbiota of healthy controls and different treatment groups of rheumatoid arthritis (RA) patients. The triangle represents the median value.

As a first approach, we compared the gut microbiota composition of the HCs with that of RA patients free of therapy. This analysis revealed that the relative abundance of the microbial phyla was almost unchanged (Figure 2A), while significant differences between the two groups were found at lower taxonomic levels. The most striking alterations were a five-fold increase in the class of Bacilli (Figure 2B) and a seventeen-fold increase in the order of Lactobacillales (Figure 2C) found in RA patients with respect to the controls (2.89 ± 3.19 vs. 0.58 ± 0.39; $p = 0.035$, and 2.69 ± 3.15 vs. 0.15 ± 0.34; $p = 0.021$, respectively). Significant reductions of the genus *Faecalibacterium* (12.21 ± 7.4 vs. 19.72 ± 4.41; $p = 0.012$) (Figure 3B) and its cognate species *Faecalibacterium prausnitzii* (3.23 ± 3.22 vs. 7.97 ± 3.78; $p = 0.006$) (Figure 3C) were also found. Furthermore, significant changes were also observed in the genus *Flavobacterium* (Figure 3B) and the species *Blautia coccoides* (Figure 3C), which were both represented in the control group, but were not detected at all in RA naïve patients (2 ± 2.44 vs. 0 ± 0; $p = 0.013$, and 0.7 ± 0.76 vs. 0 ± 0; $p = 0.006$).

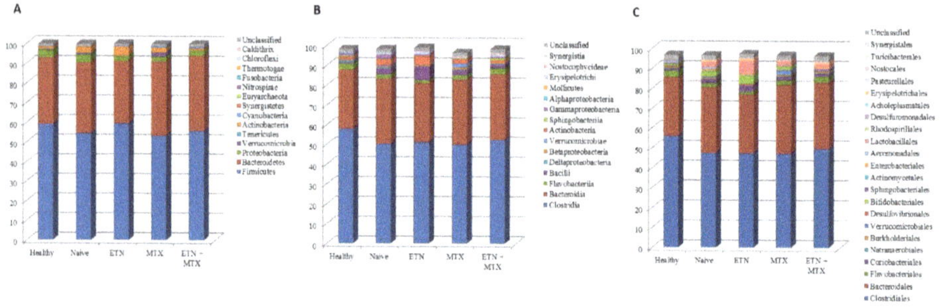

Figure 2. Microbiota composition of healthy controls and different treatment groups of RA patients at the phylum (**A**), class (**B**), and order (**C**) levels. The mean value of the eight top taxonomic classifications at each level is represented.

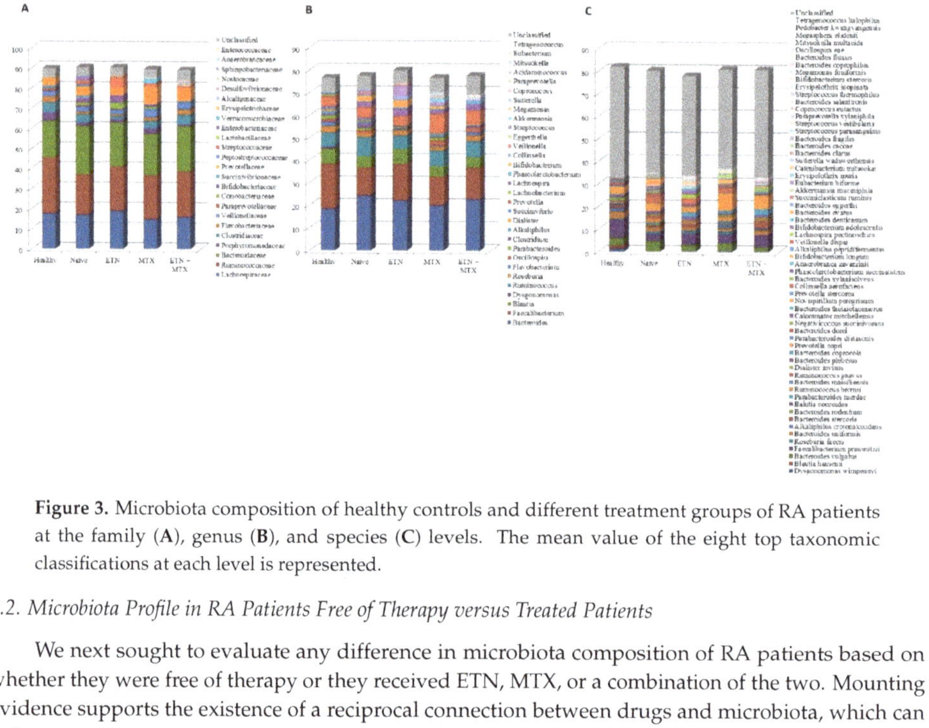

Figure 3. Microbiota composition of healthy controls and different treatment groups of RA patients at the family (**A**), genus (**B**), and species (**C**) levels. The mean value of the eight top taxonomic classifications at each level is represented.

2.2. Microbiota Profile in RA Patients Free of Therapy versus Treated Patients

We next sought to evaluate any difference in microbiota composition of RA patients based on whether they were free of therapy or they received ETN, MTX, or a combination of the two. Mounting evidence supports the existence of a reciprocal connection between drugs and microbiota, which can influence each other and have an impact on therapeutic outcomes [17]. Specifically, MTX was shown to modify microbiota composition, partly restoring the microbial balance altered by the disease [12].

When compared to naïve patients, major changes were observed in the ETN group. The Cyanobacteria significantly increased (0.49 ± 0.5 vs. 0.08 ± 0.07; $p = 0.016$) (Figure 2A), and the same increase was observed in the Nostocophycideae class (Figure 2B) and the Nostocales order (0.35 ± 0.5 vs. 0 ± 0; $p = 0.031$) (Figure 2C), which both belong to the phylum of Cyanobacteria. In detail, Nostocophycideae and Nostocales, which were not represented among the naïve subjects, were instead detected in four out of ten ETN patients. In addition, the class of Deltaproteobacteria (0.07 ± 0.23 vs. 0.57 ± 0.72; $p = 0.05$) (Figure 2B) and the family of Clostridiaceae (1.51 ± 1.76 vs. 3.97 ± 3.4; $p = 0.05$) (Figure 3A) significantly decreased in the ETN group as compared to the naïve. The only statistically significant alteration found in the MTX group was a decrease in the relative abundance of Enterobateriales (0.07 ± 0.24 vs. 0.85 ± 1.22; *p* = 0.05) (Figure 2C), while no significant changes were observed in RA patients upon ETN plus MTX therapy.

2.3. Association of Microbiota Profile with Clinical Pathological Features in RA Patients

Finally, we wondered whether microbiota composition could be associated to clinical parameters (i.e., sex, age, disease duration, disease activity Score on 28 joints (DAS-28), rheumatoid factor (RF), anti-cyclic citrullinated peptides antibodies (ACPA), erythrocyte sedimentation rate (ESR) and C-reactive protein (CRP) and lifestyle factors (diet and smoking habits) of the RA patients. For this purpose, correlations were analyzed between microorganisms at each taxonomic level and all the above described parameters (Figure 4).

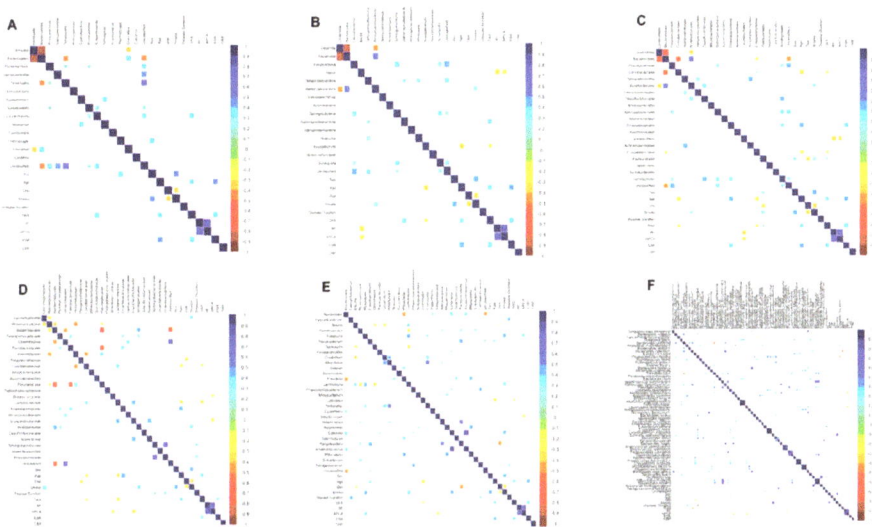

Figure 4. Association of gut microbiota profile with clinical pathological features in RA patients at the phylum (**A**), class (**B**), order (**C**), family (**D**), genus (**E**), and species (**F**) levels.

The Spearman correlation analysis revealed a direct association between the male sex and the abundance of Pasteurellales microbes, while the age of the patients was directly correlated with Enterobacteriales, Enterobacteriaceae, Flavobacterium, *Parabacteroides distasonis*, and *Bacteroides ovatus*, and inversely correlated to Erysipelotrichi, Coriobacteriales, Erysipelotrichales, Coriobacteriaceae, Lactobacillaceae, *Collinsella*, and *Collinsella aerofaciens*. The disease duration result was positively associated with the species *Bacteroides caccae*, while it was negatively correlated with *Parabacteroides merdae*. Interestingly, a direct correlation between DAS and Euryarchaeota, Gammaproteobacteria, Pasteurellales, and *Anaerobranca zavarzinii* was found, while Erysipelotrichi, Erysipelotrichales, Coriobacteriales, Coriobacteriaceae, Lactobacillaceae, *Collinsella*, *Bacteroides rodentium*, and *Collinsella aerofaciens* were inversely associated with this score. A certain number of correlations were shared by RF and ACPA positivity. In detail, both factors were positively associated with *Roseburia* and negatively with Bacilli, Lactobacillales, and *Streptococcus vestibularis*. In addition, ACPA positivity was indirectly correlated with Streptococcaceae, Erysipelotrichaceae, *Streptococcus*, *Bacteroides xylanisolvens*, and *Lachnospira pectinoschiza*. Direct correlations between ESR and Enterobacteriales, *Roseburia faecis*, and *Streptococcus parasanguinis*, and between CRP and *Parabacteroides distasonis* emerged from the analysis. Regarding lifestyle factors, a varied and well-balanced diet was inversely associated with Pasteurellales, Paraprevotellaceae, *Paraprevotella*, *Blautia*, *Blautia coccoides*, and *Bacteroides eggerthi*, while smoking was positively correlated with Betaproteobacteria, Burkholderiales, Pasteurellales, Lachnospiraceae, Alcaligenaceae, *Roseburia*, *Lachnospira*, *Sutterella*, *Lachnospira pectinoschiza*, *Bacteroides denticanum*, and *Sutterella wadsworthensis*.

Additionally, since the variables affecting the microbiota composition in RA are numerous and can be interconnected, a multivariate approach was followed for a more complete understanding of these interactions. This analysis revealed that independent factors affecting the disease were DAS and Euryarchaeota at the phylum level, DAS and Erysipelotrichi at the class level, and only DAS at the order level. On the contrary, no independent factors were found to correlate with the disease at the family, genus, and species levels (Supplementary Material).

3. Discussion

In our pilot study, we applied 16S analysis to characterize the gut microbiota of RA patients, with a particular interest in the effect of synthetic and biotechnological therapies on its composition. Any significant difference in the Shannon index and in the number of species between healthy and diseased subjects was observed in our study population. No change was observed in richness and diversity when patients were classified on the basis of the treatment they received.

A comparison of the gut microbial populations between healthy and affected individuals pointed out the role of Bacilli in the pathogenesis of RA. Our data are in line with previous studies, in which the related taxa of Lactobacillaceae and *Lactobacillus* were significantly more abundant in RA animal models and patients than in controls. A study by Liu et al. [18] demonstrated that the quantity and variety of lactobacilli in RA patients was higher than in HCs. A few years later, the same authors described an increase of the Lactobacillaceae family and the *Lactobacillus* genus in mice susceptible to developing collagen-induced arthritis, with respect to mice resistance, thus suggesting these bacteria as a predisposing factor of the disease [19]. Moreover, Zhang et al. observed an over-representation of *Lactobacillus salivarius* in the gut and mouth of RA patients, with the highest levels found in people most severely affected [12]. Bacilli (especially *Lactobacillus*) are generally regarded as friendly bacteria for the host; as such, they are among the most commonly used probiotics. Indeed, the administration of *L. casei* and *L. delbrueckii* was shown to alleviate RA symptoms in experimental models [19–22]; on the other hand, *L. rhamnosus* GG and *L. reuteri* administration failed to ameliorate the disease in patients [23–25] suggesting that different *Lactobacillus* species may act differently on RA.

The decreased abundance of *Faecalibacterium* found in our analysis is in agreement with previous studies carried out on RA [26,27] and other inflammatory conditions [28–30]. The bacteria belonging to this genus are well-known butyrate producers, help in maintaining the integrity and health of the gut epithelial barrier, and exhibit anti-inflammatory properties [28–30]; thus, their decrease may contribute to the onset of an inflammatory status. No previous association of *Blautia coccoides* (which was depleted in our naïve group) with RA was reported; nonetheless, it was shown that enriching the gut microbiota of systemic lupus erythematosus patients with *Blautia coccoides*, together with *Ruminococcus obeum* and *Bifidobacterium bifidum*, improved the inflammatory status by inducing the production of the immunosuppressive regulatory T cells (Tregs) [31].

As reported by the latest EULAR recommendations, MTX should be considered the first immunosuppressive treatment strategy in patients with RA; in the case of an inadequate response, TNF-α inhibitors or other biotechnological therapies should be started [16]. Zhang et al. previously reported that MTX can affect microbiota composition, partly reversing disease-related dysbiosis [12]. As of now, data on the effect of microbiota in the outcome of patients receiving immunosuppressive biotechnological therapies are limited and only refer to IBD patients. For this reason, we next characterized the gut microbiota of RA patients on different immunosuppressant treatment strategies (ETN, MTX, or ETN plus MTX) and compared it with that of treatment-naïve patients.

Interestingly, significant changes were found in patients receiving ETN. The phylum of Cyanobacteria and its cognate Nostocophycideae and Nostocales were enriched in the ETN group. Little is known about the role of these microorganisms in health and disease; nevertheless, Cyanobacteria produce secondary metabolites with multiple bioactivities, including anti-inflammatory and immunosuppressant activities [32] which may benefit RA patients. Also, the drop in Deltaproteobacteria caused by ETN could be potentially beneficial if we consider that these microorganisms were found enriched in patients suffering from ulcerative colitis [33] and that Proteobacteria in general are abundant in both intestinal and extra-intestinal inflammatory diseases [34]. Moreover, we observed a decrease in Clostridiaceae upon ETN treatment which could be potentially beneficial since these bacteria were previously found enriched in patients with RA and IBD-associated arthropathy [35]. In patients treated with MTX, our analysis revealed a significant decrease in Enterobacteriales, whose lipopolysaccharides may contribute to inflammation [36], and which were associated with increased intestinal permeability [37], a condition that can be found in RA patients [38].

The results discussed so far further support the evidence of a link between gut microbiota and RA, and show, for the first time, that anti-TNF-α therapy can have a beneficial impact on the microbiota composition.

With the aim of establishing any association between microbial taxa and clinical parameters of the disease, correlation analyses were performed grouping all forty-two RA patients. Among the most remarkable results, the pro-inflammatory Gammaproteobacteria and its cognate order of Pasteurellales displayed a direct correlation with disease activity (DAS-28), while the order of Enterobacteriales showed a positive association with ESR. Interestingly, the phylum of Euryarchaeota was directly correlated with DAS and emerged as an independent risk factor in RA when a multivariate analysis was performed. The function of these microorganisms in humans is still poorly explored, but their increase was observed in another autoimmune disorder, i.e., multiple sclerosis [39].

A positive association between *B. caccae* and disease duration was also found. A membrane protein of *B. caccae*, namely outer membrane protein W (OmpW), was described as a target of the immune response associated with IBD. Intriguingly, this protein is structurally related to a protein of *P. gingivalis* [40], against which increased autoantibody production was discovered in RA [41].

In addition to the clinical characteristics, some demographic and lifestyle factors of patients were taken into account. Enterobacteriales and Enterobacteriaceae (belonging to Gammaproteobacteria) were found to be associated with increasing age, while a number of taxa belonging to Betaproteobacteria (Alcaligenaceae, Burkholderiales, *Sutterella*, and *S. wadsworthensis*) were positively correlated with the habit of smoking.

When compared to previous reports, this study presents the advantage of having evaluated and compared, for the first time, the effects induced by synthetic and anti-TNF-α agents, in monotherapy and combination therapy, on gut dysbiosis in RA patients.

A limit to the current study is that the cross-sectional design can allow us to assess the presence of gut dysbiosis in RA patients who are treatment-naïve, under ETN, and/or MTX therapy; however, it does not give information on the predictive value of these changes in relation to RA clinical outcome and structural progression.

Overall, the current study revealed that RA is characterized by gut dysbiosis, some of which is associated to the inflammatory status of the disease, suggesting that the microbiota may play an important role in the promotion and clinical course of RA. Moreover, the partial restoration of a beneficial microbiota induced mainly by the anti-TNF-α ETN can contribute to the clinical efficacy of this agent. A deeper understanding of the alterations occurring in the gut microbiota of patients on different therapeutic regimens could help set up individualized and supportive therapeutic strategies providing patients with more effective and safe care.

4. Materials and Methods

4.1. Study Population

Forty-two RA patients, according to the European League Against Rheumatism (EULAR)/American College of Rheumatology (ACR) classification criteria [42] were recruited at the outpatient Division of Immunology and Rheumatology, S. Andrea Hospital, Sapienza University of Rome. Patients were divided into four groups according to current therapy: 11 patients were naïve to immunosuppressants, 11 patients were receiving MTX, 10 patients were receiving ETN, and 10 patients were receiving ETN plus MTX. Ten healthy subjects were used as controls (HCs).

The study was conducted according to the ethical guidelines of the 1975 Declaration of Helsinki. An informed consent was obtained by all the patients and the study was approved by the local ethical Committee (43/2013). All patients were receiving current therapy for at least three months and had to be naïve to other biotechnological drugs. Steroids and non-steroidal anti-inflammatory drugs (NSAIDs) had to be stopped at least seven days before the exams.

Any patients or HCs on antibiotics, consuming probiotics, or having a known history of inflammatory bowel disease or other autoimmune diseases were excluded.

DAS-28, ESR, CRP, RF, ACPA, and dietary and smoking habits were assessed the same day of stool sample collection.

Patients' clinical data are described in Table 1.

4.2. Sample Collection and DNA Extraction

Each participant collected a fresh stool sample in a collection tube filled with a DNA stabilization buffer (Canvax Biotech, Voden Medical Instruments, Meda, Italy). Then, 250 µL of each sample was processed for microbial DNA extraction using the QIAamp DNA Stool Mini Kit (Qiagen, Milan, Italy) according to the manufacturer's protocol. DNA concentration and purity were assessed using a NanoDrop spectrophotometer (Thermo Scientific, Meda, Italy).

4.3. Next-Generation Sequencing of Bacterial 16S Ribosomal RNA Gene

The Illumina 16S Metagenomic Sequencing Library Preparation instructions were followed for high-throughput sequencing. Firstly, 12.5 ng of each DNA extract was employed for the amplification of the V3–V4 hypervariable regions of the bacterial 16S ribosomal RNA (rRNA) gene, using the following primers with Illumina adapters (underlined): forward primer: 5′-TCGTCGGCAGCGTCAGATGTGTATAAGAGACAGCCTACGGGNGGCWGCAG, reverse primer: 5′-GTCTCGTGGGCTCGGAGATGTGTATAAGAGACAGGACTACHVGGGTATCTAATCC, selected from Klindworth et al. [43]. The amplification reaction was carried out in the presence of the 2× KAPA HiFi HotStart Ready Mix (Roche, Milan, Italy) under the following conditions: initial denaturation at 95 °C for 3 min, followed by 25 cycles of denaturation at 95 °C for 30 s, primer annealing at 55 °C for 30 s, extension at 72 °C for 30 s, with a final elongation at 72 °C for 5 min. PCR amplicons were then purified by means of Agencourt AMPure XP beads (Beckman Coulter, Milan, Italy). The purified DNA products were then subjected to a further PCR to attach dual Illumina indices (Nextera XT Index Kit, Illumina Inc., San Diego, CA, USA) necessary for multiplexing. The reaction was performed under the following conditions: initial denaturation at 95 °C for 3 min, followed by eight cycles of denaturation at 95 °C for 30 s, primer annealing at 55 °C for 30 s, extension at 72 °C for 30 s, with a final elongation at 72 °C for 5 min. Following a further PCR purification, the eluted DNA products were quantified using the Qubit dsDNA BR Kit assay, diluted to a concentration of 4 nM, and pooled in equal proportion into a single library. Paired-end sequencing (2 × 300 cycles) was carried out on an Illumina MiSeq device (Illumina Inc.) according to the manufacturer's instructions. Sequences were demultiplexed based on index sequences, and FASTQ files were generated.

4.4. Bioinformatic Analysis

Sequence data were analyzed using the 16S Metagenomics App provided by BaseSpace software (version 1.0.1, Illumina Inc.) which performs taxonomic classification based on the Greengenes database (available online: http://greengenes.secondgenome.com/downloads/database/13_5). For each sample, the relative abundance of the top eight taxonomic classifications at each level (from phylum to species) was considered for statistical analysis. Moreover, the software calculated the Shannon index (α-diversity) and the number of species (richness) found in each sample.

4.5. Statistical Analysis

Continuous variables are expressed as means ± standard deviation (SD). Two-group comparisons were calculated using the Student's *t*-test. Correlation analyses were performed using Spearman rank correlation. Multiple logistic regression analyses with backward variable selection were applied to assess independent correlates of subject status (healthy/pathological). All statistical tests were two-tailed and $p < 0.05$ was considered statistically significant. Statistical analyses were performed by using the R software, version 3.1.0 (10 April 2014)-B Spring Dance Copyright © 2014 The R Foundation for Statistical Computing.

Supplementary Materials: Supplementary materials can be found at http://www.mdpi.com/1422-0067/19/10/2938/s1.

Author Contributions: A.P.-D. and V.P. conceived the study; A.P.-D., C.P., V.P. and R.D. designed the experiments; C.P. performed the experiments; G.S., C.P., A.P.-D. and V.P. analyzed the data; A.P.-D., F.T. and V.P. contributed reagents/materials/analysis tools; S.S., M.L.S., B.L., M.S. and R.D.R. performed the medical examination of the RA patients; C.P., A.T., A.P.-D. and V.P. wrote the paper.

Funding: This research was supported by the "Ricerca Corrente RC1703GA31" and the "Ricerca Corrente RC1803GA30" granted by the Italian Ministry of Health to V.P.

Acknowledgments: We thank Riccardo Pracella for technical help.

Conflicts of Interest: The authors declare no conflict of interest.

References

1. Ursell, L.K.; Haiser, H.J.; Van Treuren, W.; Garg, N.; Reddivari, L.; Vanamala, J.; Dorrestein, P.C.; Turnbaugh, P.J.; Knight, R. The intestinal metabolome: An intersection between microbiota and host. *Gastroenterology* **2014**, *146*, 1470–1476. [CrossRef] [PubMed]

2. Maslowski, K.M.; Vieira, A.T.; Ng, A.; Kranich, J.; Sierro, F.; Yu, D.; Schilter, H.C.; Rolph, M.S.; Mackay, F.; Artis, D.; et al. Regulation of inflammatory responses by gut microbiota and chemoattractant receptor GPR43. *Nature* **2009**, *461*, 1282–1286. [CrossRef] [PubMed]

3. Rogier, R.; Koenders, M.I.; Abdollahi-Roodsaz, S. Toll-like receptor mediated modulation of T cell response by commensal intestinal microbiota as a trigger for autoimmune arthritis. *J. Immunol. Res.* **2015**, *2015*, 527696. [CrossRef] [PubMed]

4. Stecher, B.; Hardt, W.D. Mechanisms controlling pathogen colonization of the gut. *Curr. Opin. Microbiol.* **2011**, *14*, 82–91. [CrossRef] [PubMed]

5. Petersen, C.; Round, J.L. Defining dysbiosis and its influence on host immunity and disease. *Cell Microbiol.* **2014**, *16*, 1024–1033. [CrossRef] [PubMed]

6. Picchianti-Diamanti, A.; Rosado, M.M. D'Amelio, R. Infectious Agents and Inflammation: The Role of Microbiota in Autoimmune Arthritis. *Front. Microbiol.* **2018**, *8*, 2696. [CrossRef] [PubMed]

7. Asquith, M.; Elewaut, D.; Lin, P.; Rosenbaum, J.T. The role of the gut and microbes in the pathogenesis of spondyloarthritis. *Best Pract. Res. Clin. Rheumatol.* **2014**, *28*, 687–702. [CrossRef] [PubMed]

8. Ciccia, F.; Bombardieri, M.; Rizzo, A.; Principato, A.; Giardina, A.R.; Raiata, F.; Peralta, S.; Ferrante, A.; Drago, S.; Cottone, M.; et al. Over-expression of paneth cell-derived anti-microbial peptides in the gut of patients with ankylosing spondylitis and subclinical intestinal inflammation. *Rheumatology* **2010**, *49*, 2076–2083. [CrossRef] [PubMed]

9. Picchianti Diamanti, A.; Lagana, B.; Cox, M.C.; Pilozzi, E.; Amodeo, R.; Bove, M.; Markovic, M.; di Rosa, R.; Salemi, S.; Sorgi, M.L.; et al. TCD4$_{pos}$ lymphocytosis in rheumatoid and psoriatic arthritis patients following TNFα blocking agents. *J. Transl. Med.* **2017**, *15*, 38. [CrossRef] [PubMed]

10. Ciccia, F.; Ferrante, A.; Guggino, G.; Triolo, G. The role of the gastrointestinal tract in the pathogenesis of rheumatic diseases. *Best Pract. Res. Clin. Rheumatol.* **2016**, *30*, 889–900. [CrossRef] [PubMed]

11. Panebianco, C.; Andriulli, A.; Pazienza, V. Pharmacomicrobiomics: Exploiting the drug-microbiota interactions in anticancer therapies. *Microbiome* **2018**, *6*, 92. [CrossRef] [PubMed]

12. Zhang, X.; Zhang, D.; Jia, H.; Feng, Q.; Wang, D.; Liang, D.; Wu, X.; Li, J.; Tang, L.; Li, Y.; et al. The oral and gut microbiomes are perturbed in rheumatoid arthritis and partly normalized after treatment. *Nat. Med.* **2015**, *21*, 895–905. [CrossRef] [PubMed]

13. Enright, E.F.; Gahan, C.G.; Joyce, S.A.; Griffin, B.T. The impact of the gut microbiota on drug metabolism and clinical outcome. *Yale J. Biol. Med.* **2016**, *89*, 37.

14. Quirke, A.M.; Lugli, E.B.; Wegner, N.; Hamilton, B.C.; Charles, P.; Chowdhury, M.; Ytterberg, A.J.; Zubarev, R.A.; Potempa, J.; Culshaw, S.; et al. Heightened immune response to autocitrullinated *Porphyromonas gingivalis* peptidylarginine deiminase: A potential mechanism for breaching immunologic tolerance in rheumatoid arthritis. *Ann. Rheum. Dis.* **2014**, *73*, 263–269. [CrossRef] [PubMed]

15. Wegner, N.; Wait, R.; Sroka, A.; Eick, S.; Nguyen, K.A.; Lundberg, K.; Kinloch, A.; Culshaw, S.; Potempa, J.; Venables, P.J. Peptidylarginine deiminase from *Porphyromonas gingivalis* citrullinates human fibrinogen and alpha-enolase: Implications for autoimmunity in rheumatoid arthritis. *Arthritis Rheum.* **2010**, *62*, 2662–2672. [CrossRef] [PubMed]

16. Smolen, J.S.; Landewe, R.; Bijlsma, J.; Burmester, G.; Chatzidionysiou, K.; Dougados, M.; Nam, J.; Ramiro, S.; Voshaar, M.; van Vollenhoven, R.; et al. EULAR recommendations for the management of rheumatoid arthritis with synthetic and biological disease-modifying antirheumatic drugs: 2016 Update. *Ann. Rheum. Dis.* **2017**, *76*, 960–977. [CrossRef] [PubMed]

17. Bhat, M.; Pasini, E.; Copeland, J.; Angeli, M.; Husain, S.; Kumar, D.; Renner, E.; Teterina, A.; Allard, J.; Guttman, D.S.; et al. Impact of immunosuppression on the metagenomic composition of the intestinal microbiome: A systems biology approach to post-transplant diabetes. *Sci. Rep.* **2017**, *7*, 10277. [CrossRef] [PubMed]

18. Liu, X.; Zou, Q.; Zeng, B.; Fang, Y.; Wei, H. Analysis of fecal *Lactobacillus* community structure in patients with early rheumatoid arthritis. *Curr. Microbiol.* **2013**, *67*, 170–176. [CrossRef] [PubMed]

19. Liu, X.; Zeng, B.; Zhang, J.; Li, W.; Mou, F.; Wang, H.; Zou, Q.; Zhong, B.; Wu, L.; Wei, H.; et al. Role of the gut microbiome in modulating arthritis progression in mice. *Sci Rep.* **2016**, *6*, 30594. [CrossRef] [PubMed]

20. Alipour, B.; Homayouni-Rad, A.; Vaghef-Mehrabany, E.; Sharif, S.K.; Vaghef-Mehrabany, L.; Asghari-Jafarabadi, M.; Nakhjavani, M.R.; Mohtadi-Nia, J. Effects of *Lactobacillus casei* supplementation on disease activity and inflammatory cytokines in rheumatoid arthritis patients: A randomized double-blind clinical trial. *Int. J. Rheum. Dis.* **2014**, *17*, 519–527. [PubMed]

21. Amdekar, S.; Singh, V.; Singh, R.; Sharma, P.; Keshav, P.; Kumar, A. *Lactobacillus casei* reduces the inflammatory joint damage associated with collagen-induced arthritis (CIA) by reducing the pro-inflammatory cytokines: *Lactobacillus casei*: COX-2 inhibitor. *J. Clin. Immunol.* **2011**, *31*, 147–154. [CrossRef] [PubMed]

22. Kano, H.; Kaneko, T.; Kaminogawa, S. Oral intake of *Lactobacillus delbrueckii* subsp. bulgaricus OLL1073R-1 prevents collagen-induced arthritis in mice. *J. Food Prot.* **2002**, *65*, 153–160. [CrossRef] [PubMed]

23. So, J.S.; Kwon, H.K.; Lee, C.G.; Yi, H.J.; Park, J.A.; Lim, S.Y.; Hwang, K.C.; Jeon, Y.H.; Im, S.H. *Lactobacillus casei* suppresses experimental arthritis by down-regulating T helper 1 effector functions. *Mol. Immunol.* **2008**, *45*, 2690–2699. [CrossRef] [PubMed]

24. Hatakka, K.; Martio, J.; Korpela, M.; Herranen, M.; Poussa, T.; Laasanen, T.; Saxelin, M.; Vapaatalo, H.; Moilanen, E.; Korpela, R. Effects of probiotic therapy on the activity and activation of mild rheumatoid arthritis—A pilot study. *Scand. J. Rheumatol.* **2003**, *32*, 211–215. [CrossRef] [PubMed]

25. Pineda Mde, L.; Thompson, S.F.; Summers, K.; de Leon, F.; Pope, J.; Reid, G. A randomized, double-blinded, placebo-controlled pilot study of probiotics in active rheumatoid arthritis. *Med. Sci. Monit.* **2011**, *17*, CR347–CR354. [PubMed]

26. Chen, J.; Wright, K.; Davis, J.M.; Jeraldo, P.; Marietta, E.V.; Murray, J.; Nelson, H.; Matteson, E.L.; Taneja, V. An expansion of rare lineage intestinal microbes characterizes rheumatoid arthritis. *Genome Med.* **2015**, *8*, 43. [CrossRef] [PubMed]

27. Wu, X.; Liu, J.; Xiao, L.; Lu, A.; Zhang, G. Alterations of gut microbiome in rheumatoid arthritis. *Osteoarthr. Cartil.* **2017**, *25*, S287–S288. [CrossRef]

28. Arvonen, M.; Berntson, L.; Pokka, T.; Karttunen, T.J.; Vahasalo, P.; Stoll, M.L. Gut microbiota-host interactions and juvenile idiopathic arthritis. *Pediatr. Rheumatol. Online J.* **2016**, *14*, 44. [CrossRef] [PubMed]

29. Cao, Y.; Shen, J.; Ran, Z.H. Association between *Faecalibacterium prausnitzii* reduction and inflammatory bowel disease: A meta-analysis and systematic review of the literature. *Gastroenterol. Res. Pract.* **2014**, *2014*, 872725. [CrossRef] [PubMed]

30. Sokol, H.; Pigneur, B.; Watterlot, L.; Lakhdari, O.; Bermudez-Humaran, L.G.; Gratadoux, J.J.; Blugeon, S.; Bridonneau, C.; Furet, J.P.; Corthier, G.; et al. *Faecalibacterium prausnitzii* is an anti-inflammatory commensal bacterium identified by gut microbiota analysis of Crohn disease patients. *Proc. Natl. Acad. Sci. USA* **2008**, *105*, 16731–16736. [CrossRef] [PubMed]

31. Lopez, P.; de Paz, B.; Rodriguez-Carrio, J.; Hevia, A.; Sanchez, B.; Margolles, A.; Suarez, A. Th17 responses and natural IgM antibodies are related to gut microbiota composition in systemic lupus erythematosus patients. *Sci. Rep.* **2016**, *6*, 24072. [CrossRef] [PubMed]

32. Vijayakumar, S.; Menakha, M. Pharmaceutical applications of cyanobacteria—A review. *J. Acute Med.* **2015**, *5*, 15–23. [CrossRef]

33. Roediger, W.E.; Moore, J.; Babidge, W. Colonic sulfide in pathogenesis and treatment of ulcerative colitis. *Dig. Dis. Sci.* **1997**, *42*, 1571–1579. [CrossRef] [PubMed]

34. Rizzatti, G.; Lopetuso, L.R.; Gibiino, G.; Binda, C.; Gasbarrini, A. Proteobacteria: A common factor in human diseases. *BioMed Res. Int.* **2017**, *2017*, 9351507. [CrossRef] [PubMed]

35. Muniz-Pedrogo, D.A.; Chen, J.; Hillmann, B.M.; Jeraldo, P.; Saffouri, G.; Al-Ghalith, G.A.; Friton, J.; Taneja, V.; Davis, J.M.; Knights, D.; et al. Gut microbial markers of arthritis including inflammatory bowel disease associated arthropathy. *Gastroenterology* **2018**, *154*, S–586. [CrossRef]

36. Ramos-Romero, S.; Hereu, M.; Atienza, L.; Casas, J.; Jauregui, O.; Amezqueta, S.; Dasilva, G.; Medina, I.; Nogues, M.R.; Romeu, M.; et al. Mechanistically different effects of fat and sugar on insulin resistance, hypertension, and gut microbiota in rats. *Am. J. Physiol. Endocrinol. Metab.* **2018**, *314*, E552–E563. [CrossRef] [PubMed]

37. Pedersen, C.; Ijaz, U.Z.; Gallagher, E.; Horton, F.; Ellis, R.J.; Jaiyeola, E.; Duparc, T.; Russell-Jones, D.; Hinton, P.; Cani, P.D.; et al. Fecal *Enterobacteriales* enrichment is associated with increased in vivo intestinal permeability in humans. *Physiol. Rep.* **2018**, *6*, e13649. [CrossRef] [PubMed]

38. Bjarnason, I.; Williams, P.; So, A.; Zanelli, G.D.; Levi, A.J.; Gumpel, J.M.; Peters, T.J.; Ansell, B. Intestinal permeability and inflammation in rheumatoid arthritis: Effects of non-steroidal anti-inflammatory drugs. *Lancet* **1984**, *2*, 1171–1174. [CrossRef]

39. Jangi, S.; Gandhi, R.; Cox, L.M.; Li, N.; von Glehn, F.; Yan, R.; Patel, B.; Mazzola, M.A.; Liu, S.; Glanz, B.L.; et al. Alterations of the human gut microbiome in multiple sclerosis. *Nat. Commun.* **2016**, *7*, 12015. [CrossRef] [PubMed]

40. Wei, B.; Dalwadi, H.; Gordon, L.K.; Landers, C.; Bruckner, D.; Targan, S.R.; Braun, J. Molecular cloning of a *Bacteroides caccae* TonB-linked outer membrane protein identified by an inflammatory bowel disease marker antibody. *Infect. Immun.* **2001**, *69*, 6044–6054. [CrossRef] [PubMed]

41. Johansson, L.; Sherina, N.; Kharlamova, N.; Potempa, B.; Larsson, B.; Israelsson, L.; Potempa, J.; Rantapaa-Dahlqvist, S.; Lundberg, K. Concentration of antibodies against *Porphyromonas gingivalis* is increased before the onset of symptoms of rheumatoid arthritis. *Arthritis Res. Ther.* **2016**, *18*, 201. [CrossRef] [PubMed]

42. Aletaha, D.; Neogi, T.; Silman, A.J.; Funovits, J.; Felson, D.T.; Bingham, C.O., III; Birnbaum, N.S.; Burmester, G.R.; Bykerk, V.P.; Cohen, M.D.; et al. 2010 rheumatoid arthritis classification criteria: An american college of rheumatology/European league against rheumatism collaborative initiative. *Ann. Rheum. Dis.* **2010**, *69*, 1580–1588. [CrossRef] [PubMed]

43. Klindworth, A.; Pruesse, E.; Schweer, T.; Peplies, J.; Quast, C.; Horn, M.; Glockner, F.O. Evaluation of general 16S ribosomal RNA gene PCR primers for classical and next-generation sequencing-based diversity studies. *Nucleic Acids Res.* **2013**, *41*, e1. [CrossRef] [PubMed]

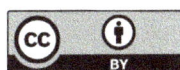

International Journal of
Molecular Sciences

MDPI

Review

The Interplay between Immunity and Microbiota at Intestinal Immunological Niche: The Case of Cancer

Rossella Cianci [1],*, Laura Franza [1], Giovanni Schinzari [2], Ernesto Rossi [2], Gianluca Ianiro [3], Giampaolo Tortora [2], Antonio Gasbarrini [3], Giovanni Gambassi [1] and Giovanni Cammarota [3]

[1] Department of Internal Medicine, Università Cattolica del Sacro Cuore, Fondazione Policlinico Universitario A. Gemelli IRCCS, Largo A. Gemelli, 8, 00168 Roma, Italy; laura.franza01@icatt.it (L.F.); giovanni.gambassi@unicatt.it (G.G.)
[2] Department of Medical Oncology, Università Cattolica del Sacro Cuore, Fondazione Policlinico Universitario A. Gemelli IRCCS, Largo A. Gemelli, 8, 00168 Roma, Italy, giovanni.schinzari@unicatt.it (G.S.); ernestorossi.rm@gmail.com (E.R.); giampaolo.tortora@policlinicogemelli.it (G.T.)
[3] Department of Gastroenterology, Università Cattolica del Sacro Cuore, Fondazione Policlinico Universitario A. Gemelli IRCCS, Largo A. Gemelli, 8, 00168 Roma, Italy; gianluca.ianiro@hotmail.it (G.I.); antonio.gasbarrini@unicatt.it (A.G.); giovanni.cammarota@unicatt.it (G.C.)
* Correspondence: rossellacianci@gmail.com; Tel.: +39-06-3015-5928; Fax: +39-06-3550-2775

Received: 21 December 2018; Accepted: 21 January 2019; Published: 24 January 2019

Abstract: The gut microbiota is central to the pathogenesis of several inflammatory and autoimmune diseases. While multiple mechanisms are involved, the immune system clearly plays a special role. Indeed, the breakdown of the physiological balance in gut microbial composition leads to dysbiosis, which is then able to enhance inflammation and to influence gene expression. At the same time, there is an intense cross-talk between the microbiota and the immunological niche in the intestinal mucosa. These interactions may pave the way to the development, growth and spreading of cancer, especially in the gastro-intestinal system. Here, we review the changes in microbiota composition, how they relate to the immunological imbalance, influencing the onset of different types of cancer and the impact of these mechanisms on the efficacy of traditional and upcoming cancer treatments.

Keywords: gut microbiota; immunological niche; dysbiosis; cancer; immune system

1. Introduction

Mounting evidence has conclusively established that the gut microbiota is involved in the pathogenesis of several medical conditions, such as inflammatory [1,2], liver [3,4], pancreatic [5], and pulmonary diseases [6], neurological [7] and skin disorders [8], and cancer [9–11].

Gut microbiota comprises all of the microorganisms residing in the human intestine, including bacteria, viruses, fungi, archea and protozoa. It contains more than 1000 different bacterial species, over 100 times more than the total number of host cells [12].

Germ-free mice models have shown that the gut microbiota plays some pivotal functions in the development and modulation of several organs and systems, such as the immune and endocrine system, blood, liver and lungs [13]. In the intestine, gut microbiota is able to maintain epithelial homeostasis to support the development of gut associated lymphoid tissue (GALT). Microbiota also enhances epithelial cytokine production, which regulates the action of T and B lymphocytes, macrophages and polimorphs [14,15]. Cytokines, such as interleukin (IL)-1β, tumor necrosis factor (TNF)-α, IL-2, IL-6, IL-15, IL-21, IL-23, can determine an inflammatory response, while others, such as IL-10 and transforming growth factor (TGF)-β, have anti-inflammatory effect. The balance between these two classes is responsible for the overall inflamed or homeostatic status of the gut [16].

In a healthy state, there is a perfect balance between gut microbiota and immune system at gut interface [17]. The breakdown of this physiological balance in microbial composition precipitates a pathological state known as 'gut dysbiosis', contributing to the overgrowth of pathogen bacteria in the intestinal lumen. Dysbiosis is considered a common effector in the different pathogenetic pathways involved in several human diseases [18–20]. Many factors, such as age, hormonal perturbations, diet composition and supplement intake, antibiotic therapies, lifestyle and physical activity exert an impact on gut microbiome and equilibrium [21,22]. Dysbiosis can also be a consequence of an inflammatory status: In genetically susceptible patients, dietary compounds, toxins and antibiotics can start a low-grade inflammation, leading to dysbiosis. In patients suffering from IBD, for example, high calorie and high fat diets, typical of the western world, have been shown to determine a worsening of the inflammatory status of the gut [23].

There appears to be a bidirectional relationship between host immunity and gut microbiota. On one hand, the development of host immunity is mediated by microbiota but, on the other hand, the microbiota itself is constantly modulated by host immunity. This permanent cross-talk between mucosal immunity and gut microbiota is responsible, for example, for the anergy of host immune cells against its own antigens and dietary ones. In fact, microbiota-driven dendritic cells (DC), particularly the CD103+ subset, can induce expression of a subset of T cells with regulatory functions (T-regs) and their related anti-inflammatory cytokines. As well, B-regulatory cells (B-regs) take part in this process, suppressing effector T cells and contributing to the overall process of immune tolerance to food antigens [24].

Here, we review the complex interaction between immune system and microbiota at the gut 'immunological niche' interface and its role in development, growth and spreading of different types of gastro-intestinal cancers.

2. Immune System and Cancer

Cancer and the immune system are inextricably linked. A similar strong interaction between gut microbiota and innate and adaptive immunity has also been established. A complex network of cytokines regulates the interplay between bacteria, viruses, parasites and fungi and mucosal immune cells [12] (Figure 1).

Toll like receptors (TLRs) are a component of innate immunity. They are germline-encoded type I transmembrane receptors, expressed on epithelial cells (e.g., intestinal cells) and on various immune system-related cells (e.g., T-lymphocytes, macrophages and dendritic cells, DCs). TLRs serve as pathogen recognition receptors (PRRs) and recognize pathogen-associated molecular patterns (PAMPs) that are specific and essential for microbes [25]. Among the different TLRs, TLR3 and TLR4 are able to activate both the transcription nuclear factor kappa-light-chain-enhancer of activated B cells (NF-κB) and the interferon regulatory factor 3 (IRF3) that induces interferon-beta (IFN-beta) production [26]. Many others TLRs also lead to the activation of mitogen-activated protein (MAP) kinases p38. This, in turn, increases the expression of many pro-inflammatory genes, via adaptor molecules, such as Myeloid differentiation primary response gene 88 (MyD88), which is able to recruit IRAKs (IL-1R-associated kinase family). The activation of MAP3 kinases follows and determines the activation of NF-κB, c-Jun N-terminal kinase (JNK) and MAP kinases p38.

Studies on MyD88-deficient mice have documented that TLRs' response to PAMPs of commensal bacteria plays a fundamental role in epithelial cell homeostasis [27], induction of antimicrobial peptides [28,29], and in the modulation of the adaptive immune response [30,31]. In contrast, bacteria-activated TLRs may mediate inflammation and carcinogenesis. Indeed, cancer cells present high expression of TLRs [32], while, MyD88-deficient mice are less prone to develop tumors [33]. In this respect, several recent studies [34,35] have pointed towards a tumor promoting function, due to the activation of pro-oncogenic Ras by JNK signaling. This inhibits apoptosis and enhances expression of metallo-proteinases [36].

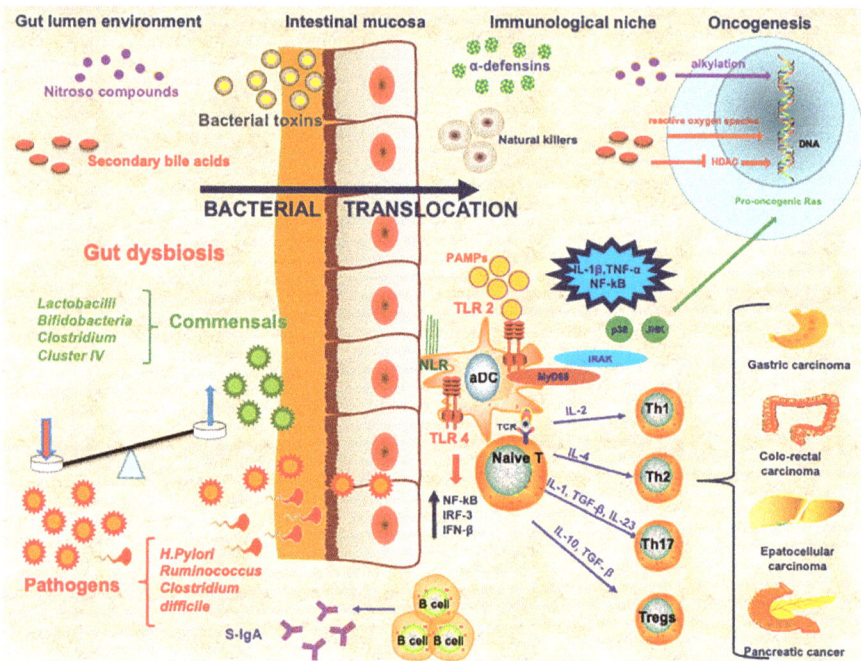

Figure 1. The complex interplay among gut lumen environment, mucosal barrier, immunological niche in oncogenesis. The failure of maintaining homeostatic equilibrium between commensals and pathogens at gut lumen level leads to dysbiosis. The bacterial products enhance the gut permeability leading to bacterial and toxins translocation. Toll-like receptors (TLRs) expressed on activated dendritic cells (aDC) are able to recognize pathogen-associated molecular patterns (PAMPs) and can activate the NF-κB, JNK and p38 mitogen-activated protein kinases. JNK promotes the activation of pro-oncogenic *Ras*. Other receptors situated on several types of immune cells are represented by nucleotide-binding oligomerization domain-like receptors (NLRs), which are pattern recognition receptors (PRRs) that can activate NF-κB and promote inflammasomes. Other carcinogenetic agents, like nitrous compounds and secondary bile acids, can act respectively as alkylating mediators or via reactive oxygen species at a DNA level. Furthermore, high doses of butyrate inhibit histone deacetylase (HDAC) that is able to inactivate many oncogenic signaling pathways. The presence of pro-inflammatory T-cells can induce pro-inflammatory cytokines at tumor site. The concomitant action of T-regs creates a state of immunosuppression at tumor level.

In the 1800s, Virchow described for the first time a large number of lymphocytes (lymphocytes infiltrating tumor or TILs), present at the tumor site [37]. Based on this observation, he hypothesized a role of the immune system in cancer development, growth and spreading.

Only many years later, thanks to technological advances, it was possible to isolate TILs and CD8+ cytotoxic T-lymphocytes (CTLs) from peripheral blood in neoplastic patients. CD8+ CTLs play a pivotal role against cancer because they are able to kill malignant cells upon recognition by T-cell receptor (TCR) of specific antigenic peptides present on the surface of target cells [16]. The existence of a tumor-specific CTLs response was further supported by the identification of tumor-associated antigens (TAA) and by the detection of TAA-specific CD8+ T-cells in spontaneously regressing tumors. Moreover, it has been recently demonstrated that, in colorectal cancer, TILs are predominantly CD4+ T cells and produce pro-inflammatory cytokines, such as IFNγ and IL-17. On the other hand, there is also a subset of CD4+ cells producing IL-4, which appear to favor Th2 phenotype, which seems to favor oncogenesis [38]. Another subset of immune cells presents itself at tumor a site in longer surviving neoplastic patients and is represented by natural killers (NK). These cells are able to trigger tumor apoptosis and inhibit cell proliferation [39].

On the other hand, many studies have shown that at the site of the tumor there is an overall immunosuppressed state. Such condition is obtained by cancer cells themselves through the production of immunosuppressive factors (e.g., TGF-β) and/or by recruiting regulatory immune cells with immunosuppressive functions (e.g., T regulatory cells, T-regs). The prevalence of T-regs and the prognosis of tumors are inversely correlated [40]. T-regs modulate tumor-specific effector T-lymphocytes by producing immunosuppressive cytokines, such as IL-10 and TGF-β, consuming IL-2 or expressing the inhibitory molecule cytotoxic T-lymphocyte associated protein 4 (CTLA-4 or CD 152). T-regs can also inhibit the proliferation of pro-inflammatory subsets of CD4+-T lymphocytes (T-helper or Th) and stimulate B lymphocytes to produce specific immunoglobulins. Th17 and signal transducer and activator of transcription 3 (STAT3) have been implicated in carcinogenesis of various human systems [41,42] by increasing cell proliferation and inhibiting apoptosis [16,43,44]. Th17 produces pro-inflammatory cytokines, such as IL-17 and IL-23 that promote tumor growth [45]. Moreover, Th17 can induce production of Th1-related pro-inflammatory cytokines, chemokine (C-X-C motif) ligand 9 and 10 (CXCL9 and CXCL10), at the tumor site. Th17 cells have similar characteristics to stem cells and are able to renew themselves and, at the same time, they can stimulate the production of Th1-like effectors. The cytokinic environment present at the tumor site influences the different patterns of expression of Th17 cells: In colorectal, hepatocellular and pancreatic cancers, Th17 is associated to a worse prognosis, as it favors immune tolerance towards the tumor, while in ovarian cancer it improves patients' life expectancy [40,46]. In cancer patients, T cells, persistently stimulated by tumor antigens, tend to lose their ability to express cytokines or attack target cells. This phenomenon is known as T-cell exhaustion and is probably the most common mechanism of immune escape [47]. When such condition ensues, the tumor is able to continue growing regardless of the initial immune response [48,49].

3. The Role of Gut Microbiota in Cancer

A growing body of evidence supports the notion that gut microbiota is able to interfere both with cancer development and with response to anti-cancer therapies (Table 1).

Gut microbiota can generate signaling molecules and microbial products, which are potentially toxic for the intestinal mucosal surface [15]. These products increase gut permeability to foreign antigens [5], and a leaky gut facilitates carcinogenesis, mainly, by enhancing inflammation and by influencing gene expression [32]. There is evidence, for example, that the quantity and quality of gut microbial species changes in genetically-predisposed individuals and/or in individuals affected by pre-neoplastic inflammatory disorders [50]. Furthermore, a gut dysbiosis has been documented in association to several tumors. On the other hand, germ-free animal models display a noteworthy reduced cancer incidence and this seems related to the absence of gut dysbiosis and mucosal inflammation [51].

Another important mechanism through which microbiota exerts an anti-neoplastic action is through dietary fibers. Dietary fibers are not metabolized and represent the substrate of saccharolytic fermentation with production of short/chain fatty acids (SCFAs), such as butyrate, propionate and acetate. SCFAs are able to suppress inflammation and expression of pro-carcinogenics and to downregulate tumor growth [52,53]. Lactobacilli and bifidobacteria maintain homeostasis in the gastrointestinal tract [54] and are the principal actors in the fiber fermentation process [55].

Yet, SCFAs are able to bind other bacterial metabolites, like secondary bile acids, that can promote and/or enhance the inflammation, oxidative DNA damage and subsequent carcinogenesis [56] and cancer growth. The different effects of butyrate are determined by its concentration. When present in large quantities, it is able to inhibit cancer cell proliferation, independently from the Warburg effect, through inhibition of histone deacetylase (HDAC), that is able to inactivate many oncogenic signaling pathways [15] and lower doses of butyrate are, instead, capable of inducing histone acetylation and not act as a HDAC inhibitor. Humphreys et al. [57] have demonstrated that butyrate supplementation reduces the level of pro-oncogenic miRNA, such as miR-17-92, in rectal biopsies. Moreover, it promotes the expression of TLR4, MAPK and NF-κB phosphorylation [58]. Butyrate is also linked to the capability to promote the T-regs proliferation and has an immune-modulating role [59,60], overall leading to some controversy on its effect [15]. Other data suggest that colonic cell response to SCFAs may be determined by the expression of caspase and peroxisome proliferator-activated receptor γ (PPARγ), implying that interactions between gut microbiota and the host are heavily influenced by the individual's genetics [61].

Microbiota and host genetics undergo a complex cross-talk, which determines for example that patients with a genetic predisposition may more easily face dysbiosis and have fewer SCFAs-producing bacteria [62].

Gut microbiota composition varies largely with age, lifestyle and lifelong dietary intake but it also modified by medications, especially antimicrobials [63]. The relation between use of antibiotics and development of cancer remains quite controversial. In fact, in an experimental murine model, antibiotics have been shown to arrest tumor progression [32]. On the contrary, recent data lends support to the hypothesis that repeated antibiotic use leads to alteration in microbiota composition, with subsequent pro-carcinogenetic modifications [64] in the gut, mostly pancreas and intestine, but also elsewhere. Penicillin use, in particular, appears to be a risk factor for the insurgence of esophagus, stomach and pancreas malignancies [65].

4. Esophageal and Stomach Cancer

The microbiota of the esophagus is more similar to the oral microbiota than to the intestinal one. In physiological conditions, the esophageal microbial population is characterized by *Firmicutes*, *Bacteroides*, *Actinobacteria*, *Proteobacteria*, *Fusobacteria* and *TM7* and is dominated by the genus *Streptococcus*. Instead, in patients with gastro-esophageal reflux and Barrett esophagus, for example, there is a higher presence of *Bacteroides*, *Proteobacteria* and *Fusobacterium*, and an overall increased diversity, finally resembling more the stomach microbiome [66].

Helicobacter pylori (*Hp*) is considered a class 1 human carcinogen for gastric adenocarcinoma [67]. In gastric samples and in the serum of mice with *Hp* associated gastric cancer, there are increased levels of IL-1, IL-17 and TNF-α, highlighting an enhanced Th17 response [40]. *Hp* has also been associated to low grade gastric mucosa associated lymphoid tissue (MALT) lymphoma and it seems that treating *Hp* in patients with a MALT lymphoma can determine a remission of the lymphoma itself [68,69]. Bacterial overgrowth is typically present in gastric tumors not *Hp*-related [70]. In these patients the continuous cross-talk between different species, particularly *Pasteurella stomatis*, *Dialister pneumosintes*, *Slakia exigua*, *Parvimonas micra* and *Streptococcus anginosus*, probably plays a key role in disease progression [71]. Surprisingly, *Hp* exerts a protective action in esophageal cancer [69]. Although not conclusively explained, this protection could be due to the reduced gastric acid secretion it induces [72].

In general, patients suffering from esophageal and gastric cancer present higher amount of T-regs compared to healthy subjects, especially among patients at advanced stage of disease or with the worst prognosis [73,74]. A recent study has shown that Enterobacteriaceae, in particular *Ruminococcus*, are significantly higher in patients with stomach cancer [56], and it could represent the initial trigger for the altered immunologic status in these patients.

5. Colorectal Cancer

Chen et al. have reported that an imbalance in gut microbiota composition is associated with colorectal cancer [75].

For example, Lactobacillaceae decrease in number in colon cancer patients, while they increase after anti-neoplastic treatment [56]. Indeed, *Lactobacilli* have been shown to block the growth of colon carcinoma [76]. Bifidobacteriaceae are also reduced in patients with rectal tumor and this could lead to a reduced folate synthesis, possibly favoring chromosomal instability. In addition, *Bifidobacterium* exerts a competitive action against pathogens and regulate immune system cells [77].

The pathogens that appear to be primarily involved in the pathogenesis of colorectal cancer [78] are *Streptococcus bovis* (*S. bovis*) [79], *Hp* [80], *Bacteroides fragilis* (*B. fragilis*) [81], *Enterococcus faecalis* (*E. faecalis*) [82], *Clostridium septicum* (*C. septicum*) [83], *Fusobacterium* spp. [84] and *Escherichia coli* (*E. coli*) [85]. Some of these bacteria have a direct carcinogenic effect. This is true for *Hp* or for some strains of *Escherichia coli* that produce colibactin, a genotoxin implicated in the onset of colorectal cancer [86]. Other microbial species act in more subtle ways. Enterotoxigenic *B. fragilis*, for example, appears to play a role in the development of colorectal carcinoma through immune-modulation via Th17. On the other hand, *B. fragilis* can determine metaplasia through the STAT-3 pathway and the strain that produces the *B. fragilis* toxin (BFT) activates the WNT and NF-κB signaling pathways, leading to a chronic inflammatory status [87,88]. *S. bovis* increases the tumors capacity of immunologic escape but it also creates a symbiotic relationship with neoplastic cells, favoring their growth [89]. The role of *E. faecalis* in cancerogenesis is ambiguous: On the one hand it reportedly increases in patients with colorectal cancer [90] and causes an inflammatory status that benefits the tumor through production of ROS, which has a damaging effect on the DNA [91]. On the other hand, it has recently been suggested that the association between colorectal cancer and *E. faecalis* is prevalently due to an altered intestinal environment in patients with colorectal cancer. In this scenario, *E. faecalis* may benefit from an already compromised situation, which allows it to grow undisturbed and uncontrolled, determining an increased virulence, which can further damage the epithelial tissue [92].

Overall, gut dysbiosis acts as a colorectal cancer promoter through a series of mechanisms, which involve immune-modulation, toxins production, metabolic activities and increased oxidative stress and inflammation in the intestinal environment [78].

6. Hepatocellular Carcinoma

The liver does not have its own microbiome and is influenced by gut microbiota metabolites through the entero-hepatic circulation [93].

Although it cannot be formally described as liver microbiota, there are microbial species capable to colonize it, most specifically hepatotropic viruses, such as *hepatitis B virus* (*HBV*) and *hepatitis C virus* (*HCV*). Such viruses increase considerably the risk of developing hepatocellular carcinoma [94]. At least part of this increased risk is explained by a direct action on liver cells through epigenetic mechanisms. *HBV* modifies methylation on p16 (INK4A), glutathione S-transferase P 1 (GSTP1), CDH1 (E-cadherin), *Ras association domain containing protein 1* (RASSF1A), *p21* (WAF1/CIP1) genes, while *HCV* alters methylation on suppressor of cytokine signaling 1 (SOCS-1), growth arrest and damage inducible beta (Gadd45β), O^6-alkylguaniline DNA alkyltransferase (MGMT), STAT1 and antigen presenting cells (APC). As well, effects on histone proteins, chromatin, and noncoding RNAs have been described [95]. In addition, *HCV* is a well-known immune-modulator; in murine models, for example, it increases FAS-mediated apoptosis of T lymphocytes [96]. At the same time, both *HCV* and *HBV* appear to determine gut dysbiosis, that contributes to disease progression [97].

Hepatocellular carcinoma is often a late evolution of a chronic liver disease. Certain gut microbial species seem to either facilitate or slow down such process [98,99]. Bacteria belonging to the *Helicobacter spp* (*pylori* and *hepaticus*, in particular) have been linked to an increased risk of liver cancer. There appear to be various mechanisms through which *H. hepaticus* is able to determine a carcinogenic effect. Not only it can directly damage DNA, activating the WNT and NF-κB signaling pathways in tumor cells, but it also appears to be able to suppress intra-tumor immunity in aflatoxin- and *hepatitis C virus*-induced HCC [100,101]. *Escherichia coli* has also been linked to the development of hepatocellular carcinoma; cirrhotic patients who developed a hepatocellular carcinoma have a microbiome enriched with *E. coli*, when compared to those who did not develop the tumor [102].

It is noteworthy that a leaky gut increases the number of toxins and bacteria potentially reaching the liver. The related state of chronic inflammation can promote non-alcoholic liver disease and fibrosis and could trigger the development of tumors [103]. For example, in obese patients the microbiota is characterized by an increase in *Firmicutes/Bacteroidetes* ratio and by an overall reduction of the number of bacterial species [104,105]. This dysbiosis favors fat storage, leading to a fatty liver and a metabolic syndrome, both established risk factors for hepatocellular carcinoma [106,107].

One of the most studied risk factors for hepatocellular carcinoma is alcohol consumption. Alcohol has a direct toxicity on the liver, but it also has important effects on gut microbiome [108]. Some studies even suggest that restoring and maintaining a normal eubiosis is able to, at least, slow down the progression of alcohol-related liver disease [109]. Yet, evidence is still scarce and further investigations are necessary. On the other hand, *Lactobacillus* species, *Bifidobacterium* species, *Parabacteroides* species, and *Oscillibacter* species, appear to have a protective effect on the liver, through their immune-modulating properties [110].

7. Pancreatic Cancer

Pancreatic adenocarcinoma remains one of the most lethal tumors overall. Several reports have proposed a pathogenetic role of *Helicobacter pylori* in pancreatic cancer [111]. *Helicobacter* seems to activate the NF-κB pathway and its lipopolysaccharide triggers *KRAS* gene mutation, which is present in 90% of pancreatic adenocarcinomas [112–114]. As well, *Hp* may enhance the activator of signal transducer and activator of transcription3 (STAT3) implicated in carcinogenesis through its capacity to promote cellular proliferation and, conversely, inhibit apoptosis [115,116]. Despite this supportive evidence, a recent meta-analysis, based on prospective epidemiologic studies, has not documented a strong association between *Hp* infection and pancreatic cancer [117].

As for the liver, the pancreas does not have its own microbiota. As such, it is foreseeable that the pancreas is influenced by the gut and oral microbiota [118].

In colon samples of patients with pancreatic carcinoma, for example, Youssef et al. have found reduced levels of *Lactobacilli* and *Parabacteroides* [56]. These species have a proven anticancer function, as they reduce TLR4 signaling pathway [119]. Moreover, levels of *Lactobacilli* are restored after anticancer treatment. Another study has linked pancreatic adenocarcinomas to decreased gut microbiota diversity, caused by an increase of LPS-producing bacteria and a decrease of both alpha diversity and butyrate-producing bacteria [63].

Geller et al. found increased levels of Enterobacteriaceae, Pseudomonadaceae, Moraxellaceae and Enterococcaceae in pancreatic cancer tissue [120]. Furthermore, Mei et al. studying the duodenal microbiota of patients with pancreatic cancer identified mostly *Acinetobacter, Aquabacterium, Oceanobacillus, Rahnella, Massilia, Delftia, Deinococcus,* and *Sphingobium*, while healthy controls harbored *Porphyromonas, Escherichia, Shigella* and *Pseudomonas* [111].

More recently, pancreatic cancer has been associated to a particular salivary microbiota. The presence of periodontal pathogens, such as *Porphyromonas gingivalis* (strain ATCC 53978) has been associated with an increased risk of pancreatic cancer, while the opposite is true for the presence of *Neisseria elongate* and *Streptococcus mitis* [121]. Furthermore, Gammaproteobacteria have been linked to pancreatic cancer and when transferred to mice, these bacteria induced gemcitabine resistance [122].

8. The Role of Microbiota in Cancer Therapy

The ability of gut microbiota to modulate the response to cancer chemotherapy and immunotherapy has been first observed in mice [123]. Recently, evidence has emerged revealing that certain clusters of gut microbiota may be related to chemotherapy outcome in several human epithelial solid tumors, such as lung and renal carcinomas, and melanoma [123]. The effects of microbiota on cancer treatment are unlikely due to a single specie but rather to changes in the ecology and metabolism of gut microbiota impacting cancer immunity altogether [124].

Patients who undergo chemotherapy have a higher risk of developing a leaky gut as a direct consequence of chemotherapy itself [125]. Leaky gut and dysbiosis appear to decrease the efficacy of platinum compounds [126]. As well, the effect of other anti-neoplastic agents is modified by gut microbiota composition. *Mycoplasma hyorhinis* and cytidine-deaminase-positive Proteobacteria are able to metabolize and modify gemcitabine, impairing its anti-tumor action and such effect is reversed with antibiotic therapy [120,127]. Likewise, the action of cyclophosfamide is influenced by gut microbiota composition. Bacterial translocation creates an inflamed environment that promotes IFN-γ-producing γδ-T-cells migration in the tumor area [128].

Microbiota appears to also modulate the response to radiotherapy as germ free mice are less susceptible to the toxicity of radiation than conventionally raised mice [126]. Gut microbiota might influence the outcomes of cancer patients who are treated surgically with effects ranging from altered wound healing to permanent dysbiosis, to selection of resistant and virulent microbial species [129].

Anti-neoplastic immunotherapies have been successfully used in melanoma and aim at activating and expanding tumor-specific CTLs, with the goal of destroying primary cancer cells and metastases [130]. The most promising current cancer immunotherapies, utilized not only in melanoma but in several solid epithelial tumors, act on immune checkpoint molecules anti-programmed death 1 (PD-1) and anti-CTLA-4 immunotherapies. PD-1 is an immuno-inhibitory lymphocyte receptor involved in the maintenance of peripheral tolerance to self. The interaction of PD-1 with its ligands, above all PD-L1 (CD274), causes the inhibition of CD8+T cell proliferation, survival and effector functions, and induces the CD4+ to Foxp3 T-cell differentiation increasing immune tolerance. CTLA-4, on the other hand, binds to CD80 or CD86 expressed on the surface of T-lymphocytes, and it causes a state of anergy in these cells. Some tumors (e.g., melanoma, prostate, kidney, lung) have the capacity to stimulate the exhaustion and anergy pathways, which is the main cause of immunologic escape capacity of these malignancies [131]. The PD-1/PD-L1 and the CTLA-4/B7 blockade has been shown to at least partly reverse immune alterations that determine T-cells exhaustion and anergy [132].

Even though these therapies are extremely promising, not all patients respond and some even experience severe side effects [133]. One of the main suspects of the very high variability in patient response is gut microbiome [134]. Marinelli et al. [135] have suggested that different bacterial species are involved in patients' response to immunotherapy. In this respect, germ free mice, for example, are not able to respond to CTLA-4 blockage [136].

Another aspect that needs to be considered is host genetics, which is an important element in determining whether the patient will respond or not to immunotherapy. Patients with a genetically determined T-cell impairment, for example, do not respond well to immunotherapies [137]. Polymorphysms of TLR4 are linked to different outcomes in patients with breast tumors, while other immune-related loci (e.g., TNF-α, NF-κB, Janus kinases (JAK)/STAT proteins, Fc receptors FcγRIII (CD16), nucleotide-binding oligomerization domain-containing protein 2 (NOD2), autophagy related protein 16 (ATG16) and inflammasome pathway proteins) have also been linked to differences in the response to immunotherapy against cancer. Overall, the immune status of the host proves to be the primary factor in determining the response to all anti-neoplastic therapies, both directly and also indirectly through alterations of the gut microbiota [138].

Immunotherapy can increase potentially dangerous bacterial species. Most specifically, it appears to increase the number of *Clostridiales*, and to decrease the number of *Bacteroidales* and *Burkholderiales*, which play a pivotal role in a correct response to therapy. Another central role played by gut microbiota is in the modulation of side effects from immunotherapy. For example, the presence of *Bacteroidetes phylum* appears to have a protective effect against checkpoint-blockade-induced colitis [139]. Overall, CTLA-4 blockage requires the presence of specific bacteria to work, while anti-PD-1 drugs appear to interact only partially with gut microbiota [140].

9. Conclusions

A healthy gut microbiota is fundamental in maintaining homeostasis in the immune system, which is also key in cancer development and response. Still, the full extent of the actions of gut microbiota is not yet completely understood. As we have reported in our review, there are both immune-modulated and direct effects it plays in carcinogenesis of the gastro intestinal tract, not only in districts such as the intestine, but also in the liver and the pancreas, which are not directly colonized by the various microbial species. While some microbial species promote a healthy gut and the correct development of the various components of the immune system, others are even capable of determining malignancies. The importance of gut microbiota has also been demonstrated in the response to therapy, as the metabolic pathways it favors or suppresses can severely affect patients' outcomes. Many studies underline the importance of microbiota in modulating different drugs' effects and, in some cases, being necessary for the chemotherapy agent to have any effect whatsoever. Therapeutic strategies such as surgery and radiotherapy are also influenced by the presence of a healthy gut microbiota.

Overall, modulating the gut microbiota could be beneficial not only for those patients who have cancer, but also as a preventive strategy in the general population. Gut microbiota is a key player in many different diseases and could be targeted specifically in each patient through a precision medicine approach, so to maximize individual benefit, choosing the best therapeutic strategy and taking into account host and tumor characteristics [141].

Table 1. An overview on the most studied gut microbioma species involved in GI cancer.

	Site	Effect	Mechanism	References
Neisseria elongate	Oral	↓↓↓ pancreatic tumor	Promotes oral homeostasis.	[121]
Streptococcus mitis	Oral	↓↓↓ pancreatic tumor	Promotes oral homeostasis.	[121]
Porphyromonas gingivalis (strain ATCC 53978)	Oral	↑↑↑ pancreatic tumor	Promotes oral dysbiosis and inflammation.	[121]
Helicobacter pylori	Stomach, liver, intestine	↑↑↑ gastric liver pancreatic colorectal tumor; ↓↓↓ esophageal tumor	Immune-modulating effect through Th17 pathway; promoting factor for dysbiosis; not clear protective properties in esophageal tumor.	[67,80,97,111,142]
Helicobacter hepaticus	Liver	↑↑↑ liver tumor	Directly damages DNA, through WNT and NF-κB signaling pathways in tumor cells; suppresses intra-tumor immunity in aflatoxin- and hepatitis C virus-induced HCC.	[97,100,101]
Streptococcus bovis	Intestine	↑↑↑ colorectal tumor	Immune-modulating effect; symbiotic relation with tumor cells.	[79,89]
Bacteroidesfragilis	Intestine	↑↑↑ progression colorectal tumor	Immune-modulating effect through TH17 pathway; promotion of WNT, NF-κB and STS-3 pathways; direct effect of BFT toxin.	[87,88,134,143]
Enterococcus faecalis	Intestine	↑↑↑ colorectal tumor	Inflammatory effect through ROS production; increases risk of epithelial damage	[82,92]
Clostridium septicum	Intestine	↑↑↑ colorectal tumor	Inflammatory effect; increases risk of infectious complications.	[83]
Fusobacterium spp.	Intestine	↓↓↓ colorectal tumor; ↑↑↑ esophageal tumor.	Immune-modulating effect. Esophageal dysbiosis marker.	[66,84,144]
Escherichia coli	Intestine, pancreas	↑↑↑ colorectal and liver tumor; ↓↓ pancreatic tumor	Direct epithelial invasion; production of nitrous compounds through eme-metabolism; promotes dysbiosis.	[85,86,102,145]
Lactobacillum spp.	Gastro intestinal apparatus	↓↓↓↓ malignancies	Promotes gut homeostasis; anti-inflammatory effects.	[54–56,76,110]
Bifidobacter spp.	Gastro intestinal apparatus	↓↓↓↓ malignancies; ↓↓ immunotherapy side-effects	Promotes gut homeostasis through competition with pathogens; anti-inflammatory effects.	[54,55,77,110]
Clostridium cluster IV	Gastro intestinal apparatus	↓↓↓↓ malignancies	Promotes gut homeostasis; anti-inflammatory effects.	[55]

Author Contributions: R.C., L.F., G.G., G.C. conceived, planned and wrote the review. G.S., E.R., G.I., G.T., A.G. critically revised the manuscript.

Funding: This research received no external funding.

Conflicts of Interest: The authors declare that there is no conflict of interest regarding the publication of this paper.

References

1. Cammarota, G.; Ianiro, G.; Cianci, R.; Bibbo, S.; Gasbarrini, A.; Curro, D. The involvement of gut microbiota in inflammatory bowel disease pathogenesis: Potential for therapy. *Pharmacol. Ther.* **2015**, *149*, 191–212. [CrossRef] [PubMed]
2. Lopetuso, L.R.; Petito, V.; Graziani, C.; Schiavoni, E.; Paroni Sterbini, F.; Poscia, A.; Gaetani, E.; Franceschi, F.; Cammarota, G.; Sanguinetti, M.; et al. Gut Microbiota in Health, Diverticular Disease, Irritable Bowel Syndrome, and Inflammatory Bowel Diseases: Time for Microbial Marker of Gastrointestinal Disorders. *Dig. Dis.* **2018**, *36*, 56–65. [CrossRef] [PubMed]
3. Bibbo, S.; Ianiro, G.; Dore, M.P.; Simonelli, C.; Newton, E.E.; Cammarota, G. Gut Microbiota as a Driver of Inflammation in Nonalcoholic Fatty Liver Disease. *Mediat. Inflamm.* **2018**, *2018*, 9321643. [CrossRef] [PubMed]
4. Targher, G.; Lonardo, A.; Byrne, C.D. Nonalcoholic fatty liver disease and chronic vascular complications of diabetes mellitus. *Nat. Reviews. Endocrinol.* **2018**, *14*, 99–114. [CrossRef]
5. Pagliari, D.; Saviano, A.; Newton, E.E.; Serricchio, M.L.; Dal Lago, A.A.; Gasbarrini, A.; Cianci, R. Gut Microbiota-Immune System Crosstalk and Pancreatic Disorders. *Mediat. Inflamm.* **2018**, *2018*, 7946431. [CrossRef] [PubMed]
6. Pragman, A.A.; Lyu, T.; Baller, J.A.; Gould, T.J.; Kelly, R.F.; Reilly, C.S.; Isaacson, R.E.; Wendt, C.H. The lung tissue microbiota of mild and moderate chronic obstructive pulmonary disease. *Microbiome* **2018**, *6*, 7. [CrossRef] [PubMed]
7. Cox, L.M.; Weiner, H.L. Microbiota Signaling Pathways that Influence Neurologic Disease. *Neurother. J. Am. Soc. Exp. Neurother.* **2018**, *15*, 135–145. [CrossRef]
8. Abdallah, F.; Mijouin, L.; Pichon, C. Skin Immune Landscape: Inside and Outside the Organism. *Mediat. Inflamm.* **2017**, *2017*, 5095293. [CrossRef]
9. York, A. Microbiome: Gut microbiota sways response to cancer immunotherapy. *Nat. Reviews. Microbiol.* **2018**. [CrossRef]
10. Mao, Q.; Jiang, F.; Yin, R.; Wang, J.; Xia, W.; Dong, G.; Ma, W.; Yang, Y.; Xu, L.; Hu, J. Interplay between the lung microbiome and lung cancer. *Cancer Lett.* **2018**, *415*, 40–48. [CrossRef]
11. Fan, X.; Alekseyenko, A.V.; Wu, J.; Peters, B.A.; Jacobs, E.J.; Gapstur, S.M.; Purdue, M.P.; Abnet, C.C.; Stolzenberg-Solomon, R.; Miller, G.; et al. Human oral microbiome and prospective risk for pancreatic cancer: A population-based nested case-control study. *Gut* **2018**, *67*, 120–127. [CrossRef] [PubMed]
12. Pagliari, D.; Gambassi, G.; Piccirillo, C.A.; Cianci, R. The Intricate Link among Gut "Immunological Niche," Microbiota, and Xenobiotics in Intestinal Pathology. *Mediat. Inflamm.* **2017**, *2017*, 8390595. [CrossRef] [PubMed]
13. Al-Asmakh, M.; Zadjali, F. Use of Germ-Free Animal Models in Microbiota-Related Research. *J. Microbiol. Biotechnol.* **2015**, *25*, 1583–1588. [CrossRef] [PubMed]
14. Geem, D.; Medina-Contreras, O.; McBride, M.; Newberry, R.D.; Koni, P.A.; Denning, T.L. Specific microbiota-induced intestinal Th17 differentiation requires MHC class II but not GALT and mesenteric lymph nodes. *J. Immunol.* **2014**, *193*, 431–438. [CrossRef] [PubMed]
15. Yoon, K.; Kim, N. The Effect of Microbiota on Colon Carcinogenesis. *J. Cancer Prev.* **2018**, *23*, 117–125. [CrossRef] [PubMed]
16. Cianci, R.; Pagliari, D.; Pietroni, V.; Landolfi, R.; Pandolfi, F. Tissue infiltrating lymphocytes: The role of cytokines in their growth and differentiation. *J. Biol. Regul. Homeost. Agents* **2010**, *24*, 239–249. [PubMed]
17. Pagliari, D.; Piccirillo, C.A.; Larbi, A.; Cianci, R. The Interactions between Innate Immunity and Microbiota in Gastrointestinal Diseases. *J. Immunol. Res.* **2015**, *2015*, 898297. [CrossRef] [PubMed]
18. de Oliveira, G.L.V.; Leite, A.Z.; Higuchi, B.S.; Gonzaga, M.I.; Mariano, V.S. Intestinal dysbiosis and probiotic applications in autoimmune diseases. *Immunology* **2017**, *152*, 1–12. [CrossRef]

19. Weiss, G.A.; Hennet, T. Mechanisms and consequences of intestinal dysbiosis. *Cell. Mol. Life Sci.* **2017**, *74*, 2959–2977. [CrossRef]
20. Zeng, M.Y.; Inohara, N.; Nunez, G. Mechanisms of inflammation-driven bacterial dysbiosis in the gut. *Mucosal Immunol.* **2017**, *10*, 18–26. [CrossRef]
21. Mondot, S.; de Wouters, T.; Dore, J.; Lepage, P. The human gut microbiome and its dysfunctions. *Dig. Dis.* **2013**, *31*, 278–285. [CrossRef]
22. Tetel, M.J.; de Vries, G.J.; Melcangi, R.C.; Panzica, G.; O'Mahony, S.M. Steroids, Stress, and the Gut Microbiome-Brain Axis. *J. Neuroendocrinol.* **2017**. [CrossRef] [PubMed]
23. Reddavide, R.; Rotolo, O.; Caruso, M.G.; Stasi, E.; Notarnicola, M.; Miraglia, C.; Nouvenne, A.; Meschi, T.; De' Angelis, G.L.; Di Mario, F.; et al. The role of diet in the prevention and treatment of Inflammatory Bowel Diseases. *Acta Bio-Med. Atenei Parm.* **2018**, *89*, 60–75. [CrossRef]
24. Satitsuksanoa, P.; Jansen, K.; Globinska, A.; van de Veen, W.; Akdis, M. Regulatory Immune Mechanisms in Tolerance to Food Allergy. *Front. Immunol.* **2018**, *9*, 2939. [CrossRef] [PubMed]
25. Janeway, C.A., Jr. The immune system evolved to discriminate infectious nonself from noninfectious self. *Immunol. Today* **1992**, *13*, 11–16. [CrossRef]
26. Kobe, B.; Deisenhofer, J. A structural basis of the interactions between leucine-rich repeats and protein ligands. *Nature* **1995**, *374*, 183–186. [CrossRef] [PubMed]
27. Rakoff-Nahoum, S.; Paglino, J.; Eslami-Varzaneh, F.; Edberg, S.; Medzhitov, R. Recognition of commensal microflora by toll-like receptors is required for intestinal homeostasis. *Cell* **2004**, *118*, 229–241. [CrossRef]
28. Vaishnava, S.; Behrendt, C.L.; Ismail, A.S.; Eckmann, L.; Hooper, L.V. Paneth cells directly sense gut commensals and maintain homeostasis at the intestinal host-microbial interface. *Proc. Natl. Acad. Sci. USA* **2008**, *105*, 20858–20863. [CrossRef] [PubMed]
29. Menendez, A.; Willing, B.P.; Montero, M.; Wlodarska, M.; So, C.C.; Bhinder, G.; Vallance, B.A.; Finlay, B.B. Bacterial stimulation of the TLR-MyD88 pathway modulates the homeostatic expression of ileal Paneth cell alpha-defensins. *J. Innate Immun.* **2013**, *5*, 39–49. [CrossRef] [PubMed]
30. Schnare, M.; Barton, G.M.; Holt, A.C.; Takeda, K.; Akira, S.; Medzhitov, R. Toll-like receptors control activation of adaptive immune responses. *Nat. Immunol.* **2001**, *2*, 947–950. [CrossRef] [PubMed]
31. Medzhitov, R.; Preston-Hurlburt, P.; Kopp, E.; Stadlen, A.; Chen, C.; Ghosh, S.; Janeway, C.A., Jr. MyD88 is an adaptor protein in the hToll/IL-1 receptor family signaling pathways. *Mol. Cell* **1998**, *2*, 253–258. [CrossRef]
32. Schwabe, R.F.; Jobin, C. The microbiome and cancer. *Nat. Rev. Cancer* **2013**, *13*, 800–812. [CrossRef] [PubMed]
33. Rakoff-Nahoum, S.; Medzhitov, R. Regulation of spontaneous intestinal tumorigenesis through the adaptor protein MyD88. *Science* **2007**, *317*, 124–127. [CrossRef] [PubMed]
34. Apidianakis, Y.; Pitsouli, C.; Perrimon, N.; Rahme, L. Synergy between bacterial infection and genetic predisposition in intestinal dysplasia. *Proc. Natl. Acad. Sci. USA* **2009**, *106*, 20883–20888. [CrossRef] [PubMed]
35. Dzutsev, A.; Goldszmid, R.S.; Viaud, S.; Zitvogel, L.; Trinchieri, G. The role of the microbiota in inflammation, carcinogenesis, and cancer therapy. *Eur. J. Immunol.* **2015**, *45*, 17–31. [CrossRef] [PubMed]
36. von Frieling, J.; Fink, C.; Hamm, J.; Klischies, K.; Forster, M.; Bosch, T.C.G.; Roeder, T.; Rosenstiel, P.; Sommer, F. Grow With the Challenge—Microbial Effects on Epithelial Proliferation, Carcinogenesis, and Cancer Therapy. *Front. Microbiol.* **2018**, *9*, 2020. [CrossRef] [PubMed]
37. Balkwill, F.; Mantovani, A. Inflammation and cancer: Back to Virchow? *Lancet* **2001**, *357*, 539–545. [CrossRef]
38. Niccolai, E.; Ricci, F.; Russo, E.; Nannini, G.; Emmi, G.; Taddei, A.; Ringressi, M.N.; Melli, F.; Miloeva, M.; Cianchi, F.; et al. The Different Functional Distribution of "Not Effector" T Cells (Treg/Tnull) in Colorectal Cancer. *Front. Immunol.* **2017**, *8*, 1900. [CrossRef] [PubMed]
39. Zhang, M.; Wen, B.; Anton, O.M.; Yao, Z.; Dubois, S.; Ju, W.; Sato, N.; DiLillo, D.J.; Bamford, R.N.; Ravetch, J.V. IL-15 enhanced antibody-dependent cellular cytotoxicity mediated by NK cells and macrophages. *Proc. Natl. Acad. Sci. USA* **2018**. [CrossRef] [PubMed]
40. Pandolfi, F.; Cianci, R.; Pagliari, D.; Landolfi, R.; Cammarota, G. Cellular mediators of inflammation: Tregs and TH17 cells in gastrointestinal diseases. *Mediat. Inflamm.* **2009**, *2009*, 132028. [CrossRef]
41. Shahmarvand, N.; Nagy, A.; Shahryari, J.; Ohgami, R.S. Mutations in the signal transducer and activator of transcription family of genes in cancer. *Cancer Sci.* **2018**, *109*, 926–933. [CrossRef] [PubMed]
42. Hurtado, C.G.; Wan, F.; Housseau, F.; Sears, C.L. Roles for Interleukin 17 and Adaptive Immunity in Pathogenesis of Colorectal Cancer. *Gastroenterology* **2018**. [CrossRef] [PubMed]

43. Francescone, R.; Hou, V.; Grivennikov, S.I. Microbiome, inflammation, and cancer. *Cancer J.* **2014**, *20*, 181–189. [CrossRef] [PubMed]

44. Pandolfi, F.; Cianci, R.; Pagliari, D.; Casciano, F.; Bagala, C.; Astone, A.; Landolfi, R.; Barone, C. The immune response to tumors as a tool toward immunotherapy. *Clin. Dev. Immunol.* **2011**, *2011*, 894704. [CrossRef] [PubMed]

45. Kryczek, I.; Wei, S.; Szeliga, W.; Vatan, L.; Zou, W. Endogenous IL-17 contributes to reduced tumor growth and metastasis. *Blood* **2009**, *114*, 357–359. [CrossRef] [PubMed]

46. Johnson, M.O.; Wolf, M.M.; Madden, M.Z.; Andrejeva, G.; Sugiura, A.; Contreras, D.C.; Maseda, D.; Liberti, M.V.; Paz, K.; Kishton, R.J.; et al. Distinct Regulation of Th17 and Th1 Cell Differentiation by Glutaminase-Dependent Metabolism. *Cell* **2018**, *175*, 1780–1795. [CrossRef] [PubMed]

47. McCaw, T.R.; Li, M.; Starenki, D.; Cooper, S.J. The expression of MHC class II molecules on murine breast tumors delays T-cell exhaustion, expands the T-cell repertoire, and slows tumor growth. *Cancer Immunol. Immunother.* **2018**. [CrossRef] [PubMed]

48. Wherry, E.J. T cell exhaustion. *Nat. Immunol.* **2011**, *12*, 492–499. [CrossRef] [PubMed]

49. Gupta, P.K.; Godec, J.; Wolski, D.; Adland, E.; Yates, K.; Pauken, K.E.; Cosgrove, C.; Ledderose, C.; Junger, W.G.; Robson, S.C.; et al. CD39 Expression Identifies Terminally Exhausted CD8$^+$ T Cells. *PLoS Pathog.* **2015**, *11*, e1005177. [CrossRef]

50. Bhatt, A.P.; Redinbo, M.R.; Bultman, S.J. The role of the microbiome in cancer development and therapy. *A Cancer J. Clin.* **2017**, *67*, 326–344. [CrossRef]

51. Vannucci, L.; Stepankova, R.; Kozakova, H.; Fiserova, A.; Rossmann, P.; Tlaskalova-Hogenova, H. Colorectal carcinogenesis in germ-free and conventionally reared rats: Different intestinal environments affect the systemic immunity. *Int. J. Oncol.* **2008**, *32*, 609–617. [CrossRef] [PubMed]

52. Louis, P.; Hold, G.L.; Flint, H.J. The gut microbiota, bacterial metabolites and colorectal cancer. *Nat. Rev. Microbiol.* **2014**, *12*, 661–672. [CrossRef] [PubMed]

53. O'Keefe, S.J.; Li, J.V.; Lahti, L. Fat, fibre and cancer risk in African Americans and rural Africans. *Nat. Commun.* **2015**, *6*, 6342. [CrossRef] [PubMed]

54. Zou, S.; Fang, L.; Lee, M.H. Dysbiosis of gut microbiota in promoting the development of colorectal cancer. *Gastroenterol. Rep.* **2018**, *6*, 1–12. [CrossRef] [PubMed]

55. Brownawell, A.M.; Caers, W.; Gibson, G.R.; Kendall, C.W.; Lewis, K.D.; Ringel, Y.; Slavin, J.L. Prebiotics and the health benefits of fiber: Current regulatory status, future research, and goals. *J. Nutr.* **2012**, *142*, 962–974. [CrossRef] [PubMed]

56. Youssef, O.; Lahti, L.; Kokkola, A.; Karla, T.; Tikkanen, M.; Ehsan, H.; Carpelan-Holmstrom, M.; Koskensalo, S.; Bohling, T.; Rautelin, H.; et al. Stool Microbiota Composition Differs in Patients with Stomach, Colon, and Rectal Neoplasms. *Dig. Dis. Sci.* **2018**. [CrossRef] [PubMed]

57. Humphreys, K.J.; Cobiac, L.; Le Leu, R.K.; Van der Hoek, M.B.; Michael, M.Z. Histone deacetylase inhibition in colorectal cancer cells reveals competing roles for members of the oncogenic miR-17-92 cluster. *Mol. Carcinog.* **2013**, *52*, 459–474. [CrossRef] [PubMed]

58. Xiao, T.; Wu, S.; Yan, C.; Zhao, C.; Jin, H.; Yan, N.; Xu, J.; Wu, Y.; Li, C.; Shao, Q.; et al. Butyrate upregulates the TLR4 expression and the phosphorylation of MAPKs and NK-kappaB in colon cancer cell in vitro. *Oncol. Lett.* **2018**, *16*, 4439–4447. [CrossRef]

59. Furusawa, Y.; Obata, Y.; Fukuda, S.; Endo, T.A.; Nakato, G.; Takahashi, D.; Nakanishi, Y.; Uetake, C.; Kato, K.; Kato, T.; et al. Commensal microbe-derived butyrate induces the differentiation of colonic regulatory T cells. *Nature* **2013**, *504*, 446–450. [CrossRef]

60. Chen, J.; Vitetta, L. Inflammation-Modulating Effect of Butyrate in the Prevention of Colon Cancer by Dietary Fiber. *Clin. Colorectal Cancer* **2018**, *17*, e541–e544. [CrossRef]

61. Tylichova, Z.; Strakova, N.; Vondracek, J.; Vaculova, A.H.; Kozubik, A.; Hofmanova, J. Activation of autophagy and PPARgamma protect colon cancer cells against apoptosis induced by interactive effects of butyrate and DHA in a cell type-dependent manner: The role of cell differentiation. *J. Nutr. Biochem.* **2017**, *39*, 145–155. [CrossRef] [PubMed]

62. Chu, H. Host gene-microbiome interactions: Molecular mechanisms in inflammatory bowel disease. *Genome Med.* **2017**, *9*, 69. [CrossRef] [PubMed]

63. Rea, D.; Coppola, G.; Palma, G.; Barbieri, A.; Luciano, A.; Del Prete, P.; Rossetti, S.; Berretta, M.; Facchini, G.; Perdona, S.; et al. Microbiota effects on cancer: From risks to therapies. *Oncotarget* **2018**, *9*, 17915–17927. [CrossRef] [PubMed]

64. Ianiro, G.; Tilg, H.; Gasbarrini, A. Antibiotics as deep modulators of gut microbiota: Between good and evil. *Gut* **2016**, *65*, 1906–1915. [CrossRef] [PubMed]

65. Boursi, B.; Mamtani, R.; Haynes, K.; Yang, Y.X. Recurrent antibiotic exposure may promote cancer formation—Another step in understanding the role of the human microbiota? *Eur. J. Cancer* **2015**, *51*, 2655–2664. [CrossRef] [PubMed]

66. Yang, L.; Chaudhary, N.; Baghdadi, J.; Pei, Z. Microbiome in reflux disorders and esophageal adenocarcinoma. *Cancer J.* **2014**, *20*, 207–210. [CrossRef] [PubMed]

67. Vogiatzi, P.; Cassone, M.; Luzzi, I.; Lucchetti, C.; Otvos, L., Jr.; Giordano, A. Helicobacter pylori as a class I carcinogen: Physiopathology and management strategies. *J. Cell. Biochem.* **2007**, *102*, 264–273. [CrossRef] [PubMed]

68. Begum, S.; Sano, T.; Endo, H.; Kawamata, H.; Urakami, Y. Mucosal change of the stomach with low-grade mucosa-associated lymphoid tissue lymphoma after eradication of Helicobacter pylori: Follow-up study of 48 cases. *J. Med Investig.* **2000**, *47*, 36–46.

69. Cammarota, G.; Fedeli, P.; Bianchi, A.; Cianci, R.; Martino, A.; Fedeli, G.; Gasbarrini, G. Regression of EI2-stage low-grade gastric MALT-lymphoma after H. pylori eradication. *Hepato-Gastroenterol.* **2005**, *52*, 975–977.

70. Wang, L.; Zhou, J.; Xin, Y.; Geng, C.; Tian, Z.; Yu, X.; Dong, Q. Bacterial overgrowth and diversification of microbiota in gastric cancer. *Eur. J. Gastroenterol. Hepatol.* **2016**, *28*, 261–266. [CrossRef] [PubMed]

71. Coker, O.O.; Dai, Z.; Nie, Y.; Zhao, G.; Cao, L.; Nakatsu, G.; Wu, W.K.; Wong, S.H.; Chen, Z.; Sung, J.J.Y.; et al. Mucosal microbiome dysbiosis in gastric carcinogenesis. *Gut* **2018**, *67*, 1024–1032. [CrossRef] [PubMed]

72. Rubenstein, J.H.; Inadomi, J.M.; Scheiman, J.; Schoenfeld, P.; Appelman, H.; Zhang, M.; Metko, V.; Kao, J.Y. Association between Helicobacter pylori and Barrett's esophagus, erosive esophagitis, and gastroesophageal reflux symptoms. *Clin. Gastroenterol. Hepatol. Off. Clin. Pract. J. Am. Gastroenterol. Assoc.* **2014**, *12*, 239–245. [CrossRef] [PubMed]

73. Kono, K.; Kawaida, H.; Takahashi, A.; Sugai, H.; Mimura, K.; Miyagawa, N.; Omata, H.; Fujii, H. CD4(+)CD25high regulatory T cells increase with tumor stage in patients with gastric and esophageal cancers. *Cancer Immunol. Immunother. Cii* **2006**, *55*, 1064–1071. [CrossRef] [PubMed]

74. Ichihara, F.; Kono, K.; Takahashi, A.; Kawaida, H.; Sugai, H.; Fujii, H. Increased populations of regulatory T cells in peripheral blood and tumor-infiltrating lymphocytes in patients with gastric and esophageal cancers. *Clin. Cancer Res. Off. J. Am. Assoc. Cancer Res.* **2003**, *9*, 4404–4408.

75. Chen, J.; Domingue, J.C.; Sears, C.L. Microbiota dysbiosis in select human cancers: Evidence of association and causality. *Semin. Immunol.* **2017**, *32*, 25–34. [CrossRef] [PubMed]

76. Chen, G.Y. The Role of the Gut Microbiome in Colorectal Cancer. *Clin. Colon Rectal Surg.* **2018**, *31*, 192–198. [CrossRef] [PubMed]

77. O'Callaghan, A.; van Sinderen, D. Bifidobacteria and Their Role as Members of the Human Gut Microbiota. *Front. Microbiol.* **2016**, *7*, 925. [CrossRef] [PubMed]

78. Gagnière, J.; Raisch, J.; Veziant, J.; Barnich, N.; Bonnet, R.; Buc, E.; Bringer, M.-A.; Pezet, D.; Bonnet, M. Gut microbiota imbalance and colorectal cancer. *World J. Gastroenterol.* **2016**, *22*, 501–518. [CrossRef] [PubMed]

79. Klein, R.S.; Recco, R.A.; Catalano, M.T.; Edberg, S.C.; Casey, J.I.; Steigbigel, N.H. Association of Streptococcus bovis with carcinoma of the colon. *N. Engl. J. Med.* **1977**, *297*, 800–802. [CrossRef] [PubMed]

80. Zumkeller, N.; Brenner, H.; Zwahlen, M.; Rothenbacher, D. Helicobacter pylori infection and colorectal cancer risk: A meta-analysis. *Helicobacter* **2006**, *11*, 75–80. [CrossRef] [PubMed]

81. Housseau, F.; Sears, C.L. Enterotoxigenic *Bacteroides fragilis* (ETBF)-mediated colitis in Min ($Apc^{+/-}$) mice: A human commensal-based murine model of colon carcinogenesis. *Cell Cycle* **2010**, *9*, 3–5. [CrossRef] [PubMed]

82. Balamurugan, R.; Rajendiran, E.; George, S.; Samuel, G.V.; Ramakrishna, B.S. Real-time polymerase chain reaction quantification of specific butyrate-producing bacteria, Desulfovibrio and Enterococcus faecalis in the feces of patients with colorectal cancer. *J. Gastroenterol. Hepatol.* **2008**, *23*, 1298–1303. [CrossRef] [PubMed]

83. Kwong, T.N.Y.; Wang, X.; Nakatsu, G.; Chow, T.C.; Tipoe, T.; Dai, R.Z.W.; Tsoi, K.K.K.; Wong, M.C.S.; Tse, G.; Chan, M.T.V.; et al. Association Between Bacteremia From Specific Microbes and Subsequent Diagnosis of Colorectal Cancer. *Gastroenterology* **2018**, *155*, 383–390.e388. [CrossRef] [PubMed]

84. Kostic, A.D.; Chun, E.; Robertson, L.; Glickman, J.N.; Gallini, C.A.; Michaud, M.; Clancy, T.E.; Chung, D.C.; Lochhead, P.; Hold, G.L.; et al. Fusobacterium nucleatum potentiates intestinal tumorigenesis and modulates the tumor-immune microenvironment. *Cell Host Microbe* **2013**, *14*, 207–215. [CrossRef] [PubMed]

85. Khan, A.A.; Khan, Z.; Malik, A.; Kalam, M.A.; Cash, P.; Ashraf, M.T.; Alshamsan, A. Colorectal cancer-inflammatory bowel disease nexus and felony of Escherichia coli. *Life Sci.* **2017**, *180*, 60–67. [CrossRef] [PubMed]

86. Arthur, J.C.; Perez-Chanona, E.; Muhlbauer, M.; Tomkovich, S.; Uronis, J.M.; Fan, T.J.; Campbell, B.J.; Abujamel, T.; Dogan, B.; Rogers, A.B.; et al. Intestinal inflammation targets cancer-inducing activity of the microbiota. *Science* **2012**, *338*, 120–123. [CrossRef] [PubMed]

87. Sears, C.L. Enterotoxigenic Bacteroides fragilis: A rogue among symbiotes. *Clin. Microbiol. Rev.* **2009**, *22*, 349–369. [CrossRef] [PubMed]

88. Wu, S.; Rhee, K.J.; Albesiano, E.; Rabizadeh, S.; Wu, X.; Yen, H.R.; Huso, D.L.; Brancati, F.L.; Wick, E.; McAllister, F.; et al. A human colonic commensal promotes colon tumorigenesis via activation of T helper type 17 T cell responses. *Nat. Med.* **2009**, *15*, 1016–1022. [CrossRef]

89. Boleij, A.; Tjalsma, H. The itinerary of Streptococcus gallolyticus infection in patients with colonic malignant disease. *Lancet Infect. Dis.* **2013**, *13*, 719–724. [CrossRef]

90. Zhou, Y.; He, H.; Xu, H.; Li, Y.; Li, Z.; Du, Y.; He, J.; Zhou, Y.; Wang, H.; Nie, Y. Association of oncogenic bacteria with colorectal cancer in South China. *Oncotarget* **2016**, *7*, 80794–80802. [CrossRef]

91. Tjalsma, H.; Boleij, A.; Marchesi, J.R.; Dutilh, B.E. A bacterial driver-passenger model for colorectal cancer: Beyond the usual suspects. *Nat. Rev. Microbiol.* **2012**, *10*, 575–582. [CrossRef] [PubMed]

92. de Almeida, C.V.; Taddei, A.; Amedei, A. The controversial role of Enterococcus faecalis in colorectal cancer. *Ther. Adv. Gastroenterol.* **2018**, *11*. [CrossRef] [PubMed]

93. Adolph, T.E.; Grander, C.; Moschen, A.R.; Tilg, H. Liver-Microbiome Axis in Health and Disease. *Trends Immunol.* **2018**, *39*, 712–723. [CrossRef] [PubMed]

94. Akram, N.; Imran, M.; Noreen, M.; Ahmed, F.; Atif, M.; Fatima, Z.; Bilal Waqar, A. Oncogenic Role of Tumor Viruses in Humans. *Viral Immunol.* **2017**, *30*, 20–27. [CrossRef] [PubMed]

95. Rongrui, L.; Na, H.; Zongfang, L.; Fanpu, J.; Shiwen, J. Epigenetic mechanism involved in the HBV/HCV-related hepatocellular carcinoma tumorigenesis. *Curr. Pharm. Des.* **2014**, *20*, 1715–1725. [CrossRef] [PubMed]

96. Hahn, C.S.; Cho, Y.G.; Kang, B.S.; Lester, I.M.; Hahn, Y.S. The HCV core protein acts as a positive regulator of fas-mediated apoptosis in a human lymphoblastoid T cell line. *Virology* **2000**, *276*, 127–137. [CrossRef] [PubMed]

97. Fox, J.G.; Feng, Y.; Theve, E.J.; Raczynski, A.R.; Fiala, J.L.; Doernte, A.L.; Williams, M.; McFaline, J.L.; Essigmann, J.M.; Schauer, D.B.; et al. Gut microbes define liver cancer risk in mice exposed to chemical and viral transgenic hepatocarcinogens. *Gut* **2010**, *59*, 88–97. [CrossRef] [PubMed]

98. Yu, L.X.; Schwabe, R.F. The gut microbiome and liver cancer: Mechanisms and clinical translation. *Nat. Rev. Gastroenterol. Hepatol.* **2017**, *14*, 527–539. [CrossRef]

99. Mima, K.; Nakagawa, S.; Sawayama, H.; Ishimoto, T.; Imai, K.; Iwatsuki, M.; Hashimoto, D.; Baba, Y.; Yamashita, Y.I.; Yoshida, N.; et al. The microbiome and hepatobiliary-pancreatic cancers. *Cancer Lett.* **2017**, *402*, 9–15. [CrossRef]

100. Krüttgen, A.; Horz, H.-P.; Weber-Heynemann, J.; Vucur, M.; Trautwein, C.; Haase, G.; Luedde, T.; Roderburg, C. Study on the association of helicobacter species with viral hepatitis-induced hepatocellular carcinoma. *Gut Microbes* **2012**, *3*, 228–233. [CrossRef]

101. Sandler, N.G.; Koh, C.; Roque, A.; Eccleston, J.L.; Siegel, R.B.; Demino, M.; Kleiner, D.E.; Deeks, S.G.; Liang, T.J.; Heller, T.; et al. Host response to translocated microbial products predicts outcomes of patients with HBV or HCV infection. *Gastroenterology* **2011**, *141*, 1220–1230. [CrossRef] [PubMed]

102. Grąt, M.; Wronka, K.M.; Krasnodębski, M.; Masior, Ł.; Lewandowski, Z.; Kosińska, I.; Grąt, K.; Stypułkowski, J.; Rejowski, S.; Wasilewicz, M.; et al. Profile of Gut Microbiota Associated With the Presence of Hepatocellular Cancer in Patients With Liver Cirrhosis. *Transplant. Proc.* **2016**, *48*, 1687–1691. [CrossRef] [PubMed]

103. Boursier, J.; Diehl, A.M. Nonalcoholic Fatty Liver Disease and the Gut Microbiome. *Clin. Liver Dis.* **2016**, *20*, 263–275. [CrossRef] [PubMed]

104. Marengo, A.; Rosso, C.; Bugianesi, E. Liver Cancer: Connections with Obesity, Fatty Liver, and Cirrhosis. *Annu. Rev. Med.* **2016**, *67*, 103–117. [CrossRef] [PubMed]

105. Brandi, G.; De Lorenzo, S.; Candela, M.; Pantaleo, M.A.; Bellentani, S.; Tovoli, F.; Saccoccio, G.; Biasco, G. Microbiota, NASH, HCC and the potential role of probiotics. *Carcinogenesis* **2017**, *38*, 231–240. [CrossRef] [PubMed]

106. Bäckhed, F.; Ding, H.; Wang, T.; Hooper, L.V.; Koh, G.Y.; Nagy, A.; Semenkovich, C.F.; Gordon, J.I. The gut microbiota as an environmental factor that regulates fat storage. *Proc. Natl. Acad. Sci. USA* **2004**, *101*, 15718–15723. [CrossRef] [PubMed]

107. Zhou, X.; Han, D.; Xu, R.; Li, S.; Wu, H.; Qu, C.; Wang, F.; Wang, X.; Zhao, Y. A Model of Metabolic Syndrome and Related Diseases with Intestinal Endotoxemia in Rats Fed a High Fat and High Sucrose Diet. *PLoS ONE* **2014**, *9*, e115148. [CrossRef] [PubMed]

108. Lowe, P.P.; Gyongyosi, B.; Satishchandran, A.; Iracheta-Vellve, A.; Ambade, A.; Kodys, K.; Catalano, D.; Ward, D.V.; Szabo, G. Alcohol-related changes in the intestinal microbiome influence neutrophil infiltration, inflammation and steatosis in early alcoholic hepatitis in mice. *PLoS ONE* **2017**, *12*, e0174544. [CrossRef]

109. Hartmann, P.; Seebauer, C.T.; Schnabl, B. Alcoholic liver disease: The gut microbiome and liver cross talk. *Alcohol. Clin. Exp. Res.* **2015**, *39*, 763–775. [CrossRef] [PubMed]

110. Arpaia, N.; Campbell, C.; Fan, X.; Dikiy, S.; van der Veeken, J.; deRoos, P.; Liu, H.; Cross, J.R.; Pfeffer, K.; Coffer, P.J.; et al. Metabolites produced by commensal bacteria promote peripheral regulatory T-cell generation. *Nature* **2013**, *504*, 451. [CrossRef] [PubMed]

111. Mei, Q.X.; Huang, C.L.; Luo, S.Z.; Zhang, X.M.; Zeng, Y.; Lu, Y.Y. Characterization of the duodenal bacterial microbiota in patients with pancreatic head cancer vs. healthy controls. *Pancreatol. Off. J. Int. Assoc. Pancreatol.* **2018**, *18*, 438–445. [CrossRef] [PubMed]

112. Armstrong, H.; Bording-Jorgensen, M.; Dijk, S.; Wine, E. The Complex Interplay between Chronic Inflammation, the Microbiome, and Cancer: Understanding Disease Progression and What We Can Do to Prevent It. *Cancers* **2018**, *10*, 83. [CrossRef] [PubMed]

113. di Magliano, M.P.; Logsdon, C.D. Roles for KRAS in pancreatic tumor development and progression. *Gastroenterology* **2013**, *144*, 1220–1229. [CrossRef]

114. Huang, H.; Daniluk, J.; Liu, Y.; Chu, J.; Li, Z.; Ji, B.; Logsdon, C.D. Oncogenic K-Ras requires activation for enhanced activity. *Oncogene* **2014**, *33*, 532–535. [CrossRef] [PubMed]

115. Yu, H.; Pardoll, D.; Jove, R. STATs in cancer inflammation and immunity: A leading role for STAT3. *Nat. Rev. Cancer* **2009**, *9*, 798–809. [CrossRef] [PubMed]

116. Meng, C.; Bai, C.; Brown, T.D.; Hood, L.E.; Tian, Q. Human Gut Microbiota and Gastrointestinal Cancer. *Genom. Proteom. Bioinform.* **2018**, *16*, 33–49. [CrossRef] [PubMed]

117. Liu, H.; Chen, Y.T.; Wang, R.; Chen, X.Z. Helicobacter pylori infection, atrophic gastritis, and pancreatic cancer risk: A meta-analysis of prospective epidemiologic studies. *Medicine* **2017**, *96*, e7811. [CrossRef] [PubMed]

118. Ertz-Archambault, N.; Keim, P.; Von Hoff, D. Microbiome and pancreatic cancer: A comprehensive topic review of literature. *World J. Gastroenterol.* **2017**, *23*, 1899–1908. [CrossRef]

119. Koh, G.Y.; Kane, A.; Lee, K.; Xu, Q.; Wu, X.; Roper, J.; Mason, J.B.; Crott, J.W. Parabacteroides distasonis attenuates toll-like receptor 4 signaling and Akt activation and blocks colon tumor formation in high-fat diet-fed azoxymethane-treated mice. *Int. J. Cancer* **2018**. [CrossRef]

120. Geller, L.T.; Straussman, R. Intratumoral bacteria may elicit chemoresistance by metabolizing anticancer agents. *Mol. Cell. Oncol.* **2018**, *5*, e1405139. [CrossRef]

121. Michaud, D.S.; Izard, J.; Wilhelm-Benartzi, C.S.; You, D.-H.; Grote, V.A.; Tjønneland, A.; Dahm, C.C.; Overvad, K.; Jenab, M.; Fedirko, V.; et al. Plasma antibodies to oral bacteria and risk of pancreatic cancer in a large European prospective cohort study. *Gut* **2013**, *62*, 1764–1770. [CrossRef] [PubMed]

122. Geller, L.T.; Barzily-Rokni, M. Potential role of intratumor bacteria in mediating tumor resistance to the chemotherapeutic drug gemcitabine. *Science* **2017**, *357*, 1156–1160. [CrossRef] [PubMed]

123. Vetizou, M.; Trinchieri, G. Anti-PD1 in the wonder-gut-land. *Cell Res.* **2018**. [CrossRef] [PubMed]

124. Alexander, J.L.; Wilson, I.D.; Teare, J.; Marchesi, J.R.; Nicholson, J.K.; Kinross, J.M. Gut microbiota modulation of chemotherapy efficacy and toxicity. *Nat. Rev. Gastroenterol. Hepatol.* **2017**, *14*, 356. [CrossRef] [PubMed]

125. Wardill, H.R.; Bowen, J.M. Chemotherapy-induced mucosal barrier dysfunction: An updated review on the role of intestinal tight junctions. *Curr. Opin. Supportive Palliat. Care* **2013**, *7*, 155–161. [CrossRef] [PubMed]

126. Roy, S.; Trinchieri, G. Microbiota: A key orchestrator of cancer therapy. *Nat. Rev. Cancer* **2017**, *17*, 271. [CrossRef] [PubMed]

127. Lehouritis, P.; Cummins, J.; Stanton, M.; Murphy, C.T.; McCarthy, F.O.; Reid, G.; Urbaniak, C.; Byrne, W.L.; Tangney, M. Local bacteria affect the efficacy of chemotherapeutic drugs. *Sci. Rep.* **2015**, *5*, 14554. [CrossRef] [PubMed]

128. Daillere, R.; Vetizou, M.; Waldschmitt, N.; Yamazaki, T.; Isnard, C.; Poirier-Colame, V.; Duong, C.P.M.; Flament, C.; Lepage, P.; Roberti, M.P.; et al. Enterococcus hirae and Barnesiella intestinihominis Facilitate Cyclophosphamide-Induced Therapeutic Immunomodulatory Effects. *Immunity* **2016**, *45*, 931–943. [CrossRef] [PubMed]

129. Guyton, K.; Alverdy, J.C. The gut microbiota and gastrointestinal surgery. *Nat. Rev. Gastroenterol. Hepatol.* **2016**, *14*, 43. [CrossRef]

130. Eggermont, A.M.M.; Dummer, R. The 2017 complete overhaul of adjuvant therapies for high-risk melanoma and its consequences for staging and management of melanoma patients. *Eur. J. Cancer* **2017**, *86*, 101–105. [CrossRef]

131. Buchbinder, E.I.; Desai, A. CTLA-4 and PD-1 Pathways: Similarities, Differences, and Implications of Their Inhibition. *Am. J. Clin. Oncol.* **2016**, *39*, 98–106. [CrossRef] [PubMed]

132. Farkona, S.; Diamandis, E.P.; Blasutig, I.M. Cancer immunotherapy: The beginning of the end of cancer? *Bmc Med.* **2016**, *14*, 73. [CrossRef] [PubMed]

133. Carbonnel, F.; Soularue, E.; Coutzac, C.; Chaput, N.; Mateus, C.; Lepage, P.; Robert, C. Inflammatory bowel disease and cancer response due to anti-CTLA-4: Is it in the flora? *Semin. Immunopathol.* **2017**, *39*, 327–331. [CrossRef] [PubMed]

134. Routy, B.; Le Chatelier, E.; Derosa, L.; Duong, C.P.M.; Alou, M.T.; Daillere, R.; Fluckiger, A.; Messaoudene, M.; Rauber, C.; Roberti, M.P.; et al. Gut microbiome influences efficacy of PD-1-based immunotherapy against epithelial tumors. *Science* **2018**, *359*, 91–97. [CrossRef] [PubMed]

135. Marinelli, L.; Tenore, G.C.; Novellino, E. Probiotic species in the modulation of the anticancer immune response. *Semin. Cancer Biol.* **2017**, *46*, 182–190. [CrossRef] [PubMed]

136. Vétizou, M.; Pitt, J.M.; Daillère, R.; Lepage, P.; Waldschmitt, N.; Flament, C.; Rusakiewicz, S.; Routy, B.; Roberti, M.P.; Duong, C.P.M.; et al. Anticancer immunotherapy by CTLA-4 blockade relies on the gut microbiota. *Science* **2015**, *350*, 1079–1084. [CrossRef] [PubMed]

137. Jenkins, R.W.; Barbie, D.A.; Flaherty, K.T. Mechanisms of resistance to immune checkpoint inhibitors. *Br. J. Cancer* **2018**, *118*, 9–16. [CrossRef] [PubMed]

138. Chen, D.S.; Mellman, I. Elements of cancer immunity and the cancer-immune set point. *Nature* **2017**, *541*, 321–330. [CrossRef]

139. Dubin, K.; Callahan, M.K.; Ren, B.; Khanin, R.; Viale, A.; Ling, L.; No, D.; Gobourne, A.; Littmann, E.; Huttenhower, C.; et al. Intestinal microbiome analyses identify melanoma patients at risk for checkpoint-blockade-induced colitis. *Nat. Commun.* **2016**, *7*, 10391. [CrossRef]

140. Sivan, A.; Corrales, L.; Hubert, N.; Williams, J.B.; Aquino-Michaels, K.; Earley, Z.M.; Benyamin, F.W.; Man Lei, Y.; Jabri, B.; Alegre, M.-L.; et al. Commensal *Bifidobacterium* promotes antitumor immunity and facilitates anti–PD-L1 efficacy. *Science* **2015**, *350*, 1084–1089. [CrossRef]

141. Amedei, A.; Boem, F. I've Gut A Feeling: Microbiota Impacting the Conceptual and Experimental Perspectives of Personalized Medicine. *Int. J. Mol. Sci.* **2018**, *19*, 3756. [CrossRef] [PubMed]

142. Castro, C.; Peleteiro, B.; Lunet, N. Modifiable factors and esophageal cancer: A systematic review of published meta-analyses. *J. Gastroenterol.* **2018**, *53*, 37–51. [CrossRef] [PubMed]

143. Donaldson, G.P.; Ladinsky, M.S. Gut microbiota utilize immunoglobulin A for mucosal colonization. *Science* **2018**, *360*, 795–800. [CrossRef] [PubMed]

144. Browne, H.P.; Neville, B.A.; Forster, S.C.; Lawley, T.D. Transmission of the gut microbiota: Spreading of health. *Nat. Rev. Microbiol.* **2017**, *15*, 531–543. [CrossRef] [PubMed]

145. Gamage, S.M.K.; Dissabandara, L.; Lam, A.K.; Gopalan, V. The role of heme iron molecules derived from red and processed meat in the pathogenesis of colorectal carcinoma. *Crit. Rev. Oncol. Hematol.* **2018**, *126*, 121–128. [CrossRef] [PubMed]

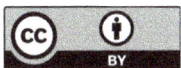

International Journal of
Molecular Sciences

MDPI

Review

Microbiota: Overview and Implication in Immunotherapy-Based Cancer Treatments

Giovanni Brandi * and Giorgio Frega *

Department of Experimental, Diagnostic and Specialty Medicine, Sant'Orsola-Malpighi Hospital, University of Bologna, 40138 Bologna, Italy
* Correspondence: giovanni.brandi@unibo.it (G.B.); giorgio.frega2@unibo.it (G.F.); Tel.: +39-051-2143-838 (G.B.)

Received: 6 March 2019; Accepted: 26 May 2019; Published: 31 May 2019

Abstract: During the last few years, the gut microbiota has gained increasing attention as a consequence of its emerging role as a modulator of the immune system. With the advent of the era of checkpoint inhibitors immunotherapy and adoptive cell transfer (ACT) in oncology, these findings became of primary relevance in light of experimental data that suggested the microbiota involvement as a plausible predictor of a good or poor response. These remarks justify the efforts to pinpoint the specific actions of the microbiota and to identify new strategies to favorably edit its composition.

Keywords: microbiota; microbiome; immunotherapy; adoptive cell transfer (ACT); CAR T-cell; TCR; TIL; checkpoint inhibitors; immuno-oncology; cancer; diet

1. Introduction

In the last two decades, intestinal microbiota, a silent and forgotten, but capital player of health, has finally been recognized in its own role concerning human physiology and pathology.

Initially hypothesized to be limited to the gastrointestinal tract, its role is now suggested to be much larger, including immune-modulatory effects outside the gut and even impacting on several brain functions.

Meanwhile, we experienced the dawn of immunotherapy in the treatment of hematological and solid tumors. The immunotherapies already approved, and the new concept ones, such as cutting-edge types of adoptive cell transfer (ACT) therapy, are promising to gain an ever-increasing relevance within the landscape of cancer treatments.

Here we summarize some general aspects of human microbiome, focusing on specific immunomodulatory functions and on its emerging role as modulator of response to cancer immunotherapies.

2. The Human Microbiota: Overview

Only recently the concept of humans as not merely autonomous eukaryotic organisms, but rather as 'holobiots' (the host plus his connected microbial network) reached the spotlights [1,2].

All in all the human microbiota has been estimated to contain near to 1×10^{14} colonizing bacteria, over one hundred and sixty bacterial species in each individual (of more than one thousand identified), and millions of genes [3–6].

This huge bacterial population may reside within and colonize the gastrointestinal tract (i.e., autochthonous bacteria) or pass transiently through the gastrointestinal tract (i.e., allochthonous bacteria). Autochthonous bacteria should be considered dominant ($>10^7$ CFU/g) or subdominant ($<10^7$ CFU/g) depending on their concentration [7,8]. This is significant because the effect on the host relies on the amount of producing bacteria, especially if mediated by bacterial metabolites [8].

In the large bowel, the anaerobic–aerobic ratio varies, being lower on the mucosal surface and higher in the lumen [9]. The intestine in newborns is sterile, but bacterial colonization quickly occurs with pioneer facultative anaerobes bacteria, coming from the environment and the mother. These microbes burn out the oxygen in the colonic lumen, thereby creating propitious environmental conditions for the spread of strict anaerobes. Actually, the anaerobes will then become the vast majority (dominant population), while the other bacteria will be only metabolically minor players; however, their role in immune regulation cannot be excluded [10,11].

The early colonization and composition of the gut microbiota play a relevant role in shaping the immune system and have delayed consequences, affecting the risk of developing several diseases such as asthma, allergies, and inflammatory bowel disease (IBD) [12]. The real impact of these early-in-life events on risk and treatment of neoplastic diseases has not been completely clarified yet.

The adult human gut tract, as mentioned, hosts an extremely complex and dynamic microbial ecosystem playing a crucial role in the regulation of both enteric and systemic homeostasis. Its composition has been studied by traditional cultural methods for centuries. However, traditional bacterial culture methods permit the culture of a limited portion (<50%) of bacteria [13,14].

Recently, molecular techniques with 16S rRNA or DNA/sequencing/metagenomics approaches provided greater information about both taxonomy and the whole genome of microbiota (so-called microbiome), unraveling several potential functions of gut microbes. The 16S rRNA technique relies on the isolation and sequencing of the 16S rRNA gene, which encodes for the 16 rRNA, the structural component of the small ribosomal subunit. The 16S rRNA gene contains hypervariable regions which lead to a sequence peculiarity among bacterial species [15]. Metagenomics analysis relies on the study of the nucleic acids of a community of organisms extracted from the environment [16]. Metagenomics approaches can be "targeted" to the analysis of a specific region (such as the 16S rRNA gene sequence) or "untargeted" (or "shotgun"), namely on the basis of the sequencing of all microbial genetic material contained in the specimen [17,18]. Unfortunately, these non-culture-based approaches also suffered for several limitations, mainly linked to their specific methods. Furthermore, the molecular approaches do not allow bacterial strains for in vivo experiments using gnotobiotic animal models. In summary, on the one hand, less than 20% of bacteria grown from stool are detectable with metagenomics [19]; on the other hand, a large number of bacteria detected in feces are nonviable. In this context, improved culture methods are still an absolute necessity.

More recently, culturomics approaches that couple cultivation of living bacteria using several culture media with MALDI-TOF for rapid identification of the strain, increase the number of species detectable in the human gut [20]. The definition of taxonomic hierarchy by the operational taxonomic unit (OTU) shows that microbiota is organized along several levels of similarity (from phyla to strains), going from >99% of sequence similarity for bacterial strains to <90% of similarity for phyla levels.

Only limited types of bacteria can colonize the gut. The majority of human bacteria belong to at least four phyla: *Firmicutes*, *Bacteroidetes*, *Actinobacteria*, and *Proteobacteria* [21,22], and to six genera of strict anaerobes: *Bacteroides*, *Eubacteria*, *Bifidobacteria*, *Clostridia*, *Peptostreptococci*, and *Ruminococci*. *Firmicutes* and *Bacteroidetes* are the dominant phyla [22].

Notwithstanding a unique and distinct microbial pattern that every subject has, like an adjunctive fingerprint, intestinal microbiota seems not built in a random fashion, but stratified along main clusters (enterotypes) based on *Bacteroides*, *Prevotella*, and *Ruminococcus* genera. Subdominant bacteria support metabolic profiles of enterotypes, because defined functions are shared among different bacteria indifferently, by their numerousness [23].

A further key point concerns the relationship of the human gut microbiota and the gastrointestinal tract, in terms of both its anatomical distribution and relationships with the mucosa. These aspects are very different in humans and in rodents, and this suggests caution in translating data generated in rodents to human beings [24].

Actually, the bacterial density in the human small bowel is relatively low, increasing from the duodenum ($\approx 10^{1-3}$ CFU/mL) to the ileocecal valve ($\approx 10^{10}$ CFU/mL) and reaching the highest concentration in the colon ($\approx 10^{11-12}$ CFU/mL) [25–27]. Conversely, in rodents, the number of endoluminal bacteria along the whole alimentary tract is less variable. Even the relationship between the microbiota and the intestinal epithelium is different between rodents and humans. First of all, the anatomy of the intestinal tract is significantly dissimilar between the two species. There is a discrepancy in terms of the relative extent of the digestive tract (in relation to the whole body size) [24]. Furthermore, even if the ratio between the entire intestinal surface and the whole body surface is similar [28], it is not the same when focusing on distinct tracts of the gut [29]. The small intestine:colon length ratio and the small intestine:colon surface ratio are more than two times and more than twenty times higher in humans than in mice, respectively [28–30]. There are also great differences in terms of length of the intestinal villi and anatomical structure of the intestinal wall [29]. As in humans, two distinct layers of mucus line the mouse colon epithelium [31]. Much less is known about the bacterial–epithelium interaction in the murine small intestine [32]. Undoubtedly, the epithelial RegIIIγ secretion plays a cardinal role in preserving a spatial separation (approximately 50 μm) between the epithelium and the microbes, as shown by pieces of evidence in Myd88−/−mice [33]. Nevertheless, focusing on this research, it is important to bear in mind that also in wild-type mice the mucosa-associated microbes are not completely absent, even if they are in a significantly lower amount when compared with cohoused Myd88−/− littermates [33].

In rodents, there is probably an intimate relationship between the intestinal mucosa and a large number of bacteria, often found to cluster over the mucus gel or in direct contact with epithelial cells. In humans, such great proximity is lacking.

In particular, human colonic epithelium beneath the mucus layer remains overwhelmingly germ-free under normal conditions [34]. We described this aspect using a scanning electron microscope, afterwards confirmed by different techniques, nearly twenty years ago [35] (Figure 1).

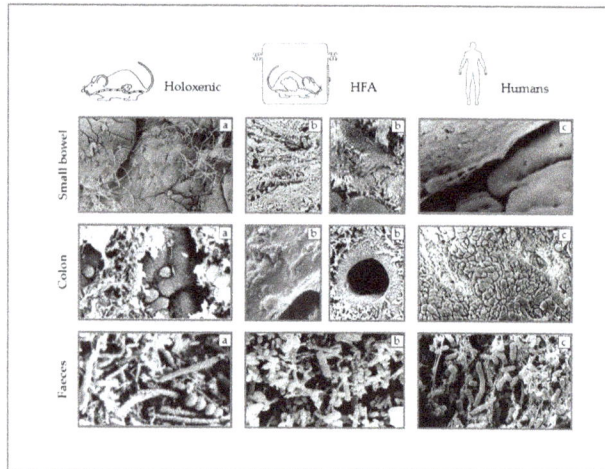

Figure 1. Scanning electron microscopy images of small bowel mucosa, colon mucosa, and fecal bacteria in holoxenic (i.e., raised under conventional circumstances) mice (**a**), HFA (human-flora-associated mice) mice, namely germ-free mice inoculated with components of the human flora (**b**), and humans (**c**).

Intraluminal bacteria are stratified through the existence of a mucous layer and the activity of immunoglobulins (IgA) yielded by plasma cells in the lamina propria and transferred within the gut lumen by transcytoses [36].

The mucus occurs in two distinct physical forms: a thin layer of stable, insoluble mucus gel firmly adhering to the intestinal mucosal surface and a soluble mucus, quite viscous, but that mixes with the luminal juice and plays a crucial role in regulating the relationships between bacteria and the colonic mucosa [31]. The inner stable mucus is impervious for bacteria that, conversely, can be found in the outer loose mucus layer [37]. This latter mucus is continuously secreted and then shed, discarded, or digested by specific bacteria [38].

Moreover, the thickness of mucus in humans (50–450 mm) is approximately double that in rodents. It is the mucus layer, together with the innate immune system that, at least in mice, actively contains microbiota, mainly in the lumen, limiting penetration into the mucosa and avoiding excessive pro-inflammatory signaling [39]. FISH analysis of colon biopsies of healthy subjects confirmed that the number of bacteria on the mucosa is also lower (<10^7 CFU) than in feces and large zones of the mucus layer are often free from bacteria [40–43].

Clearly, it will be impossible and counterproductive (as showed by germ-free animal experiments) to obtain persistent and complete isolation along of the entire size of the intestinal surface. Physiologically, commensals can induce the secretion of mucin and antibacterial peptide (such as defensins) by epithelial cells, the recruitment of immune cells to the mucosa, and the maturation of GALT (Gut-Associated Lymphoid Tissue) [25,44]. These microbes can also sometimes reach the lamina propria, where they are sampled and removed by means of macrophages or dendritic-cells-mediated phagocytosis.

Bacteria can persist alive within dendritic cells and induce a mucosal IgA immune response [45]. Live-carried bacteria can induce a stronger IgA plasma cells response than killed ones [25]. Loaded dendritic cells are then confined by mesenteric lymph nodes and cannot roll in the other systemic secondary lymphoid tissues [25,45].

Mucus likely plays an indirect role also in microbiota-related GALT genesis and even in immunity response at distance from the GI tract. The immune system is organized at various levels (molecular, cellular, and systemic) in order to discriminate among a range of stimuli [46], some of which are able to provoke or activate a response leading to immunity (for pathogens, neoplastic, and grafted cells) and inhibit some others, leading to tolerance for both normal microbiota and dietary antigens.

3. Microbiota: Physiological Fluctuations and Induced Disruptions

The microbiota has different characteristics during life, and these changes, in physiological conditions, are mainly driven by diet changes. During childhood, *Bifidobacteria* initially dominate the microbiota [47,48], countering the pro-inflammatory environment typical of the gastrointestinal (GI) tract at this stage of life. In adults, the microbiota is mainly represented by *Firmicutes* and *Bacteroides*, able to provide SCFA (short-chain fatty acids) to the host, digesting plant polysaccharides (otherwise indigestible), thus increasing the ability to extract energy from the diet [49].

In old age, there is a progressive loss of bacterial biodiversity, with an increase in pathobionts (as *Fusobacteria*) and a rearrangement of bacteria producing butyrate (*F. prausnitzii/Roseburia* vs. *Eubacterium limosum*) [50]. In centenarians, bacterial clusters are selected that potentially may interfere with the immune response (*Akkermansia* and *Christensenellaceae*) [51,52].

Although these physiological changes in microbiota composition during life are related to diet changes, recently it has been suggested that other factors may be involved: the geographic origin of the subject and ethnicity [53,54].

Finally, additional conditions may induce dysbiosis, such as the use of antibiotics. The latter deeply impacts the bacterial ecology of the gut. A five-day treatment with broad-spectrum antibiotics, administered to healthy subjects, may induce depletion of some bacterial strains (*Bifidobacteria*) and an explosion of pathobionts (*E. faecalis* and *F. nucleatum*) [55]. The same authors also reported that more than a month is required to restore a near-previous composition and a few common species remain undetectable longer [55]. These disruptions can probably strongly interfere with the systemic immune response [56].

4. Digest on Immuno-Oncology Landscape

Immunoescape is one of the hallmarks of cancers [57]. Cancer cells are able to generate an immunosuppressive microenvironment that allows them to grow and to avoid immune destruction. Nevertheless, the immune system does not have a passive role in tumor evolution. The immunoediting hypothesis (elimination, equilibrium, escape) confers to the immunity the ability to sculpt the immunologic phenotype of the tumor [58]. According to this, cancers acquire an immuno-imprinted habitus that confers them an evolving ability to suppress or to escape from the immune system [58].

Since the first FDA (Food and Drug Administration) approval of ipilimumab in melanoma patients in 2011, checkpoint inhibitors revolutionized the landscape of cancer treatments. These treatments basically target proteins that physiologically suppress the immune system, avoiding abnormal immune responses. In addition to the already approved anti-CTL4-mAb and anti-PD-1/PD-L1-mAbs, other innovative agents aimed at activating the antitumor T-cell response or targeting other inhibitory receptors (e.g., Tim-3, VISTA or Lag-3) are currently under investigation in solid tumors [59,60].

Unfortunately, despite the exciting, durable response sometimes obtainable, not all patients and not all malignancies are susceptible to immunotherapy to date.

The reasons for the lack of response of some tumors are not completely understood, even if probably it mostly depends on defects in antigenicity and adjuvanticity, which are keys factor in shaping the immunogenicity of tumor cells [61]. To date, several biomarkers (PD-L1 expression, tumor-infiltrating lymphocytes, mutational burden, immune gene signatures, etc.) have been proposed, even if they are not always predictive alone due to lack of sensibility or sensitivity [62]. The level of somatic mutations seems to be a crucial factor. Tumors with a high number of somatic mutations (i.e., melanomas and smoking lung cancers) are more responsive than low rate ones (i.e., gastrointestinal cancers and breast) [63].

Adoptive cell therapy (ACT) is a new and promising strategy to immunologically fight cancer. Only a few months ago, the FDA approved autologous T cells (elaborated to express a chimeric anti CD-19 B lymphocyte antigen) for the treatment of diffuse large B-cell lymphoma and acute lymphoblastic leukemia (children and young adults) in relapsed or refractory setting [64].

This groundbreaking weapon lies in the patient's leukapheresis, T-cell engineering on the bench to express a chimeric antigen receptor (CAR) specific against a defined tumoral antigen, and finally reinfusion, usually after preconditioning lymphodepletion. A similar strategy consists of reinfusion of T-cell receptor (TCR)-engineered T cells, which possess a genetically modified receptor brought against tumoral antigens and comparable to a natural T-cell receptor (Figure 2).

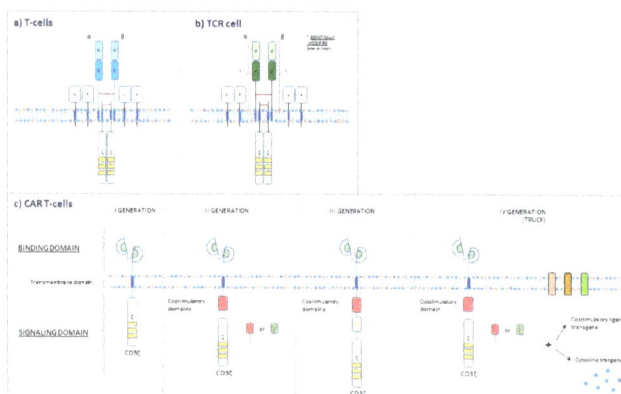

Figure 2. (a) T-cell receptor on the surface of T cell, (b) engineered T-cell receptor on the surface of engineered T cell (TCR cell), (c) Four generations of chimeric antigen receptor (CAR) T cells. I generation: the intracellular signaling domain alone (CD3 ζ-chain). II generation: one costimulatory domain and the intracellular signaling domain. III generation: two costimulatory domains and the intracellular signaling domain. IV generation: costimulatory domain(s), the intracellular signaling domain, and activity enhancing factors (e.g., cytokines, co-stimulatory ligands).

The availability of ever-honed gene-editing technologies promises to lead to further evolutions, such as the development of allogeneic T cells generated by healthy donors [65]. Furthermore, newly developed CAR T cells such as tandem CAR T cell (which harbor two ligand-binding domains), multi-CAR T cells (which harbor different chimeric antigen receptors), built-in-CAR T cells (which are modified to release anti-PD-L1 antibodies within the tumor), and many others have already been generated, mainly with the aim to potentiate the efficacy or reduce the toxicities [66–68].

Unfortunately, this approach seems not to be equally effective in hematological and nonhematological malignancies, mainly due to the absence of properly tumoral-specific antigens and to surface cellular antigens heterogeneity [69]. Moreover, even achieving a potent antitumoral efficacy, there remains the issue of serious adverse events, notably in brain tumors [70]. Despite that, the advances in the knowledge of cancers immunogenetics, tumoral antigens, and the advent of new technologies to curtail side effects will favor the advent of these therapeutic approaches.

Further cell therapies, based on the reinfusion of autologous tumoral-infiltrating lymphocytes (TIL) or autologous/engineered natural killer cells (NK) expanded in vitro after patient's systemic lymphodepletion, showed encouraging results in some cancer types and appear more promising in the foreseeable future, even if the proper sequence and the real gain with respect to other disposable immunotherapies will have to be defined [71,72].

Adoptive therapy with tumoral-infiltrating lymphocytes, screened for their activity against mutant cancer proteins, and then amplified, seems to be able to achieve striking responses in selected patients, even if these therapies are at the dawn [73,74].

Furthermore, the considerable researches that foster these approaches are allowing unique somatic mutations (specific of each singular malignancy and hardly ever shared between and also within distinct cancer types) to be identified that can lead an anti-tumoral response [75].

Finally, along the lines of what happens with checkpoint inhibitors, not all subjects respond well to these futuristic treatments to date and some patients explore relevant toxicities [76,77].

5. Microbiota: Implications in Immuno-Oncology

As mentioned above, the intestinal immune system probably has the heaviest and the most fragile task within the entire host immune system, facing a huge amount of alimentary and microbial antigens during the entire lifetime.

The vast majority of the current knowledge on microbiota as an immune system modulator originates from germ-free animal model studies. These animals are raised under sterile conditions and the following exposure to single or small microbial communities (gnotobiotic animals) allow the investigations on the interactions between each species and the host [36].

Data obtained by this type of research showed how some bacteria (*Clostridium* cluster 4 and 14) may enhance the anti-inflammatory branches of the adaptive immune system, inducing a peripheral expansion of Foxp3+ Tregs [78,79]. These regulatory T cells (Tregs) are able to produce IL-10 (and other molecules such as CTLA-4, IL-2, IL-10, TGF-β, IL-35, and more) thus leading to immune-tolerance and immunosuppression [80,81]. In light of this, these lymphocytes play a key role in maintaining the immunological self-tolerance, preventing autoimmunity [81]. By way of example, Tregs-derived IL-10 cytokine exerts a key role in safeguarding the right immune balance at the sites of environmental exposed surfaces (i.e., lung and gut) [80]. The role of Tregs in cancer is likewise crucial. Several preclinical pieces of evidence showed how these cells are able to hamper the immune response against cancer [82,83]. Consequently, Tregs are considered an attractive target for cancer immunotherapies [81]. Furthermore, a recent study suggested that PD-1+ regulatory T cells could be responsible for hyper-progression to anti–PD-1 immunotherapy [84].

Conversely, the pro-inflammatory component of GALT is induced in rodents from SFB that alone are able to replace the whole activity of microbiota for this specific characteristic [85]. These bacteria have the ability to penetrate the epithelium of both the small intestine and cecum of rodents, not only on the Peyer's patches, but also elsewhere (Figure 3).

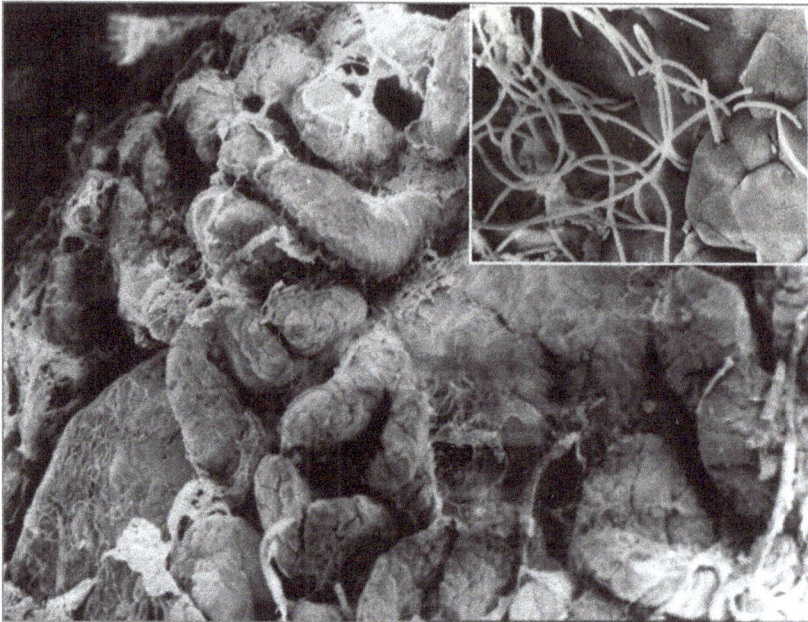

Figure 3. Scanning electron microscopy images, showing SFB (segmented filamentous bacteria) inside and outside the Peyer's patches.

In this way, they lead to IL-17, IL-23, and IL-6 release by dendritic cells, as well as to T-helper 17 recruitment. These bacteria play a pivotal role in the GALT formation in rodents, however, they have never been detected in adult human microbiota [86]. Conversely, some recent reports suggest their existence and their potential role at an early age [87].

Furthermore, the belief that organs and tumors are absolutely sterile sanctuaries has recently collapsed [88]. Some bacterial species have been established to be able to accompany the neoplastic growth of colon–rectal cancers and to migrate in metastatic sites [89]. Moreover, recent data showed that an unexpected presence of bacteria within tumor tissue, even in malignancies beyond the gastrointestinal tract, could modulate the immune response by inducing immune suppression. For instance, the endogenous microbial population in pancreatic ductal adenocarcinoma, which is more abundant than in a normal pancreas, suppresses monocytic differentiation, so inducing T-cell anergy [90]. Similarly, *Fusobacterium nucleatum* has been detected in certain colon cancers, both in primitive tumors and in liver metastases, and has been reported to correlate with a worse prognosis [91]. Furthermore, antibiotic treatments delay the tumor growth of patients' xenograft mice-derived from *F. nucleatum*-positive colon rectal tumors [89]. It has also been described that *F. nucleatum* can interact with receptors of the innate immune system (TLR4) by modulating autophagy, by decreasing apoptosis and by inducing chemoresistance [92].

The role of intratumoral bacteria as a potential reason for chemoresistance could also result from bacterial metabolic functions, as reported for gemcitabine in a colon cancer mouse model [93]. A previous study showed the ability of certain bacteria to influence (to impair but also to improve) the efficacy of chemotherapeutic agents in vitro [94]. The same authors validated the negative impact of intratumoral bacteria on the efficacy of a sample drug (i.e., gemcitabine) in vivo [94]. These findings are credibly expected to outbreak new frontiers in the fields of cancer-immune-escape mechanisms and drug resistance.

Moving on to the anti-cancer immune response, about ten years ago a group of scientists described how microbiota or, more precisely, some subdominant bacterial species can induce the recruitment of T cells within organs in mice [95]. Other studies revealed the importance of microbiota in modulating the efficacy of certain chemotherapies (i.e., oxaliplatin, cyclophosphamide) by promoting an immune response against the tumor [96,97].

Along these lines, Sivan A. and coauthors formulated the hypothesis and elegantly demonstrated how microbiota could also play a major role in shaping the anticancer immune response and tumor growth. Genetically identical mice imported from two different facilities (and consequently with different microbiota composition) displayed a dissimilar response to immunotherapy. Conversely, no differences were reported by cohousing mice. Furthermore, direct administration of *Bifidobacterium spp.* improves tumor-specific immunity and response to anti-PD-L1 immunotherapy by activating intratumoral antigen-presenting cells [98]. An analogous research revealed the lack of response to CTLA-4 blockade in antibiotic-treated or germ-free mice and allowed the identification of bacterial species (i.e., *Bacteroides fragilis*) related to the response [99].

Afterwards, three research teams confirmed these data in humans, reporting the unexpected role of specific members of the gut microbiota as a predictor of response to immunotherapy in a distinctive series of epithelial tumors (NSCLC, renal cell carcinoma, and urothelial carcinoma) and melanoma patients [100–102]. Unfortunately, the bacteria genera or species accompanied with the responder phenotype can only partially be matched among these studies [103].

Moreover, the phenotype of responders or nonresponders can be transferred by performing a fecal microbiota transplantation procedure, namely conventionalizing germ-free or antibiotic-pretreated mice with the feces of responder or nonresponder patients [100–102]. Similarly, an oral supplementation with specific bacteria (i.e., *Akkermansia muciniphila*) can restore the phenotype of responders in avatar mice obtained from non-responder patients [100].

It is interesting that bacteria involved in the response to checkpoint inhibitors resemble those eating mucin (e.g., *B. longum* or *A. muciniphila*). Theoretically, mucus-eating bacteria could expose a part of the epithelium to themselves or other bacteria, or their antigens [104], thus triggering a proinflammatory response also at a distance.

Zitvogel L. et al. [19] hypothesized different plausible mechanisms of immunostimulation by intestinal bacteria including cross-reactions between microbial and tumor antigens, stimulation of pattern-recognition receptors (PRRs), and production of bacterial metabolites that might exert systemic modulatory effects.

In light of the recent findings of the microbiota as a significant modulator of response to immune checkpoint blockers, it will be interesting to explore the impact of our gut ecosystem on the new concept T-cell-based immunotherapies. Recently, some teams are publishing pioneering works in this field. The gut microbiome and antibiotic therapy appear to impact on the response to adoptive cell therapies in murine models [105,106]. Preliminary data on hematological and solid tumor case series seems to validate this data [107].

Collectively, these and further findings could be deeply significant in order to define plausible combination therapies with microbiota-modulating drugs/foods and the optimal timeline of treatments, given that patients who access this therapy are currently highly pretreated with chemotherapies or other "microbiota-disrupting" therapies. In light of the huge impact of the microbiota on immune system functions and on systemic immune balance, the modulations of its composition or the use of bacterial bioactive compounds, once identified, might gain greater prominence as underpinning therapy to boost the efficacy, or to curtail the toxicities of already available and future immunotherapies [19].

Plausible strategies to fine-tune the microbiota encompass dietary refinement, avoiding improper use of antibiotics, fecal microbial transplantations, and the administrations of prebiotics/probiotics [19,108].

Evidence in mice and human revealed the impact of diet in modulating our microbiome. Intestinal enterotypes are profoundly shaped by long-term diet habits. A prevalence of *Bacteroides* genus and *Prevotella* genus has been associated with an animal protein/fat-based diet and with a plant carbohydrates-based diet, respectively [109]. Furthermore, modifications induced by diet variation occur in a short amount of time [110]. This could impact in modulating the amount of "good" or "bad" bacterial species.

Along these lines, variations in fiber intake can affect the production of short-chain fatty acids (SCFA) and the proportion of potentially beneficial species such as *Faecalibacterium prausnitzii* and *Roseburia spp.* [111]. In particular, SCFA can directly impact on systemic immune regulation through G protein–coupled receptor 43 (GPR43) interaction [112]. Analogously, ω-3 fatty acids can modulate inflammation and insulin sensitivity, interacting with the G protein-coupled receptor 120 (GPR120) [113,114]. These polyunsaturated fatty acids seem also able to induce a transitory increase of some SCFA-producer bacterial genera and to potentially act in restoring eubiosis [115,116].

In view of the above, other modifications of dietary compositions in terms of micro/macronutrient may directly, processed by microbiota or via secondary bacterial/hepatic metabolites, modulate the immune functions and the response to malignant or infectious diseases.

Furthermore, the potential beneficial or noxious effect of nutrients or modern diet habits and subsequently their potential in favorably or detrimentally reshaping the gut compositions will require a closer focus in view of the conceivable implications [117,118].

Preliminary data suggest how lifestyle habits, more specifically diet fiber intake, could impact in terms of odds of response to anti-PD-1 treatment [119].

A further approach could consist of administrating probiotics before, during, or after potentially "microbiota-disrupting" or "microbiota-modulated" treatments. Many trials are currently exploring the effects of these approaches in limiting treatments toxicities, modifying the intratumoral immune response and even impacting on survival outcomes [108].

Focusing on antibiotics, a recent retrospective analysis confirmed how antibiotic treatment prior to immunotherapy (but not concurrently) negatively impacts in terms of overall survival and response rate in cancer patients treated with anti-PD-1/PD-L1 checkpoint inhibitors [120]. Clearly, the infections (respiratory infections were the most common site of infection in the previous series) themselves can exert a negative impact on the outcome of patients (especially in terms of overall survival), but the effect on tumoral response and the great difference reported in terms of survival justify a greater effort to mechanistically understand the reasons of these evidences.

Finally, fecal microbiota transplantation (FMT), which has achieved promising results in the treatment of *Clostridium difficile* infections or refractory IBDs, is going to be evaluated to obtain a recovery of the microbial ecosystem after disrupting treatment such as intensive chemotherapy or allogeneic hematopoietic cell transplantation (NCT03678493), to treat patients with refractory and acute graft versus host disease (NCT03549676, NCT03492502) or to foster the response to immunotherapies in previously "nonresponders" patients (heterologous fecal transplantation from "good-responders") (NCT03353402) [121–123].

Author Contributions: G.B. and G.F. equally contributed to the review.

Funding: This research received no external funding.

Conflicts of Interest: The authors declare no conflict of interest.

Abbreviations

cfu	colony-forming unit
Tregs	Regulatory T Cells
GALT	Gut-associated lymphoid tissue
CTLA-4	CTLA-4 (Cytotoxic T-Lymphocyte Antigen 4)
PD-1	Programmed cell death protein-1
PD-L1	Programmed cell death-ligand 1
mAbs	Monoclonal antibodies
SFB	Segmented filamentous bacteria
PRRs	Pattern-recognition receptors
TLR4	Toll-like receptor 4

IBD	Inflammatory bowel disease
CAR T	Chimeric antigen receptors T-cell
TCR	T-cell receptor engineered T-cell
SCFA	short-chain fatty acids
FDA	food and drug administration

References

1. Bordenstein, S.R.; Theis, K.R. Host Biology in Light of the Microbiome: Ten Principles of Holobionts and Hologenomes. *PLoS Biol.* **2015**, *13*, e1002226. [CrossRef] [PubMed]
2. Postler, T.S.; Ghosh, S. Understanding the Holobiont: How Microbial Metabolites Affect Human Health and Shape the Immune System. *Cell Metab.* **2017**, *26*, 110–130. [CrossRef] [PubMed]
3. Sender, R.; Fuchs, S.; Milo, R. Are We Really Vastly Outnumbered? Revisiting the Ratio of Bacterial to Host Cells in Humans. *Cell* **2016**, *164*, 337–340. [CrossRef] [PubMed]
4. Qin, J.; Li, R.; Raes, J.; Arumugam, M.; Burgdorf, K.S.; Manichanh, C.; Nielsen, T.; Pons, N.; Levenez, F.; Yamada, T.; et al. A human gut microbial gene catalogue established by metagenomic sequencing. *Nature* **2010**, *464*, 59–65. [CrossRef] [PubMed]
5. Lloyd-Price, J.; Mahurkar, A.; Rahnavard, G.; Crabtree, J.; Orvis, J.; Hall, A.B.; Brady, A.; Creasy, H.H.; McCracken, C.; Giglio, M.G.; et al. Strains, functions and dynamics in the expanded Human Microbiome Project. *Nature* **2017**, *550*, 61–66. [CrossRef] [PubMed]
6. Gill, S.R.; Pop, M.; DeBoy, R.T.; Eckburg, P.B.; Turnbaugh, P.J.; Samuel, B.S.; Gordon, J.I.; Relman, D.A.; Fraser-Liggett, C.M.; Nelson, K.E. Metagenomic Analysis of the Human Distal Gut Microbiome. *Science* **2006**, *312*, 1355–1359. [CrossRef] [PubMed]
7. Mariat, D.; Firmesse, O.; Levenez, F.; Guimarães, V.; Sokol, H.; Doré, J.; Corthier, G.; Furet, J.-P. The Firmicutes/Bacteroidetes ratio of the human microbiota changes with age. *BMC Microbiol.* **2009**, *9*, 123. [CrossRef] [PubMed]
8. Bergogne-Berezin, E. *Microbial Ecology and Intestinal Infections*; Springer Science & Business Media: Berlin, Germany, 2013; ISBN 978-2-8178-0922-9.
9. Eckburg, P.B.; Bik, E.M.; Bernstein, C.N.; Purdom, E.; Dethlefsen, L.; Sargent, M.; Gill, S.R.; Nelson, K.E.; Relman, D.A. Diversity of the Human Intestinal Microbial Flora. *Science* **2005**, *308*, 1635–1638. [CrossRef]
10. Nicholson, J.K.; Holmes, E.; Kinross, J.; Burcelin, R.; Gibson, G.; Jia, W.; Pettersson, S. Host-Gut Microbiota Metabolic Interactions. *Science* **2012**, *336*, 1262–1267. [CrossRef]
11. Fanaro, S.; Chierici, R.; Guerrini, P.; Vigi, V. Intestinal microflora in early infancy: Composition and development. *Acta Paediatr.* **2003**, *92*, 48–55. [CrossRef]
12. Gensollen, T.; Iyer, S.S.; Kasper, D.L.; Blumberg, R.S. How colonization by microbiota in early life shapes the immune system. *Science* **2016**, *352*, 539–544. [CrossRef] [PubMed]
13. Goodman, A.L.; Kallstrom, G.; Faith, J.J.; Reyes, A.; Moore, A.; Dantas, G.; Gordon, J.I. Extensive personal human gut microbiota culture collections characterized and manipulated in gnotobiotic mice. *Proc. Natl. Acad. Sci. USA* **2011**, *108*, 6252–6257. [CrossRef] [PubMed]
14. Rettedal, E.A.; Gumpert, H.; Sommer, M.O.A. Cultivation-based multiplex phenotyping of human gut microbiota allows targeted recovery of previously uncultured bacteria. *Nat. Commun.* **2014**, *5*, 4714. [CrossRef] [PubMed]
15. Chakravorty, S.; Helb, D.; Burday, M.; Connell, N.; Alland, D. A detailed analysis of 16S ribosomal RNA gene segments for the diagnosis of pathogenic bacteria. *J. Microbiol. Methods* **2007**, *69*, 330–339. [CrossRef] [PubMed]
16. Hugenholtz, P.; Tyson, G.W. Microbiology: Metagenomics. *Nature* **2008**, *455*, 481–483. [CrossRef] [PubMed]
17. Quince, C.; Walker, A.W.; Simpson, J.T.; Loman, N.J.; Segata, N. Shotgun metagenomics, from sampling to analysis. *Nat. Biotechnol.* **2017**, *35*, 833–844. [CrossRef] [PubMed]
18. Amrane, S.; Raoult, D.; Lagier, J.-C. Metagenomics, culturomics, and the human gut microbiota. *Expert Rev. Anti-Infect. Ther.* **2018**, *16*, 373–375. [CrossRef] [PubMed]
19. Zitvogel, L.; Ma, Y.; Raoult, D.; Kroemer, G.; Gajewski, T.F. The microbiome in cancer immunotherapy: Diagnostic tools and therapeutic strategies. *Science* **2018**, *359*, 1366–1370. [CrossRef]

20. Lagier, J.-C.; Khelaifia, S.; Alou, M.T.; Ndongo, S.; Dione, N.; Hugon, P.; Caputo, A.; Cadoret, F.; Traore, S.I.; Seck, E.H.; et al. Culture of previously uncultured members of the human gut microbiota by culturomics. *Nat. Microbiol.* **2016**, *1*, 16203. [CrossRef]

21. Hugon, P.; Dufour, J.-C.; Colson, P.; Fournier, P.-E.; Sallah, K.; Raoult, D. A comprehensive repertoire of prokaryotic species identified in human beings. *Lancet Infect. Dis.* **2015**, *15*, 1211–1219. [CrossRef]

22. The Human Microbiome Project Consortium. Structure, Function and Diversity of the Healthy Human Microbiome. *Nature* **2012**, *486*, 207–214. [CrossRef] [PubMed]

23. Arumugam, M.; Raes, J.; Pelletier, E.; Le Paslier, D.; Yamada, T.; Mende, D.R.; Fernandes, G.R.; Tap, J.; Bruls, T.; Batto, J.-M.; et al. Enterotypes of the human gut microbiome. *Nature* **2011**, *473*, 174–180. [CrossRef] [PubMed]

24. Hugenholtz, F.; de Vos, W.M. Mouse models for human intestinal microbiota research: A critical evaluation. *Cell Mol. Life Sci.* **2018**, *75*, 149–160. [CrossRef] [PubMed]

25. Macpherson, A.J.; Harris, N.L. Interactions between commensal intestinal bacteria and the immune system. *Nat. Rev. Immunol.* **2004**, *4*, 478–485. [CrossRef] [PubMed]

26. O'Hara, A.M.; Shanahan, F. The gut flora as a forgotten organ. *EMBO Rep.* **2006**, *7*, 688–693. [CrossRef] [PubMed]

27. Kaper, J.B.; Sperandio, V. Bacterial Cell-to-Cell Signaling in the Gastrointestinal Tract. *Infect. Immun.* **2005**, *73*, 3197–3209. [CrossRef] [PubMed]

28. Casteleyn, C.; Rekecki, A.; Van der Aa, A.; Simoens, P.; Van den Broeck, W. Surface area assessment of the murine intestinal tract as a prerequisite for oral dose translation from mouse to man. *Lab. Anim.* **2010**, *44*, 176–183. [CrossRef]

29. Nguyen, T.L.A.; Vieira-Silva, S.; Liston, A.; Raes, J. How informative is the mouse for human gut microbiota research? *Dis. Models Mech.* **2015**, *8*, 1–16. [CrossRef]

30. Treuting, P.M.; Arends, M.J.; Dintzis, S.M. 12—Lower Gastrointestinal Tract. In *Comparative Anatomy and Histology*, 2nd ed.; Treuting, P.M., Dintzis, S.M., Montine, K.S., Eds.; Academic Press: San Diego, CA, USA, 2018; pp. 213–228. ISBN 978-0-12-802900-8.

31. Johansson, M.E.V.; Phillipson, M.; Petersson, J.; Velcich, A.; Holm, L.; Hansson, G.C. The inner of the two Muc2 mucin-dependent mucus layers in colon is devoid of bacteria. *Proc. Natl. Acad. Sci. USA* **2008**, *105*, 15064–15069. [CrossRef]

32. Wells, J.M.; Rossi, O.; Meijerink, M.; Baarlen, P. van Epithelial crosstalk at the microbiota–mucosal interface. *PNAS* **2011**, *108*, 4607–4614. [CrossRef]

33. Vaishnava, S.; Yamamoto, M.; Severson, K.M.; Ruhn, K.A.; Yu, X.; Koren, O.; Ley, R.; Wakeland, E.K.; Hooper, L.V. The antibacterial lectin RegIIIgamma promotes the spatial segregation of microbiota and host in the intestine. *Science* **2011**, *334*, 255–258. [CrossRef] [PubMed]

34. Swidsinski, A.; Loening-Baucke, V.; Theissig, F.; Engelhardt, H.; Bengmark, S.; Koch, S.; Lochs, H.; Dörffel, Y. Comparative study of the intestinal mucus barrier in normal and inflamed colon. *Gut* **2007**, *56*, 343–350. [CrossRef] [PubMed]

35. Ultrastructure et écologie microbienne du tube digestif humain Giovanni Brandi, . . . Annamaria Pisi, . . . Guido Biasco, . . . Brandi Giovanni. Available online: http://bibliotheque.bordeaux.fr/in/faces/details.xhtml?id=mgroup%3A9788886457132 (accessed on 13 January 2019).

36. Hooper, L.V.; Littman, D.R.; Macpherson, A.J. Interactions between the microbiota and the immune system. *Science* **2012**, *336*, 1268–1273. [CrossRef] [PubMed]

37. Juge, N. Special Issue: Gut Bacteria-Mucus Interaction. *Microorganisms* **2019**, *7*, 6. [CrossRef] [PubMed]

38. Sicard, J.-F.; Le Bihan, G.; Vogeleer, P.; Jacques, M.; Harel, J. Interactions of Intestinal Bacteria with Components of the Intestinal Mucus. *Front. Cell. Infect. Microbiol.* **2017**, *7*. [CrossRef] [PubMed]

39. Artis, D. Epithelial-cell recognition of commensal bacteria and maintenance of immune homeostasis in the gut. *Nat. Rev. Immunol.* **2008**, *8*, 411–420. [CrossRef]

40. Thompson-Chagoyán, O.C.; Maldonado, J.; Gil, A. Colonization and impact of disease and other factors on intestinal microbiota. *Dig. Dis. Sci.* **2007**, *52*, 2069–2077. [CrossRef]

41. Swidsinski, A.; Sydora, B.C.; Doerffel, Y.; Loening-Baucke, V.; Vaneechoutte, M.; Lupicki, M.; Scholze, J.; Lochs, H.; Dieleman, L.A. Viscosity gradient within the mucus layer determines the mucosal barrier function and the spatial organization of the intestinal microbiota. *Inflamm. Bowel Dis.* **2007**, *13*, 963–970. [CrossRef]

42. Zoetendal, E.G.; Ben-Amor, K.; Harmsen, H.J.M.; Schut, F.; Akkermans, A.D.L.; de Vos, W.M. Quantification of uncultured Ruminococcus obeum-like bacteria in human fecal samples by fluorescent in situ hybridization and flow cytometry using 16S rRNA-targeted probes. *Appl. Environ. Microbiol.* **2002**, *68*, 4225–4232. [CrossRef]

43. Ahmed, S.; Macfarlane, G.T.; Fite, A.; McBain, A.J.; Gilbert, P.; Macfarlane, S. Mucosa-Associated Bacterial Diversity in Relation to Human Terminal Ileum and Colonic Biopsy Samples. *Appl. Environ. Microbiol.* **2007**, *73*, 7435–7442. [CrossRef]

44. Hooper, L.V.; Macpherson, A.J. Immune adaptations that maintain homeostasis with the intestinal microbiota. *Nat. Rev. Immunol.* **2010**, *10*, 159–169. [CrossRef] [PubMed]

45. Macpherson, A.J.; Uhr, T. Induction of protective IgA by intestinal dendritic cells carrying commensal bacteria. *Science* **2004**, *303*, 1662–1665. [CrossRef] [PubMed]

46. Lewis, D.E.; Blutt, S.E. 2—Organization of the Immune System. In *Clinical Immunology*, 5th ed.; Rich, R.R., Fleisher, T.A., Shearer, W.T., Schroeder, H.W., Frew, A.J., Weyand, C.M., Eds.; Elsevier: London, UK, 2019; pp. 19–38.e1. ISBN 978-0-7020-6896-6.

47. Favier, C.F.; Vaughan, E.E.; De Vos, W.M.; Akkermans, A.D.L. Molecular monitoring of succession of bacterial communities in human neonates. *Appl. Environ. Microbiol.* **2002**, *68*, 219–226. [CrossRef] [PubMed]

48. Yoshioka, H.; Iseki, K.; Fujita, K. Development and differences of intestinal flora in the neonatal period in breast-fed and bottle-fed infants. *Pediatrics* **1983**, *72*, 317–321. [PubMed]

49. den Besten, G.; van Eunen, K.; Groen, A.K.; Venema, K.; Reijngoud, D.-J.; Bakker, B.M. The role of short-chain fatty acids in the interplay between diet, gut microbiota, and host energy metabolism. *J. Lipid Res.* **2013**, *54*, 2325–2340. [CrossRef] [PubMed]

50. Brandi, G.; De Lorenzo, S.; Candela, M.; Pantaleo, M.A.; Bellentani, S.; Tovoli, F.; Saccoccio, G.; Biasco, G. Microbiota, NASH, HCC and the potential role of probiotics. *Carcinogenesis* **2017**, *38*, 231–240. [CrossRef] [PubMed]

51. Zmora, N.; Suez, J.; Elinav, E. You are what you eat: Diet, health and the gut microbiota. *Nat. Rev. Gastroenterol. Hepatol.* **2019**, *16*, 35. [CrossRef] [PubMed]

52. Biagi, E.; Franceschi, C.; Rampelli, S.; Severgnini, M.; Ostan, R.; Turroni, S.; Consolandi, C.; Quercia, S.; Scurti, M.; Monti, D.; et al. Gut Microbiota and Extreme Longevity. *Curr. Biol.* **2016**, *26*, 1480–1485. [CrossRef] [PubMed]

53. He, Y.; Wu, W.; Zheng, H.-M.; Li, P.; McDonald, D.; Sheng, H.-F.; Chen, M.-X.; Chen, Z.-H.; Ji, G.-Y.; Zheng, Z.-D.-X.; et al. Regional variation limits applications of healthy gut microbiome reference ranges and disease models. *Nat. Med.* **2018**, *24*, 1532. [CrossRef] [PubMed]

54. Deschasaux, M.; Bouter, K.E.; Prodan, A.; Levin, E.; Groen, A.K.; Herrema, H.; Tremaroli, V.; Bakker, G.J.; Attaye, I.; Pinto-Sietsma, S.-J.; et al. Depicting the composition of gut microbiota in a population with varied ethnic origins but shared geography. *Nat. Med.* **2018**, *24*, 1526. [CrossRef] [PubMed]

55. Palleja, A.; Mikkelsen, K.H.; Forslund, S.K.; Kashani, A.; Allin, K.H.; Nielsen, T.; Hansen, T.H.; Liang, S.; Feng, Q.; Zhang, C.; et al. Recovery of gut microbiota of healthy adults following antibiotic exposure. *Nat. Microbiol.* **2018**, *3*, 1255–1265. [CrossRef] [PubMed]

56. Hathaway-Schrader, J.D.; Steinkamp, H.M.; Chavez, M.B.; Poulides, N.A.; Kirkpatrick, J.E.; Chew, M.E.; Huang, E.; Alekseyenko, A.V.; Aguirre, J.I.; Novince, C.M. Antibiotic Perturbation of Gut Microbiota Dysregulates Osteoimmune Cross Talk in Postpubertal Skeletal Development. *Am. J. Pathol.* **2019**, *189*, 370–390. [CrossRef] [PubMed]

57. Hanahan, D.; Weinberg, R.A. Hallmarks of Cancer: The Next Generation. *Cell* **2011**, *144*, 646–674. [CrossRef] [PubMed]

58. Dunn, G.P.; Bruce, A.T.; Ikeda, H.; Old, L.J.; Schreiber, R.D. Cancer immunoediting: From immunosurveillance to tumor escape. *Nat. Immunol.* **2002**, *3*, 991. [CrossRef] [PubMed]

59. Kavecansky, J. Beyond Checkpoint Inhibitors: The Next Generation of Immunotherapy in Oncology. *Am. J. Hematol./Oncol.* **2017**, *13*, 9–20.

60. Granier, C.; Guillebon, E.D.; Blanc, C.; Roussel, H.; Badoual, C.; Colin, E.; Saldmann, A.; Gey, A.; Oudard, S.; Tartour, E. Mechanisms of action and rationale for the use of checkpoint inhibitors in cancer. *ESMO Open* **2017**, *2*, e000213. [CrossRef] [PubMed]

61. Galluzzi, L.; Buqué, A.; Kepp, O.; Zitvogel, L.; Kroemer, G. Immunogenic cell death in cancer and infectious disease. *Nat. Rev. Immunol.* **2017**, *17*, 97–111. [CrossRef] [PubMed]

62. Gibney, G.T.; Weiner, L.M.; Atkins, M.B. Predictive biomarkers for checkpoint inhibitor-based immunotherapy. *Lancet Oncol.* **2016**, *17*, e542–e551. [CrossRef]

63. Australian Pancreatic Cancer Genome Initiative; ICGC Breast Cancer Consortium; ICGC MMML-Seq Consortium; ICGC PedBrain; Alexandrov, L.B.; Nik-Zainal, S.; Wedge, D.C.; Aparicio, S.A.J.R.; Behjati, S.; Biankin, A.V.; et al. Signatures of mutational processes in human cancer. *Nature* **2013**, *500*, 415–421. [CrossRef] [PubMed]

64. June, C.H.; O'Connor, R.S.; Kawalekar, O.U.; Ghassemi, S.; Milone, M.C. CAR T cell immunotherapy for human cancer. *Science* **2018**, *359*, 1361–1365. [CrossRef] [PubMed]

65. Mollanoori, H.; Shahraki, H.; Rahmati, Y.; Teimourian, S. CRISPR/Cas9 and CAR-T cell, collaboration of two revolutionary technologies in cancer immunotherapy, an instruction for successful cancer treatment. *Hum. Immunol.* **2018**, *79*, 876–882. [CrossRef] [PubMed]

66. Hartmann, J.; Schüßler-Lenz, M.; Bondanza, A.; Buchholz, C.J. Clinical development of CAR T cells—challenges and opportunities in translating innovative treatment concepts. *EMBO Mol. Med.* **2017**, *9*, 1183–1197. [CrossRef] [PubMed]

67. Yoon, D.H.; Osborn, M.J.; Tolar, J.; Kim, C.J. Incorporation of Immune Checkpoint Blockade into Chimeric Antigen Receptor T Cells (CAR-Ts): Combination or Built-In CAR-T. *Int. J. Mol. Sci.* **2018**, *19*, 340. [CrossRef] [PubMed]

68. Simon, B.; Wiesinger, M.; März, J.; Wistuba-Hamprecht, K.; Weide, B.; Schuler-Thurner, B.; Schuler, G.; Dörrie, J.; Uslu, U. The Generation of CAR-Transfected Natural Killer T Cells for the Immunotherapy of Melanoma. *Int. J. Mol. Sci.* **2018**, *19*, 2365. [CrossRef] [PubMed]

69. Newick, K.; O'Brien, S.; Moon, E.; Albelda, S.M. CAR T Cell Therapy for Solid Tumors. *Ann. Rev. Med.* **2017**, *68*, 139–152. [CrossRef] [PubMed]

70. Mount, C.W.; Majzner, R.G.; Sundaresh, S.; Arnold, E.P.; Kadapakkam, M.; Haile, S.; Labanieh, L.; Hulleman, E.; Woo, P.J.; Rietberg, S.P.; et al. Potent antitumor efficacy of anti-GD2 CAR T cells in H3-K27M + diffuse midline gliomas. *Nat. Med.* **2018**, *24*, 572. [CrossRef] [PubMed]

71. Forget, M.-A.; Haymaker, C.; Hess, K.R.; Meng, Y.J.; Creasy, C.; Karpinets, T.; Fulbright, O.J.; Roszik, J.; Woodman, S.E.; Kim, Y.U.; et al. Prospective Analysis of Adoptive TIL Therapy in Patients with Metastatic Melanoma: Response, Impact of Anti-CTLA4, and Biomarkers to Predict Clinical Outcome. *Clin. Cancer Res.* **2018**, *24*, 4416–4428. [CrossRef] [PubMed]

72. Saint-Jean, M.; Knol, A.-C.; Volteau, C.; Quéreux, G.; Peuvrel, L.; Brocard, A.; Pandolfino, M.-C.; Saiagh, S.; Nguyen, J.-M.; Bedane, C.; et al. Adoptive Cell Therapy with Tumor-Infiltrating Lymphocytes in Advanced Melanoma Patients. Available online: https://www.hindawi.com/journals/jir/2018/3530148/citations/ (accessed on 22 February 2019).

73. Zacharakis, N.; Chinnasamy, H.; Black, M.; Xu, H.; Lu, Y.-C.; Zheng, Z.; Pasetto, A.; Langhan, M.; Shelton, T.; Prickett, T.; et al. Immune recognition of somatic mutations leading to complete durable regression in metastatic breast cancer. *Nat. Med.* **2018**, *24*, 724. [CrossRef]

74. Tran, E.; Robbins, P.F.; Lu, Y.-C.; Prickett, T.D.; Gartner, J.J.; Jia, L.; Pasetto, A.; Zheng, Z.; Ray, S.; Groh, E.M.; et al. T-Cell Transfer Therapy Targeting Mutant KRAS in Cancer. *N. Engl. J. Med.* **2016**, *375*, 2255–2262. [CrossRef]

75. Rosenberg, S.A. Abstract IA14: Cell transfer immunotherapy targeting unique somatic mutations in cancer. *Cancer Immunol. Res.* **2019**, *7*. [CrossRef]

76. Brudno, J.N.; Kochenderfer, J.N. Toxicities of chimeric antigen receptor T cells: Recognition and management. *Blood* **2016**, *127*, 3321–3330. [CrossRef] [PubMed]

77. D'Aloia, M.M.; Zizzari, I.G.; Sacchetti, B.; Pierelli, L.; Alimandi, M. CAR-T cells: The long and winding road to solid tumors. *Cell Death Dis.* **2018**, *9*, 282. [CrossRef] [PubMed]

78. Atarashi, K.; Tanoue, T.; Shima, T.; Imaoka, A.; Kuwahara, T.; Momose, Y.; Cheng, G.; Yamasaki, S.; Saito, T.; Ohba, Y.; et al. Induction of Colonic Regulatory T Cells by Indigenous Clostridium Species. *Science* **2011**, *331*, 337–341. [CrossRef] [PubMed]

79. Round, J.L.; Lee, S.M.; Li, J.; Tran, G.; Jabri, B.; Chatila, T.A.; Mazmanian, S.K. The Toll-like receptor pathway establishes commensal gut colonization. *Science* **2011**, *332*, 974–977. [CrossRef] [PubMed]

80. Rubtsov, Y.P.; Rasmussen, J.P.; Chi, E.Y.; Fontenot, J.; Castelli, L.; Ye, X.; Treuting, P.; Siewe, L.; Roers, A.; Henderson, W.R.; et al. Regulatory T cell-derived interleukin-10 limits inflammation at environmental interfaces. *Immunity* **2008**, *28*, 546–558. [CrossRef]

81. Tanaka, A.; Sakaguchi, S. Regulatory T cells in cancer immunotherapy. *Cell Res.* **2017**, *27*, 109–118. [CrossRef]

82. Onizuka, S.; Tawara, I.; Shimizu, J.; Sakaguchi, S.; Fujita, T.; Nakayama, E. Tumor rejection by in vivo administration of anti-CD25 (interleukin-2 receptor alpha) monoclonal antibody. *Cancer Res.* **1999**, *59*, 3128–3133.

83. Shimizu, J.; Yamazaki, S.; Sakaguchi, S. Induction of tumor immunity by removing CD25+CD4+ T cells: A common basis between tumor immunity and autoimmunity. *J. Immunol.* **1999**, *163*, 5211–5218.

84. Kamada, T.; Togashi, Y.; Tay, C.; Ha, D.; Sasaki, A.; Nakamura, Y.; Sato, E.; Fukuoka, S.; Tada, Y.; Tanaka, A.; et al. PD-1+ regulatory T cells amplified by PD-1 blockade promote hyperprogression of cancer. *PNAS* **2019**, *116*, 9999–10008. [CrossRef]

85. Gaboriau-Routhiau, V.; Rakotobe, S.; Lécuyer, E.; Mulder, I.; Lan, A.; Bridonneau, C.; Rochet, V.; Pisi, A.; De Paepe, M.; Brandi, G.; et al. The key role of segmented filamentous bacteria in the coordinated maturation of gut helper T cell responses. *Immunity* **2009**, *31*, 677–689. [CrossRef]

86. Honda, K.; Littman, D.R. The microbiota in adaptive immune homeostasis and disease. *Nature* **2016**, *535*, 75–84. [CrossRef] [PubMed]

87. Chen, B.; Chen, H.; Shu, X.; Yin, Y.; Li, J.; Qin, J.; Chen, L.; Peng, K.; Xu, F.; Gu, W.; et al. Presence of Segmented Filamentous Bacteria in Human Children and Its Potential Role in the Modulation of Human Gut Immunity. *Front. Microbiol.* **2018**, *9*. [CrossRef] [PubMed]

88. Vieira, S.M.; Hiltensperger, M.; Kumar, V.; Zegarra-Ruiz, D.; Dehner, C.; Khan, N.; Costa, F.R.C.; Tiniakou, E.; Greiling, T.; Ruff, W.; et al. Translocation of a gut pathobiont drives autoimmunity in mice and humans. *Science* **2018**, *359*, 1156–1161. [CrossRef] [PubMed]

89. Bullman, S.; Pedamallu, C.S.; Sicinska, E.; Clancy, T.E.; Zhang, X.; Cai, D.; Neuberg, D.; Huang, K.; Guevara, F.; Nelson, T.; et al. Analysis of *Fusobacterium* persistence and antibiotic response in colorectal cancer. *Science* **2017**, *358*, 1443–1448. [CrossRef] [PubMed]

90. Pushalkar, S.; Hundeyin, M.; Daley, D.; Zambirinis, C.P.; Kurz, E.; Mishra, A.; Mohan, N.; Aykut, B.; Usyk, M.; Torres, L.E.; et al. The Pancreatic Cancer Microbiome Promotes Oncogenesis by Induction of Innate and Adaptive Immune Suppression. *Cancer Discov.* **2018**, *8*, 403–416. [CrossRef] [PubMed]

91. Mima, K.; Nishihara, R.; Qian, Z.R.; Cao, Y.; Sukawa, Y.; Nowak, J.A.; Yang, J.; Dou, R.; Masugi, Y.; Song, M.; et al. Fusobacterium nucleatum in colorectal carcinoma tissue and patient prognosis. *Gut* **2016**, *65*, 1973–1980. [CrossRef] [PubMed]

92. Yu, T.; Guo, F.; Yu, Y.; Sun, T.; Ma, D.; Han, J.; Qian, Y.; Kryczek, I.; Sun, D.; Nagarsheth, N.; et al. Fusobacterium nucleatum Promotes Chemoresistance to Colorectal Cancer by Modulating Autophagy. *Cell* **2017**, *170*, 548–563.e16. [CrossRef] [PubMed]

93. Geller, L.T.; Barzily-Rokni, M.; Danino, T.; Jonas, O.H.; Shental, N.; Nejman, D.; Gavert, N.; Zwang, Y.; Cooper, Z.A.; Shee, K.; et al. Potential role of intratumor bacteria in mediating tumor resistance to the chemotherapeutic drug gemcitabine. *Science* **2017**, *357*, 1156–1160. [CrossRef]

94. Lehouritis, P.; Cummins, J.; Stanton, M.; Murphy, C.T.; McCarthy, F.O.; Reid, G.; Urbaniak, C.; Byrne, W.L.; Tangney, M. Local bacteria affect the efficacy of chemotherapeutic drugs. *Sci. Rep.* **2015**, *5*, 14554. [CrossRef]

95. Ivanov, I.I.; Atarashi, K.; Manel, N.; Brodie, E.L.; Shima, T.; Karaoz, U.; Wei, D.; Goldfarb, K.C.; Santee, C.A.; Lynch, S.V.; et al. Induction of Intestinal Th17 Cells by Segmented Filamentous Bacteria. *Cell* **2009**, *139*, 485–498. [CrossRef]

96. Iida, N.; Dzutsev, A.; Stewart, C.A.; Smith, L.; Bouladoux, N.; Weingarten, R.A.; Molina, D.A.; Salcedo, R.; Back, T.; Cramer, S.; et al. Commensal bacteria control cancer response to therapy by modulating the tumor microenvironment. *Science* **2013**, *342*, 967–970. [CrossRef] [PubMed]

97. Viaud, S.; Saccheri, F.; Mignot, G.; Yamazaki, T.; Daillère, R.; Hannani, D.; Enot, D.P.; Pfirschke, C.; Engblom, C.; Pittet, M.J.; et al. The intestinal microbiota modulates the anticancer immune effects of cyclophosphamide. *Science* **2013**, *342*, 971–976. [CrossRef] [PubMed]

98. Sivan, A.; Corrales, L.; Hubert, N.; Williams, J.B.; Aquino-Michaels, K.; Earley, Z.M.; Benyamin, F.W.; Man Lei, Y.; Jabri, B.; Alegre, M.-L.; et al. Commensal *Bifidobacterium* promotes antitumor immunity and facilitates anti–PD-L1 efficacy. *Science* **2015**, *350*, 1084–1089. [CrossRef] [PubMed]

99. Vétizou, M.; Pitt, J.M.; Daillère, R.; Lepage, P.; Waldschmitt, N.; Flament, C.; Rusakiewicz, S.; Routy, B.; Roberti, M.P.; Duong, C.P.M.; et al. Anticancer immunotherapy by CTLA-4 blockade relies on the gut microbiota. *Science* **2015**, *350*, 1079–1084. [CrossRef] [PubMed]

100. Routy, B.; Le Chatelier, E.; Derosa, L.; Duong, C.P.M.; Alou, M.T.; Daillère, R.; Fluckiger, A.; Messaoudene, M.; Rauber, C.; Roberti, M.P.; et al. Gut microbiome influences efficacy of PD-1–based immunotherapy against epithelial tumors. *Science* **2018**, *359*, 91–97. [CrossRef] [PubMed]

101. Gopalakrishnan, V.; Spencer, C.N.; Nezi, L.; Reuben, A.; Andrews, M.C.; Karpinets, T.V.; Prieto, P.A.; Vicente, D.; Hoffman, K.; Wei, S.C.; et al. Gut microbiome modulates response to anti–PD-1 immunotherapy in melanoma patients. *Science* **2017**, *359*, 97–103. [CrossRef] [PubMed]

102. Matson, V.; Fessler, J.; Bao, R.; Chongsuwat, T.; Zha, Y.; Alegre, M.-L.; Luke, J.J.; Gajewski, T.F. The commensal microbiome is associated with anti–PD-1 efficacy in metastatic melanoma patients. *Science* **2018**, *359*, 104–108. [CrossRef] [PubMed]

103. Derosa, L.; Routy, B.; Kroemer, G.; Zitvogel, L. The intestinal microbiota determines the clinical efficacy of immune checkpoint blockers targeting PD-1/PD-L1. *OncoImmunology* **2018**, *7*, e1434468. [CrossRef]

104. Desai, M.S.; Seekatz, A.M.; Koropatkin, N.M.; Kamada, N.; Hickey, C.A.; Wolter, M.; Pudlo, N.A.; Kitamoto, S.; Terrapon, N.; Muller, A.; et al. A Dietary Fiber-Deprived Gut Microbiota Degrades the Colonic Mucus Barrier and Enhances Pathogen Susceptibility. *Cell* **2016**, *167*, 1339–1353.e21. [CrossRef] [PubMed]

105. Kuczma, M.P.; Ding, Z.-C.; Li, T.; Habtetsion, T.; Chen, T.; Hao, Z.; Bryan, L.; Singh, N.; Kochenderfer, J.N.; Zhou, G. The impact of antibiotic usage on the efficacy of chemoimmunotherapy is contingent on the source of tumor-reactive T cells. *Oncotarget* **2017**, *8*, 111931–111942. [CrossRef]

106. Uribe-Herranz, M.; Bittinger, K.; Rafail, S.; Guedan, S.; Pierini, S.; Tanes, C.; Ganetsky, A.; Morgan, M.A.; Gill, S.; Tanyi, J.L.; et al. Gut microbiota modulates adoptive cell therapy via CD8α dendritic cells and IL-12. *JCI Insight* **2018**, *3*. [CrossRef] [PubMed]

107. Smith, M. Intestinal Microbiota Composition Prior to CAR T Cell Infusion Correlates with Efficacy and Toxicity. *Blood* **2018**, *132*, 3492. [CrossRef]

108. Gopalakrishnan, V.; Helmink, B.A.; Spencer, C.N.; Reuben, A.; Wargo, J.A. The Influence of the Gut Microbiome on Cancer, Immunity, and Cancer Immunotherapy. *Cancer Cell* **2018**, *33*, 570–580. [CrossRef] [PubMed]

109. Wu, G.D.; Chen, J.; Hoffmann, C.; Bittinger, K.; Chen, Y.-Y.; Keilbaugh, S.A.; Bewtra, M.; Knights, D.; Walters, W.A.; Knight, R.; et al. Linking long-term dietary patterns with gut microbial enterotypes. *Science* **2011**, *334*, 105–108. [CrossRef] [PubMed]

110. David, L.A.; Maurice, C.F.; Carmody, R.N.; Gootenberg, D.B.; Button, J.E.; Wolfe, B.E.; Ling, A.V.; Devlin, A.S.; Varma, Y.; Fischbach, M.A.; et al. Diet rapidly and reproducibly alters the human gut microbiome. *Nature* **2014**, *505*, 559–563. [CrossRef] [PubMed]

111. Benus, R.F.J.; van der Werf, T.S.; Welling, G.W.; Judd, P.A.; Taylor, M.A.; Harmsen, H.J.M.; Whelan, K. Association between Faecalibacterium prausnitzii and dietary fibre in colonic fermentation in healthy human subjects. *Br. J. Nutr.* **2010**, *104*, 693–700. [CrossRef] [PubMed]

112. Corrêa-Oliveira, R.; Fachi, J.L.; Vieira, A.; Sato, F.T.; Vinolo, M.A.R. Regulation of immune cell function by short-chain fatty acids. *Clin. Transl. Immunol.* **2016**, *5*, e73. [CrossRef] [PubMed]

113. Maslowski, K.M.; Mackay, C.R. Diet, gut microbiota and immune responses. *Nat. Immunol.* **2010**, *12*, 5–9. [CrossRef] [PubMed]

114. Oh, D.Y.; Talukdar, S.; Bae, E.J.; Imamura, T.; Morinaga, H.; Fan, W.; Li, P.; Lu, W.J.; Watkins, S.M.; Olefsky, J.M. GPR120 is an omega-3 fatty acid receptor mediating potent anti-inflammatory and insulin-sensitizing effects. *Cell* **2010**, *142*, 687–698. [CrossRef] [PubMed]

115. Costantini, L.; Molinari, R.; Farinon, B.; Merendino, N. Impact of Omega-3 Fatty Acids on the Gut Microbiota. *Int. J. Mol. Sci.* **2017**, *18*, 2645. [CrossRef]

116. Watson, H.; Mitra, S.; Croden, F.C.; Taylor, M.; Wood, H.M.; Perry, S.L.; Spencer, J.A.; Quirke, P.; Toogood, G.J.; Lawton, C.L.; et al. A randomised trial of the effect of omega-3 polyunsaturated fatty acid supplements on the human intestinal microbiota. *Gut* **2018**, *67*, 1974–1983. [CrossRef] [PubMed]

117. Kroemer, G.; López-Otín, C.; Madeo, F.; de Cabo, R. Carbotoxicity-Noxious Effects of Carbohydrates. *Cell* **2018**, *175*, 605–614. [CrossRef] [PubMed]

118. Gu, Y.; Wang, X.; Li, J.; Zhang, Y.; Zhong, H.; Liu, R.; Zhang, D.; Feng, Q.; Xie, X.; Hong, J.; et al. Analyses of gut microbiota and plasma bile acids enable stratification of patients for antidiabetic treatment. *Nat. Commun.* **2017**, *8*, 1785. [CrossRef] [PubMed]

119. Spencer, C.N.; Gopalakrishnan, V.; McQuade, J.; Andrews, M.C.; Helmink, B.; Khan, M.A.W.; Sirmans, E.; Haydu, L.; Cogdill, A. The gut microbiome (GM) and immunotherapy response are influenced by host lifestyle factors. In Proceedings of the 110th Annual Meeting of the American Association for Cancer Research, Atlanta, GA, USA, 29 March–3 April 2019; AACR: Philadelphia, PA, USA, 2019.

120. Meeting Library|Antibiotic Treatment Prior to Immune Checkpoint Inhibitor Therapy as a Tumor-Agnostic Predictive Correlate of Response in Routine Clinical Practice. Available online: https://meetinglibrary.asco.org/record/170372/abstract (accessed on 5 May 2019).

121. van Nood, E.; Vrieze, A.; Nieuwdorp, M.; Fuentes, S.; Zoetendal, E.G.; de Vos, W.M.; Visser, C.E.; Kuijper, E.J.; Bartelsman, J.F.W.M.; Tijssen, J.G.P.; et al. Duodenal Infusion of Donor Feces for Recurrent Clostridium difficile. *N. Engl. J. Med.* **2013**, *368*, 407–415. [CrossRef] [PubMed]

122. Paramsothy, S.; Kamm, M.A.; Kaakoush, N.O.; Walsh, A.J.; van den Bogaerde, J.; Samuel, D.; Leong, R.W.L.; Connor, S.; Ng, W.; Paramsothy, R.; et al. Multidonor intensive faecal microbiota transplantation for active ulcerative colitis: A randomised placebo-controlled trial. *Lancet* **2017**, *389*, 1218–1228. [CrossRef]

123. van Lier, Y.F.; de Groot, P.F.; Nur, E.; Zeerleder, S.S.; Nieuwdorp, M.; Blom, B.; Hazenberg, M.D. Fecal Microbiota Transplantation As Safe and Successful Therapy for Intestinal Graft-Versus-Host Disease. *Blood* **2017**, *130*, 1986.

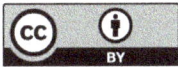

International Journal of
Molecular Sciences

MDPI

Review

The Possible Role of Gut Microbiota and Microbial Translocation Profiling During Chemo-Free Treatment of Lymphoid Malignancies

Valentina Zuccaro [1], Andrea Lombardi [1], Erika Asperges [1], Paolo Sacchi [1], Piero Marone [2], Alessandra Gazzola [1,2], Luca Arcaini [3,4] and Raffaele Bruno [1,5,*]

[1]   Infectious Diseases Unit, Fondazione IRCCS "San Matteo", 27100 Pavia, Italy; zuccaro.v@gmail.com (V.Z.);
      andrea.lombardi02@universitadipavia.it (A.L.); erika.asperges01@universitadipavia.it (E.A.);
      paolo.sacchi1962@gmail.com (P.S.); alegazzola@hotmail.it (A.G.)
[2]   U.O.C. Microbiologia e Virologia, Fondazione IRCCS Policlinico San Matteo, 27100 Pavia, Italy;
      pmarone@smatteo.pv.it
[3]   Department of Molecular Medicine, University of Pavia, 27100 Pavia, Italy; luca.arcaini@unipv.it
[4]   Department of Hematology Oncology, Fondazione IRCCS Policlinico San Matteo, 27100 Pavia, Italy
[5]   Department of Medical, Surgical, Diagnostic and Paediatric Science, University of Pavia, 27100 Pavia, Italy
*   Correspondence: raffaele.bruno@unipv.it; Tel.: +39-0382-501080

Received: 7 January 2019; Accepted: 4 April 2019; Published: 9 April 2019

Abstract: The crosstalk between gut microbiota (GM) and the immune system is intense and complex. When dysbiosis occurs, the resulting pro-inflammatory environment can lead to bacterial translocation, systemic immune activation, tissue damage, and cancerogenesis. GM composition seems to impact both the therapeutic activity and the side effects of anticancer treatment; in particular, robust evidence has shown that the GM modulates the response to immunotherapy in patients affected by metastatic melanoma. Despite accumulating knowledge supporting the role of GM composition in lymphomagenesis, unexplored areas still remain. No studies have been designed to investigate GM alteration in patients diagnosed with lymphoproliferative disorders and treated with chemo-free therapies, and the potential association between GM, therapy outcome, and immune-related adverse events has never been analyzed. Additional studies should be considered to create opportunities for a more tailored approach in this set of patients. In this review, we describe the possible role of the GM during chemo-free treatment of lymphoid malignancies.

Keywords: gut microbiota; chemo free treatment; lymphoid malignancies

1. Introduction

The use of small molecules and immune-targeted therapies has had significant impact on the prognosis of some cancers. Data have shown that gut microbiota composition may play a significant role in determining the efficacy and safety of such therapies. So far, the relationship between microbiota and hematologic malignancies is not well understood.

The aim of this review was to describe the possible role of the gut microbiota (GM) and microbial translocation profiling during chemo-free treatment of lymphoid malignancies. A web-based search of MEDLINE (PubMed) was performed from 2009 until March 2018 in order to identify pertinent articles. We structured our term search using the following keywords: "gut microbiota; chemo free treatment; lymphoid malignancies". This review first describes the characteristic of the gut microbiota and its relationship with both the immune system and inflammation and microbial translocation. Then, we report what is known about the interplay between microbiota cancer, hematologic disorders, and lymphoid malignancies.

2. Human Gut Microbiota

The human microbiota is composed of numerous micro-organisms including eukaryotes, archaea, bacteria, and viruses, which colonize the whole human body: skin surface, airways, and genital and gastrointestinal systems [1]. It consists of 10–100 trillion cells and the number of genes greatly exceeds those in the human genome [2]. Considerable effort has been invested in characterizing the human microbiota using next generation sequencing (NGS) technology: the Human Microbiome Project (HMP), launched in 2008, was designed to estimate the complexity of the microbial community at each body site to understand its potential role in human health [3].

The majority of microbes harbored in the gut (GM) are bacteria, at around 10^{13}–10^{14} bacterial cells [1]. In healthy intestines, the GM is dominated by Gram-negative *Bacteroidetes* phyla and Gram-positive *Firmicutes* phyla, with small proportions of *Actinobacteria*, *Proteobacteria*, and *Verrucomicrobia* [1,4]. The GM is a dynamic ecosystem linked to age, geographical location, human lifestyle (diet), and environmental factors [5]. For this reason, identifying a stable composition of healthy GM is difficult.

Resilience measures the extent to which, and how permanently, any kind of stress may perturb GM composition [1,6]. To better assess the community resilience, reproducible patterns of GM, called enterotypes, were identified using shotgun sequencing of fecal metagenomes from healthy individuals of European and American descent [7–10]. Three robust clusters were recognized: Enterotype 1 is rich in *Bacteroides* and *Parabacteroides* and is able to derive energy from carbohydrates and proteins (Western diet); Enterotype 2 is rich in *Prevotella* and *Desulfovibrio* and their hydrolases are specialized in the degradation of plant fibers; and Enterotype 3, the most frequent, is rich in *Ruminococcus* as well as co-occurring *Akkermansia* [5,8].

GM can influence physiological human homeostasis: it has metabolic functions, provides protection against pathogens, and modulates the immune response. GM modifications associated with disease are being increasingly frequently studied. Dysbiosis includes any condition that disrupts the stable composition of that GM. It can be caused by infection and by environmental factors such as antibiotics consumption or dietary changes [11,12]. Several human and animal studies showed a link between dysbiosis and disease, such as cancer, immune-related disorders, metabolic diseases, inflammatory bowel disease, pulmonary conditions, oral diseases, as well as skin and neurological disorders [4,12].

3. The Role of Gut Microbiota on the Immune System

The GM has multiple functions and the relationship with the host is regulated by a complex network of interactions. The GM is involved in energy harvest and storage and plays a role in generating nutrients from substrates indigestible by the host, such as starch and soluble dietary fiber. These products act as energy substrates for the host and, unfortunately, as effectors of immune responses and tumorigenesis [13,14].

The crosstalk between GM and the immune system is intense and complex. The gastrointestinal (GI) tract is one of the body niches where the external environment meets the internal one. The GI tract is composed of enterocytes covered by mucous, immunoglobulins A, and glycocalyx, which separates the luminal environment from the lymphoid tissue. To reach the lymphoid tissue, antigens pass through the cells (transcellular movement mediated by pumps and channels) or through paracellular compartments (tight junctions). The intestinal barrier then acts as a physical barrier and its integrity is crucial for maintaining the balance between health and disease [15]. The intestinal barrier consists of another structure: the immunologic barrier, which is composed of lymphoid cells and humoral factors such as dendritic cells, macrophages, granulocytes, mast cells, B and T cells, and CD4+CD25+ cells. The GM is a part of a third intestinal barrier, called the biological barrier, and it includes several antimicrobial molecules acting as a defense against pathogens [15]. For these reasons, both the GM and the intestinal barrier are defined as the "missing organs" of the human body [16].

Even in healthy intestine, commensal bacteria influence immune homeostasis. Pattern recognition receptors, like toll-like receptors (TLRs), present on the enterocytes recognize pathogen associated molecular patterns (PAMPs) of commensal bacteria, promoting the initiation of the inflammatory response [1,17] by the release of nuclear factor kappa-light-chain-enhancer of activated B cells (NF-κB), which activates a variety of genes coding for chemokines, cytokines, acute phase proteins, and other effectors of the humoral immune response [18]. Some bacteria can produce metabolites, such as short-chain fatty acids (SCFAs) and reactive oxygen species (ROS), able to activate T cells, and regulatory T cells (Tregs) versus Th17 phenotype. When dysbiosis occurs, the resultant pro-inflammatory environment can aggravate the inflammatory status, triggering the recruitment of immune effector cells and the shedding of additional pro-inflammatory cytokines [1,13]. Beyond the recruitment of immune cells, the GM shapes global immune cell repertoires by modulating the differentiation of T cell populations into different types of helper cells (Th): Th1, Th2, and Th17, or into Tregs [19,20]. SCFAs are suppressors of nuclear NF-κB, interleukein-6 (IL-6), and tumor necrosis factor α (TNF- α) and enhance the production of IL-10. Through this mechanism, SCFAs promote the generation of Th1, Th17, and IL-10+ cells and decrease the proliferation of T and B cells, whereas a specific type of SCFAs, butyrate, enhances T-cell apoptosis [19]. Next to the proinflammatory role, the GM may have also a protective role. Tregs limits the aberrant inflammatory response and several studies have reported how the microbial community promotes the differentiation of anti-inflammatory regulatory T cells: Mazmanian et al. [20] demonstrated the role of *Bacteroides fragilis* in suppressing the production of IL-17 and in protecting against potential inflammatory reactions initiated by bacterial antigens.

Several studies and animal models have demonstrated that GM composition leads to a proper maturation of the immune system and the production of haemopoietic cells [19]. *Clostridiales* species, for example, suppress immune response by promoting Tregs polarization and IL-10 production [21,22]. *Enterococcus hirae* increase the level of Th17 and then stimulate the immune response [21,23].

While there is accumulating evidence on the role of GM in gut local immunity, more data are needed to confirm the relationship between the GM and systemic immunity and inflammation. For example, Ichinohe et al. [24,25] showed how the consumption of broad-spectrum antibiotics seems to reduce the T and B cell response against intranasal infection due to the influenza virus by promoting the inflammasome-mediated induction of IL-1β and IL-18 secretion. Commensal-derived peptidoglycan seemed to improve the killing of *Streptococcus pneumoniae* and *Staphylococcus aureus* by bone-marrow derived neutrophils in a **nucleotide-binding oligomerization domain-containing protein 1** (NOD1), an intracellular pattern-recognition receptor. [24,26].

4. The Relationship Between GM and Microbial Translocation

Microbial translocation (MT) is defined as the non-physiological passage of the GI bacteria from the gut lumen to the local mesenteric lymph nodes [27]. In physiological conditions, bacteria are phagocytized before they reach the lymph nodes. If the intestinal barrier functioning is reduced with increased intestinal permeability as a result of the impairment of local immunity, such as in the case of dysbiosis, MT can occurs [28].

MT has been extensively studied in animal models and the endpoint used to quantify MT is the number of organisms cultured in the regional lymph nodes [28]. In recent years, the association between GM, MT, and immune activation was reported by several studies in humans, particularly in HIV-infected patients [27,29]. Individuals with multiple sclerosis (MS) are characterized by low-grade translocation of bacteria from the intestines into the systemic circulation. Some authors speculated on the possibility that MT contributes to the development of the disease [30]. Facultative intracellular pathogens are able to resist phagocytic killing and are mainly responsible for MT. Several MT surrogate markers are described in literature; the most relevant is lipopolysaccharide (LPS). Soluble CD14 (sCD14) is also widely used; it is a biomarker of monocyte activation not specific for MT [27]. Other surrogate

MT markers are bacterial DNA fragments and LPS binding protein (LBP), which binds to LPS and presents it to CD14 and TLR-4.

The relationship between GM and MT is important because translocating bacteria and microbial components may aggravate a pre-existing inflammatory status. To the best of our knowledge, there are no studies on the links between modifications of GM composition, MT, and inflammatory status.

5. Gut Microbiota and Cancer

Considering the above, the interest in the potential crosslink between dysbiosis and disease, in particular with cancer, is not surprising.

Several epidemiological studies demonstrated the association between intra-abdominal infections, the use of antibiotics, the consequent dysbiosis, and an increased incidence of colorectal cancer. Carcinogen-induced models of tumorigenesis highlighted the oncogenic effects of some bacterial metabolites and ROS species [11]. Oncogenic effects of dysbiosis act locally and systematically; however, it is complicated to prove these relationships. The GM not only have an effect on carcinogenesis, but also on the pharmacology and the side effects of anticancer therapies [11].

We now focus on the potential role of the GM in the response to chemo-free treatments. Chemo-free cancer therapy is a novel therapeutic approach that aims to control the malignancy by taking advantage of the immune system's physiological activity. Chemo-free agents include cytokines, checkpoint inhibitors, agonists of co-stimulatory receptors, T cells manipulators, oncolytic viruses, vaccines, and therapies directed at other cell types [31]. Currently, the most widely studied and used checkpoint inhibitors are: monoclonal antibodies (mAbs) that target programmed cell death protein 1 (PD-1) (pembrolizumab, nivolumab), its ligand PD-L1 (atezolizumab, avelumab, durvalumab), and the cytotoxic T-lymphocyte-associated protein 4 (CTLA-4) (ipilimumab, tremelimumab). These molecules are approved and indicated for different cancers, such as advanced melanoma, non-small-cell lung cancer (NSCLC), and renal cell carcinoma [31,32]. They have dramatically improved patients' survival; however, the beneficial effects were ascertained only in a subgroup of patients [33]. In a mice model, Sivan et al. [33,34] supplied robust evidence about the impact of the GM on the efficacy of PD-L1 blockage: Bifidobacterium-treated mice improved tumor control in contrast with non-Bifidobacterium-treated mice, suggesting the possibility of enhancing the anti-tumor efficacy of anti-PD-L1 with probiotics. Matson et al. [33,35] confirmed these data in human studies: they found that in patients with metastatic melanoma, ***Bifidobacterium*** *longum*, *Collinsella aerofaciens*, and *Enterococcus faecium* were more abundant in the stool samples (collected before the start of therapy) of chemo-free therapy responders, thus supporting the anti-tumor effects of the Bifidobacterium species. In another set of metastatic melanoma patients receiving anti-PD1 therapy, Wargo et al. [33,36] found that responders had a high bacterial diversity and an abundance of *Ruminococcaceae*, whereas non-responders showed a higher percentage of Bacteroidales.

Many other studies were designed with different patients to better characterize GM composition and its contribution in chemo-free therapies efficacy and toxicity [17]. The research data have increased on the potential role of GM modulation through diet, administration of probiotics, and fecal microbial translocation to improve response to therapy.

In their review, Gopalakrishnan et al. [17] summarized the ongoing and planned clinical trials designed to evaluate the possible GM manipulation to enhance responses to cancer immunotherapy. Several approaches were presented involving fecal transplantation, administration of probiotics, physical activities, and specific integration within a normal diet. Two trials investigating the role of GM in colorectal cancer have concluded and showed how patients with colon cancer harbor a distinct microbiota signature and how probiotics administration can modify the cytokines expression profile.

6. Gut Microbiota and Hematologic Disorders

GM seems to have an impact on the products of the hematopoietic systems. Although the underlying mechanisms are unclear, the pool of the bone marrow myeloid cells is strongly correlated with GM composition [19]. Balmer et al. [37] compared the number of myeloid cells, mature monocytes, and granulocyte-monocyte progenitor between germ-free mice and specific pathogen-free (SPF) mice. SCFAs also play a fundamental role in the hematological setting: the product activates several G-protein-coupled cell surface receptors, such as GPR43, GPR109a, and C4, expressed by granulocytes, some myeloid cells epithelial cells, adipocytes, macrophages, and dendritic cells. As discussed above, SCFAs promote the generation of Th1, Th17, and IL-10+ cells and decrease the proliferation of T and B cells (Figure 1) [19].

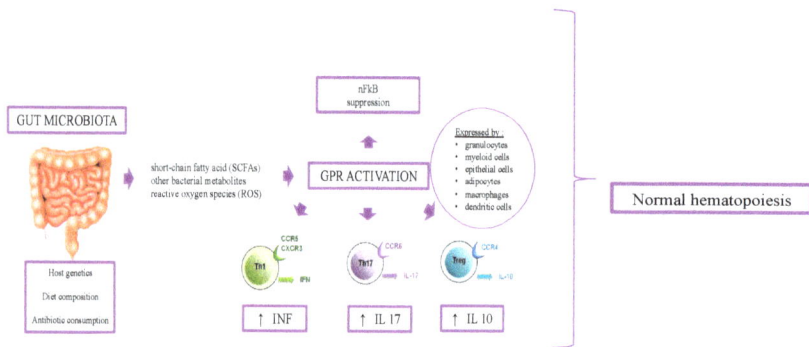

Figure 1. Gut microbiome composition in hematopoiesis. SCFAs activates several G-protein-coupled cell surface receptors, such as GPR43, GPR109a and C4, expressed by granulocytes, some myeloid cells epithelial cells, adipocytes, macrophages, and dendritic cells. SCFAs are responsible for promoting the generation of Th1, Th17, and IL-10+ cells and for decreasing the proliferation of T and B cells.

Considering the close interplay between the immune system and the GM, the lymphoid tissue is involved in the oncogenic process. One example of this is mucosal-associated lymphoid tissue (MALT) lymphoma, which is strongly associated with the presence of certain bacteria, such as *Helicobacter pylori* [38] (Table 1).

Table 1. Described associations between specific microorganisms, and lymphoid malignancies.

Disease	Microorganism	Reference
Gastric MALT	Linked to infection with *Helicobacter pylori*.	[39]
Marginal zone lymphomas	*Hepatitis C virus* (HCV) is a trigger of initial antigenic stimulus for B-cell clonal expansion.	[40]
Burkitt lymphoma	Lymphoma, especially in endemic cases in sub-Saharan Africa, is associated with EBV infection	[41]
Castleman disease	Human herpesvirus 8 (Kaposi sarcoma-associated herpes virus) sequences have been described in some cases of multicentric Castleman disease.	[42]

Modified from Manzo and Bhatt [19].

As discussed above, dysbiosis can stimulate local gut immunity and generate a pro-inflammatory environment. Among the immune effector cells that participate in local immunity, lymphocytes play a key role in responding to microbial perturbation. Bacterial metabolites, such as SCFAs, seem to influence cell type recruitment and hematopoiesis [43,44]. Given the role of GM in normal hematopoiesis, alterations in the GM composition are associated with hematologic disorders. Some GM compositions are associated with the promotion or neutralization of mutagens and oxidative stress [38]. Some enterotypes or dysbiosis can act as antigens and as chronic stimulation to immune cells, leading the potential expansion of B cells [38]. A correlation between microbial tanslocation and lymphoma and blood cancer exists: *Borrelia burgdorferi* was associated with cutaneous

B-cell non-Hodgkin lymphoma [43,45], and *Chlamydophila psittaci* was been detected in various non-gastrointestinal organs in patients with MALT [43,46].

Despite the strong rational linking gut immunity perturbation to lymphomagenesis, there is a paucity of animal models supporting this hypothesis. However, one example was provided by the inoculation of segmented filamentous bacteria in the intestine of mice, which leads to a change in T cell activity eliciting a range of responses including increases in IL-10, IL-17, and IFN-γ [47]. Another animal model showed an alternative underlying mechanism of lymphomagenesis due to GM composition: mice with a restricted microbiota showed an increase in CD8+ T cells and, consequently, a decrease in B cells in the marginal zone through a cytolytic mechanism. [38,48]. In a mouse model, Scheeren et al. [49,50] showed that high-level expression of IL-21 is critically associated with the expansion of mature B cells, leading to potential development of Hodgkin disease, multiple myeloma, chronic lymphocytic leukemia, Waldenstrom macroglobulinemia, and angioimmunoblastic T-cell lymphoma. Rajagopala et al. [51] compared GM composition in pediatric and adolescent patients with acute leukemia with that of their sibling controls. The GM profiles of both groups were dominated by *Bacteroides*, *Prevotella*, and *Faecalibacterium*, but the diversity of the patient group was significantly lower than that of the control group.

Once it was ascertained that the GM composition impacts normal hematopoiesis, researchers' efforts were directed toward understanding the role of the microbiota in mediating treatment response and the outcomes in response to therapy. Concerning lymphoid malignancies, chemo-free agents represent the newest approach in the treatment of lymphoproliferative disorders [52]. However, some patients are still not responding to chemo-free therapy, the efficacy of which could be limited by the occurrence of immune related adverse events (irAEs). Since most of the side effects of these new molecules are gut-related (i.e., colitis and diarrhea), the GM could be implicated in the genesis and development of such adverse reactions. However, to the best of our knowledge, no studies have ever explored GM alteration in patients with lymphoproliferative disorders treated with chemo-free therapies and its association with the outcome and immune-related adverse events. In a recent multicentric study conducted by Peled et al. [53], patients undergoing hematopoietic cell transplantation (HCT) at four institutions in three continents presented a similar GM composition, whereas the GM differed when compared with those of healthy people. Pre-HCT microbiota injury seemed to predict poor overall survival.

As discussed above, beyond bacterial species, almost 1500 virotypes colonize the gut lumen (10^9 virus-like particles (VLPs) per gram of human feces) [54]. This aspect is interesting when we consider the association of lymphomas with specific microorganisms. The viral infection–lymphoma relationship was described between HCV and B-cell clonal expansion, EBV and endemic Burkitt lymphoma and post-transplantation lymphoproliferative disorder (PTLD), and human herpesvirus 8 (HHV-8) and multicentric Castleman disease [19]. For this reason, more efforts should be devoted to elucidate the potential link between gut virome and disease, maybe with the creation of a human virome project [54].

7. Potential Correlation and Clinical Implication

Given what was described above, we hypothesize that the immunostimulatory and antitumor effects of BCRi in patients with lymphoid malignancies could be influenced by distinct gut microbiota compositions. Therefore, the study of the gut microbiota in these patients might be important for recognizing different enterotypes able to distinguish among patients who have and have not achieved a clinical response and those at greater risk to experience immune-related adverse events (irAEs).

8. Conclusions and Future Directions

Thanks to the progress in the fields of biotechnology, genetics, and genomics, clinicians can use the analysis of big data as an additional tool to choose the best decision-making algorithm; this is called precision medicine [16,55].

Specific gut microbiota states are reportedly associated with autoimmune disorders and, although the relationship between microbes and host immune responses suggests an association of the GM composition with lymphoma and blood cancer, mechanistic understanding of how the microbiota directly or indirectly impacts hematopoiesis is limited.

No studies have evaluated the relationship between GM and therapy outcome in patients with lymphoproliferative disorders treated with chemo-free therapies. Evidence on the relationship between GM and MT in this set of patients is lacking.

Further studies should be considered to open up the possibility for more tailored approaches, in terms of precision medicine, that consider the systemic impact of GM.

Funding: This research received no external funding.

Acknowledgments: Ricerca Corrente No. 08020418 study group Fondazione IRCCS Policlinico San Matteo. We wish to thank Elvira Calabrese for her help in reviewing the language of the manuscript.

Conflicts of Interest: The authors declare no conflict of interest.

Abbreviations

CTLA-4	cytotoxic T-lymphocyte-associated protein 4
C4	Complement component 4
EBV	Epstein-Barr virus
GM	gut microbiota
GPR41-GPR43	G protein-coupled receptors
HCT	hematopoietic cell transplantation
HCV	hepatitis C virus
HHV-8	human herpesvirus 8
HIV	human immunodeficiency virus
HMP	Human Microbiome Project
IL10	Interleukin 10
IFN	Interferon
irAEs	immune related adverse events
LBP	LPS binding protein
LPS	lipopolysaccharide
MALT	mucosal-associated lymphoid tissue
MD	Microbial translocation
MS	multiple sclerosis
NF-kB	nuclear factor kappa-light-chain-enhancer of activated B cells
NGS	next generation sequencing
NOD-1	Nucleotide-binding oligomerization domain-containing protein 1
NSCLC	non–small cell lung cancer
PAMPs	pathogen associated molecular patterns
PD-1	programmed cell death protein 1
PD-L1	programmed cell death protein 1 ligand
PTLD	post-transplantation lymphoproliferative disorder
ROS	reactive oxygen species
sCD14	soluble CD14
SCFAs	short-chain fatty acids
SPF	specific pathogen-free
TLRs	Toll-like receptors
Th1-Th17	T helper cells
Treg	regulatory T cell
VLP	virus-like particles

References

1. Glendinning, L.; Nausch, N.; Free, A.; Taylor, D.W.; Mutapi, F. The microbiota and helminths: Sharing the same niche in the human host. *Parasitology* **2014**, *141*, 1255–1271. [CrossRef]

2. Morgan, X.C.; Huttenhower, C. Chapter 12: Human Microbiome Analysis. *PLoS Comput. Biol.* **2012**, *8*, e1002808. [CrossRef] [PubMed]

3. Human Microbiome Project—Websites of Interest. Available online: https://commonfund.nih.gov/hmp/websites (accessed on 26 December 2018).

4. Lynch, S.V.; Pedersen, O. The Human Intestinal Microbiome in Health and Disease. *N. Engl. J. Med.* **2016**, *375*, 2369–2379. [CrossRef] [PubMed]

5. Requena, T.; Martínez-Cuesta, M.C.; Peláez, C. Diet and microbiota linked in health and disease. *Food Funct.* **2018**, *9*, 688–704. [CrossRef]

6. Lozupone, C.A.; Stombaugh, J.I.; Gordon, J.I.; Jansson, J.K.; Knight, R. Diversity, stability and resilience of the human gut microbiota. *Nature* **2012**, *489*, 220–230. [CrossRef] [PubMed]

7. Costea, P.I.; Hildebrand, F.; Arumugam, M.; Bäckhed, F.; Blaser, M.J.; Bushman, F.D.; de Vos, W.M.; Ehrlich, S.D.; Fraser, C.M.; Hattori, M.; et al. Enterotypes in the landscape of gut microbial community composition. *Nat. Microbiol.* **2018**, *3*, 8–16. [CrossRef]

8. Arumugam, M.; Raes, J.; Pelletier, E.; Le Paslier, D.; Yamada, T.; Mende, D.R.; Fernandes, G.R.; Tap, J.; Bruls, T.; Batto, J.-M.; et al. Enterotypes of the human gut microbiome. *Nature* **2011**, *473*, 174–180. [CrossRef]

9. Turnbaugh, P.J.; Hamady, M.; Yatsunenko, T.; Cantarel, B.L.; Duncan, A.; Ley, R.E.; Sogin, M.L.; Jones, W.J.; Roe, B.A.; Affourtit, J.P.; et al. A core gut microbiome in obese and lean twins. *Nature* **2009**, *457*, 480–484. [CrossRef]

10. Qin, J.; Li, R.; Raes, J.; Arumugam, M.; Burgdorf, K.S.; Manichanh, C.; Nielsen, T.; Pons, N.; Levenez, F.; Yamada, T.; et al. A human gut microbial gene catalog established by metagenomic sequencing. *Nature* **2010**, *464*, 59–65. [CrossRef] [PubMed]

11. Zitvogel, L.; Galluzzi, L.; Viaud, S.; Vétizou, M.; Daillère, R.; Merad, M.; Kroemer, G. Cancer and the gut microbiota: An unexpected link. *Sci. Transl. Med.* **2015**, *7*, ps1–ps271. [CrossRef]

12. Poussin, C.; Sierro, N.; Boué, S.; Battey, J.; Scotti, E.; Belcastro, V.; Peitsch, M.C.; Ivanov, N.V.; Hoeng, J. Interrogating the microbiome: Experimental and computational considerations in support of study reproducibility. *Drug Discov. Today* **2018**, *23*, 1644–1657. [CrossRef]

13. Shreiner, A.B.; Kao, J.Y.; Young, V.B. The gut microbiome in health and in disease. *Curr. Opin. Gastroenterol.* **2015**, *31*, 69–75. [CrossRef]

14. Kho, Z.Y.; Lal, S.K. The Human Gut Microbiome—A Potential Controller of Wellness and Disease. *Front. Microbiol.* **2018**, *9*. [CrossRef]

15. Novati, S.; Sacchi, P.; Cima, S.; Zuccaro, V.; Columpsi, P.; Pagani, L.; Filice, G.; Bruno, R. General issues on microbial translocation in HIV-infected patients. *Eur. Rev. Med. Pharmacol. Sci.* **2015**, *19*, 866–878. [PubMed]

16. Amedei, A.; Boem, F. I've Gut A Feeling: Microbiota Impacting the Conceptual and Experimental Perspectives of Personalized Medicine. *Int. J. Mol. Sci.* **2018**, *19*, 3756. [CrossRef] [PubMed]

17. Gopalakrishnan, V.; Helmink, B.A.; Spencer, C.N.; Reuben, A.; Wargo, J.A. The Influence of the Gut Microbiome on Cancer, Immunity, and Cancer Immunotherapy. *Cancer Cell* **2018**, *33*, 570–580. [CrossRef] [PubMed]

18. Lazar, V.; Ditu, L.-M.; Pircalabioru, G.G.; Gheorghe, I.; Curutiu, C.; Holban, A.M.; Picu, A.; Petcu, L.; Chifiriuc, M.C. Aspects of Gut Microbiota and Immune System Interactions in Infectious Diseases, Immunopathology, and Cancer. *Front. Immunol.* **2018**, *9*, 1830. [CrossRef] [PubMed]

19. Manzo, V.E.; Bhatt, A.S. The human microbiome in hematopoiesis and hematologic disorders. *Blood* **2015**, *126*, 311–318. [CrossRef]

20. Round, J.L.; Mazmanian, S.K. The gut microbiome shapes intestinal immune responses during health and disease. *Nat. Rev. Immunol.* **2009**, *9*, 313–323. [CrossRef]

21. Yi, M.; Yu, S.; Qin, S.; Liu, Q.; Xu, H.; Zhao, W.; Chu, Q.; Wu, K. Gut microbiome modulates efficacy of immune checkpoint inhibitors. *J. Hematol. Oncol.* **2018**, *11*, 47. [CrossRef]

22. Liu, D.; Wang, S.; Bindeman, W. Clinical applications of PD-L1 bioassays for cancer immunotherapy. *J. Hematol. Oncol.* **2017**, *10*, 110. [CrossRef]

23. Daillère, R.; Vétizou, M.; Waldschmitt, N.; Yamazaki, T.; Isnard, C.; Poirier-Colame, V.; Duong, C.P.M.; Flament, C.; Lepage, P.; Roberti, M.P.; et al. Enterococcus hirae and Barnesiella intestinihominis Facilitate Cyclophosphamide-Induced Therapeutic Immunomodulatory Effects. *Immunity* **2016**, *45*, 931–943. [CrossRef]

24. Belkaid, Y.; Hand, T.W. Role of the Microbiota in Immunity and Inflammation. *Cell* **2014**, *157*, 121–141. [CrossRef]

25. Ichinohe, T.; Pang, I.K.; Kumamoto, Y.; Peaper, D.R.; Ho, J.H.; Murray, T.S.; Iwasaki, A. Microbiota regulates immune defense against respiratory tract influenza A virus infection. *Proc. Natl. Acad. Sci. USA* **2011**, *108*, 5354–5359. [CrossRef]

26. Clarke, T.B.; Davis, K.M.; Lysenko, E.S.; Zhou, A.Y.; Yu, Y.; Weiser, J.N. Recognition of Peptidoglycan from the Microbiota by Nod1 Enhances Systemic Innate Immunity. *Nat. Med.* **2010**, *16*, 228–231. [CrossRef]

27. Marchetti, G.; Tincati, C.; Silvestri, G. Microbial Translocation in the Pathogenesis of HIV Infection and AIDS. *Clin. Microbiol. Rev.* **2013**, *26*, 2–18. [CrossRef]

28. Wiest, R.; Lawson, M.; Geuking, M. Pathological bacterial translocation in liver cirrhosis. *J. Hepatol.* **2014**, *60*, 197–209. [CrossRef]

29. Sacchi, P.; Cima, S.; Corbella, M.; Comolli, G.; Chiesa, A.; Baldanti, F.; Klersy, C.; Novati, S.; Mulatto, P.; Mariconti, M.; et al. Liver fibrosis, microbial translocation and immune activation markers in HIV and HCV infections and in HIV/HCV co-infection. *Dig. Liver Dis.* **2015**, *47*, 218–225. [CrossRef]

30. Mirza, A.; Mao-Draayer, Y. The gut microbiome and microbial translocation in multiple sclerosis. *Clin. Immunol.* **2017**, *183*, 213–224. [CrossRef]

31. Principles of Cancer Immunotherapy—UpToDate. Available online: https://www.uptodate.com/contents/principles-of-cancer-immunotherapy?search=cancer%20immunotherapy&source=search_result&selectedTitle=1~||150&usage_type=default&display_rank=1 (accessed on 26 December 2018).

32. Routy, B.; Le Chatelier, E.; Derosa, L.; Duong, C.P.M.; Alou, M.T.; Daillère, R.; Fluckiger, A.; Messaoudene, M.; Rauber, C.; Roberti, M.P.; et al. Gut microbiome influences efficacy of PD-1–based immunotherapy against epithelial tumors. *Science* **2018**, *359*, 91–97. [CrossRef]

33. Wang, Y.; Ma, R.; Liu, F.; Lee, S.A.; Zhang, L. Modulation of Gut Microbiota: A Novel Paradigm of Enhancing the Efficacy of Programmed Death-1 and Programmed Death Ligand-1 Blockade Therapy. *Front. Immunol.* **2018**, *9*, 374. [CrossRef] [PubMed]

34. Sivan, A.; Corrales, L.; Hubert, N.; Williams, J.B.; Aquino-Michaels, K.; Earley, Z.M.; Benyamin, F.W.; Lei, Y.M.; Jabri, B.; Alegre, M.-L.; et al. Commensal Bifidobacterium promotes antitumor immunity and facilitates anti–PD-L1 efficacy. *Science* **2015**, *350*, 1084–1089. [CrossRef]

35. Matson, V.; Fessler, J.; Bao, R.; Chongsuwat, T.; Zha, Y.; Alegre, M.-L.; Luke, J.J.; Gajewski, T.F. The commensal microbiome is associated with anti–PD-1 efficacy in metastatic melanoma patients. *Science* **2018**, *359*, 104–108. [CrossRef]

36. Gopalakrishnan, V.; Spencer, C.N.; Nezi, L.; Reuben, A.; Andrews, M.C.; Karpinets, T.V.; Prieto, P.A.; Vicente, D.; Hoffman, K.; Wei, S.C.; et al. Gut microbiome modulates response to anti–PD-1 immunotherapy in melanoma patients. *Science* **2018**, *359*, 97–103. [CrossRef]

37. Balmer, M.L.; Schürch, C.M.; Saito, Y.; Geuking, M.B.; Li, H.; Cuenca, M.; Kovtonyuk, L.V.; McCoy, K.D.; Hapfelmeier, S.; Ochsenbein, A.F.; et al. Microbiota-Derived Compounds Drive Steady-State Granulopoiesis via MyD88/TICAM Signaling. *J. Immunol.* **2014**, *193*, 5273–5283. [CrossRef]

38. Yamamoto, M.; Schiestl, R. Lymphoma Caused by Intestinal Microbiota. *Int. J. Environ. Res. Public. Health* **2014**, *11*, 9038–9049. [CrossRef]

39. Bayerdörffer, E.; Rudolph, B.; Neubauer, A.; Thiede, C.; Lehn, N.; Eidt, S.; Stolte, M. MALT Lymphoma Study Group Regression of primary gastric lymphoma of mucosa-associated lymphoid tissue type after cure of Helicobacter pylori infection. *Lancet* **1995**, *345*, 1591–1594.

40. Franco, V. Splenic marginal zone lymphoma. *Blood* **2003**, *101*, 2464–2472. [CrossRef]

41. Tao, Q.; Robertson, K.D.; Manns, A.; Hildesheim, A.; Ambinder, R.F. Epstein-Barr Virus (EBV) in Endemic Burkitt's Lymphoma: Molecular Analysis of Primary Tumor Tissue. *Blood* **1998**, *91*, 1373–1381.

42. Soulier, J.; Grollet, L.; Oksenhendler, E.; Cacoub, P.; Cazals-Hatem, D.; Babinet, P. Kaposi's Sarcoma-Associated Herpesvirus-Like DNA Sequences in Multicentric Castleman's Disease. *Blood* **1995**, *86*, 1276–1280.

43. Hildebr, G.C.; Kumari, R.; Palaniy, S. The human microbiome in hematologic malignancies. *Hematol. Transfus. Int. J.* **2016**, *2*, 00047.

44. Marsland, B.J.; Gollwitzer, E.S. Host-microorganism interactions in lung diseases. *Nat. Rev. Immunol.* **2014**, *14*, 827–835. [CrossRef]

45. Schöllkopf, C.; Melbye, M.; Munksgaard, L.; Smedby, K.E.; Rostgaard, K.; Glimelius, B.; Chang, E.T.; Roos, G.; Hansen, M.; Adami, H.-O.; et al. Borrelia infection and risk of non-Hodgkin lymphoma. *Blood* **2008**, *111*, 5524–5529. [CrossRef] [PubMed]

46. Aigelsreiter, A.; Gerlza, T.; Deutsch, A.J.A.; Leitner, E.; Beham-Schmid, C.; Beham, A.; Popper, H.; Borel, N.; Pospischil, A.; Raderer, M.; et al. Chlamydia psittaci Infection in nongastrointestinal extranodal MALT lymphomas and their precursor lesions. *Am. J. Clin. Pathol.* **2011**, *135*, 70–75. [CrossRef]

47. Gaboriau-Routhiau, V.; Rakotobe, S.; Lécuyer, E.; Mulder, I.; Lan, A.; Bridonneau, C.; Rochet, V.; Pisi, A.; De Paepe, M.; Brandi, G.; et al. The key role of segmented filamentous bacteria in the coordinated maturation of gut helper T cell responses. *Immunity* **2009**, *31*, 677–689. [CrossRef]

48. Wei, B.; Su, T.T.; Dalwadi, H.; Stephan, R.P.; Fujiwara, D.; Huang, T.T.; Brewer, S.; Chen, L.; Arditi, M.; Borneman, J.; et al. Resident enteric microbiota and CD8+ T cells shape the abundance of marginal zone B cells. *Eur. J. Immunol.* **2008**, *38*, 3411–3425. [CrossRef] [PubMed]

49. Jain, S.; Ward, J.M.; Shin, D.-M.; Wang, H.; Naghashfar, Z.; Kovalchuk, A.L.; Morse, H.C. Associations of Autoimmunity, Immunodeficiency, Lymphomagenesis, and Gut Microbiota in Mice with Knockins for a Pathogenic Autoantibody. *Am. J. Pathol.* **2017**, *187*, 2020–2033. [CrossRef]

50. Scheeren, F.A.; Diehl, S.A.; Smit, L.A.; Beaumont, T.; Naspetti, M.; Bende, R.J.; Blom, B.; Karube, K.; Ohshima, K.; van Noesel, C.J.M.; et al. IL-21 is expressed in Hodgkin lymphoma and activates STAT5: Evidence that activated STAT5 is required for Hodgkin lymphomagenesis. *Blood* **2008**, *111*, 4706–4715. [CrossRef]

51. Rajagopala, S.V.; Vashee, S.; Oldfield, L.M.; Suzuki, Y.; Venter, J.C.; Telenti, A.; Nelson, K.E. The Human Microbiome and Cancer. *Cancer Prev. Res.* **2017**, *10*, 226–234. [CrossRef] [PubMed]

52. Thanarajasingam, G.; Thanarajasingam, U.; Ansell, S.M. Immune checkpoint blockade in lymphoid malignancies. *FEBS J.* **2016**, *283*, 2233–2244. [CrossRef]

53. Peled, J.U.; Devlin, S.M.; Staffas, A.; Lumish, M.; Khanin, R.; Littmann, E.R.; Ling, L.; Kosuri, S.; Maloy, M.; Slingerland, J.B.; et al. Intestinal Microbiota and Relapse After Hematopoietic-Cell Transplantation. *J. Clin. Oncol.* **2017**, *35*, 1650–1659. [CrossRef] [PubMed]

54. Columpsi, P.; Sacchi, P.; Zuccaro, V.; Cima, S.; Sarda, C.; Mariani, M.; Gori, A.; Bruno, R. Beyond the gut bacterial microbiota: The gut virome. *J. Med. Virol.* **2016**, *88*, 1467–1472. [CrossRef] [PubMed]

55. Personalized Medicine—UpToDate. Available online: https://www.uptodate.com/contents/personalized-medicine?search=personalized%20medicine&source=search_result&selectedTitle=1~||150&usage_type=default&display_rank=1 (accessed on 26 December 2018).

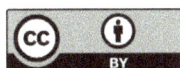

International Journal of
Molecular Sciences

MDPI

Review

Bacteriocins and Bacteriophages: Therapeutic Weapons for Gastrointestinal Diseases?

Loris Riccardo Lopetuso [1,2], **Maria Ernestina Giorgio** [1], **Angela Saviano** [1], **Franco Scaldaferri** [1,2], **Antonio Gasbarrini** [1,2] **and Giovanni Cammarota** [1,2,*]

[1]   Istituto di Patologia Speciale Medica, Università Cattolica del Sacro Cuore, 00168 Roma, Italy;
        lopetusoloris@libero.it (L.R.L.); estin.gio3@gmail.com (M.E.G.); saviange@libero.it (A.S.);
        francoscaldaferri@gmail.com (F.S.); antonio.gasbarrini@unicatt.it (A.G.)
[2]   UOC Medicina Interna E Gastroenterologia, Area Gastroenterologia ed Oncologia Medica, Dipartimento di
        Scienze Gastroenterologiche, Endocrino-Metaboliche e Nefro-Urologiche, Fondazione Policlinico
        Universitario A. Gemelli IRCCS, 00168 Roma, Italy
*   Correspondence: giovanni.cammarota@unicatt.it; Tel.: +39-063-503-310

Received: 8 December 2018; Accepted: 28 December 2018; Published: 6 January 2019

Abstract: Bacteriocins are bactericidal peptides, ribosomally synthesized, with an inhibitory activity against diverse groups of undesirable microorganisms. Bacteriocins are produced by both gram-positive and gram-negative bacteria, and to a lesser extent by some archaea. Bacteriophages are viruses that are able to infect bacterial cells and force them to produce viral components, using a lytic or lysogenic cycle. They constitute a large community in the human gut called the phageome, the most abundant part of the gut virome. Bacteriocins and bacteriophages may have an influence on both human health and diseases, thanks to their ability to modulate the gut microbiota and regulate the competitive relationship among the different microorganisms, strains and cells living in the human intestine. In this review, we explore the role of bacteriocins and bacteriophages in the most frequent gastrointestinal diseases by dissecting their interaction with the complex environment of the human gut, analyzing a possible link with extra-intestinal diseases, and speculating on their possible therapeutic application with the end goal of promoting gut health.

Keywords: bacteriocins; bacteriophages; antibiotics; gastrointestinal diseases; dysbiosis; gut barrier; gut microbiota; virus

---

1. Introduction

Bacteriocins are potent small and heat-stable bactericidal peptides [1] with antimicrobial properties against different groups of microorganisms [2].

They were first described in 1925, but the interest in their production, function and possible applications in medical areas has been growing only recently [2]. Diverse kinds of bacteriocins have been described by size, inhibitory mechanism, target cells, spectrum of action, interaction with the immune system and biochemical features [3]. Bacteriocins are produced by both gram-positive and gram-negative bacteria, and by some archaea [4]. They are synthetized by ribosomes and influenced by environmental factors (e.g., temperature, pH, and composition of the culture medium) [5,6].

Many bacteriocins are produced by the *Firmicutes* phylum, others belong to *Bacteroidetes* and the remaining percentage to the *Actinobacteria* and *Proteobacteria* phyla [7–9].

In particular, within the *Firmicutes* phylum, the major interest has involved the bacteriocins derived from the gram-positive, lactic acid bacteria (LAB), bacteria commonly used in food fermentation and well-represented both in the human gastrointestinal, respiratory and genital tract [10].

Lactic acid bacteria mainly produce two classes of bacteriocins [11]. Class I includes the modified-peptides known as "lanthionine-containing bacteriocins" (an example is nisin [12], and it can also include linaridin, azoline, cyanobactin, glycocin, sactiobiotic, thiopeptide, and lasso peptide) [3]; class II includes "non-lanthionine-containing bacteriocins" divided into four other subclasses (a,b,c,d) based on their size [12]. Subclass a (i.e., pediocin PA-1, sakacin A [13]) is active against *Lactobacillus*, *Enterococcus*, *Clostridium*, *Pediococcus* and *Leuconostoc* [14–16]. Subclass b (i.e., plantaricins E,F and J,K) [17] is made up of two antimicrobial-peptides that work only in combination (E with F and J with K) [18]. Subclass c (i.e., garvacin ML) is represented by circular bacteriocins [11], while subclass d (i.e., enterocin Q, L50) is composed of linear bacteriocins with an unknown role [11,19]. Class II also includes subclass II e (i.e., microcin E492).

Most of these bacteriocins are able to inhibit the pathogens' growth, defend the producer and to play a role in "signaling" peptides [3]. Mechanistically, they can act as pore-forming agents, or membrane perturbers [20], or they can interfere with the cellular division processes. Moreover, bacteriocins possess anti-viral, spermicidal [2], and anti-cancer properties [21], and can enhance the positive effects of probiotic bacteria [22] (i.e., bacteriocins produced by the *Bifidobacterium* strain) [3].

Most of the above-mentioned functions are shared by bacteriophages. These are viruses that infect bacterial cells and force them to produce viral components, using diverse mechanisms such as the lytic or lysogenic cycle [23,24], but also to a lesser extent the pseudo-lysogenic cycle, the cryptic life cycle [25] or chronic infection [26,27]. Abortive infections rarely occur [28].

Bacteriophages constitute a large community of the human gut microbiota [29] and, together with viruses, are considered the most abundant organisms on the planet [30]. In the human colon they represent around 10^{15} cells [31]. Bacteriophages are classified according to their DNA or RNA, morphology (filamentous, polyhedral, pleomorphic, spiral, etc.), life cycle and their habitats [32,33]. They usually act on a narrow, closed and specific range of bacteria [34]. Broad-spectrum bacteriophages are rarely described in the literature [35]. In the human gut, the bacteriophages-family of Caudovirales (Siphoviridae, Myovirididae, Podoviridae) is the most abundant, followed by Microviridae [36]. In healthy individuals the balanced and inverse correlation between Caudovirales and Microviridae ensures the maintenance of a eubiotic state. In fact, bacteriophages regulate the bacterial population (shifting the ratio of both symbionts and pathobionts), control their metabolism [37] and mediate anti-inflammatory responses. They can interact with immune cells, inducing the production of pro-inflammatory cytokines, they can down-regulate the oxidative stress, reducing the reactive oxygen species, and they carry out both protective and immuno-modulating effects on gut-lymphoid tissue [38].

In this review, we explored the multiple relationships of bacteriocins and bacteriophages with the gut barrier and their role in the most common gastrointestinal diseases.

2. Relationship of Bacteriophages and Bacteriocins with the Gut Barrier

In the gut mucosa, bacteriophages select specific bacteria by using horizontal gene transfer, influencing their rate of mutation and genetic variability, and thus modulating their abundance and diversity [39,40]. On the capsid they express Ig (Immunoglobulin)-like receptors, which interact with mucin glycoproteins and can regulate innate and acquired immunity [41]. Thus, bacteriophages can influence bacterial composition, modify their function and interaction with epithelial cells, and modulate the glycoproteic mucin layer and control other microorganism populations both directly and indirectly [38]. Moreover, they are dynamic entities that can translocate across the gut barrier and migrate into the peripheral blood and the peripheral tissue, activating the immune system [38]. They also have a complementary action on dendritic cells and can be considered both activators of inflammation and at the same time anti-inflammatory players [42]. The bacteriophages' translocation across the gut barrier has been confirmed by different metagenomics studies that revealed their presence in ascitic, urine and blood samples [42,43]. In this scenario, their actions should not only be considered to be focused on the gastrointestinal tract, but also extended to other sites.

Further, bacteriocins act both on the immune system and on the inhibition of competitive strains by directly influencing the niche competition among commensals [44]. Bacteriocins are commonly used strategically by commensals to colonize and persist in the human gut. Their activities could resemble those of a "probiotic". Indeed, they allow the survival of specific communities in the gastrointestinal tract by selecting strains that are able to resist modification by the host diet, the inhibition of natural defensins, bile salts and other killing factors, and colonization by other species, overall improving gut barrier function and the host immune response [45]. Studies on animal ilea have confirmed the potential effects of bacteriocin against pathogens, which led to positive changes in the gut microbiota composition. This is the case of Bacteriocin Abp118 [3], produced by *Lactobacillus salivarius UCC118* [13] or salivaricin P, produced by another *Lactobacillus salivarius* strain with a probiotic trait [3]. Interestingly, *Lactobacillus salivarius* expresses the srtA gene to tie it to the epithelial cell's surface, before producing protective bacteriocins [3]. Bactofencin A or bacteriocin 21 produced by *Enterococcus faecalis* are able to kill multidrug resistant-bacteria and contribute to the regulation of the niche competition among intestinal bacteria [44]. Similarly, LAB bacteriocins exert their role against *Staphylococcus Aureus* [14], some vancomycin-resistant enterococci [44], *Salmonella enteritidis* [14], *Clostridium Difficile* [46] and *Listeria monocytogenes* [14]. More studies are needed to test the therapeutic potential of these findings. At the same time, it should be noted that not all changes observed in vitro have also been registered in vivo. This discrepancy is not surprising since several perturbing factors can deeply affect bacteriocin production and their activities.

3. Role of Bacteriophages in Gastrointestinal Chronic Inflammation

The role of bacteriocins and bacteriophages in most gastrointestinal diseases remains unknown [38]. Many studies have focused on the role they play in inflammatory bowel disease (IBD), such as Crohn's disease (CD) and ulcerative colitis (UC) [31].

Recent analyses support the idea that the gut virome is involved in intestinal inflammation [47]. Bacteriophages can induce bacterial lysis leading to the release of nucleic acids, proteins and lipids, which are sources of pro-inflammatory stimuli and are able to provoke crucial dysbiotic alterations in CD and UC. An increased abundance of *Caudovirales* with a lower presence of *Coliphages* is found in IBD patients, both in CD and UC [38,48]. At the same time, bacteriophages can influence the abundance and diversity of bacteria in IBD with multifactorial and often unknown mechanisms. Usually, bacteriophages possess a narrow spectrum of action both on bacterial cells and on the immune system, which is activated by their coat proteins. They can act as antigens or ligands and can contribute to chronic intestinal inflammation [49]. This high diversity in phage-composition could represent a possible risk factor for developing IBD. On the other hand, bacteriophages could represent promising therapeutic tools to control inflammation. In this scenario, recent studies have demonstrated that bacteriophages are effective in reducing intestinal *E. coli* colonization [50,51], in particular the adherent invasive strain (AIEC) [52], which is considered to be involved in the maintenance of chronic inflammation in IBD [53]. Galtier et al. found three virulent bacteriophages that were able to replicate in ileal and colonic portions and feces from gut murine samples colonized with the prototype AIEC strain LF82. A single day of oral treatment with these bacteriophages significantly decreased the intestinal colonization of AIEC strain LF82. Furthermore, this single-dose reduced DSS-induced colitis symptoms over a 2-week period in mice colonized with LF82 [52].

In humans, a recent randomized trial of oral phage therapy in 120 children with acute bacterial diarrhea in Bangladesh did not report any adverse events, but failed to achieve intestinal amplification or improve the diarrhea outcome [54]. This could be due to low phage coverage and insufficient E. coli pathogen titers, which required higher phage doses. One should note that, since bacteriophages are part of the human commensal microbiota and because they are highly specific, they are likely to have a better safety profile than antibiotic therapy. Currently, a phase I double-blind randomized placebo-controlled trial is ongoing in quiescent CD to assess the safety of a lytic phage preparation containing seven bacteriophages targeting AIEC. This study involves participants with documented AIEC in the stool taking either a phage preparation or placebo for 2 weeks to evaluate adverse events or disease exacerbation. If safe and successful, the goal is to develop this as an adjuvant therapy in patients with CD and AIEC colonization.

Furthermore, the potential presence of bacteriophages in the blood represents a new, unexplored field. More studies are necessary to evaluate the opportunity of using bacteriophages for screening and predicting disease progression [31,55] and to understand the amount and types of bacterial species associated with a specific degree of disease. Similarly, the changes in the gut bacteriophage population, and the consequent modulation of commensal bacteria and the activation of pro-inflammatory strains in IBD require further analysis. Understanding these mechanisms could be useful to positively act on bacterial antibiotic-resistance or to calibrate the anti-inflammatory effect of specific bacteria [47,48].

4. Bacteriophages and Bacteriocins in Bacterial Food Infections

The antibacterial properties of bacteriophages and bacteriocins are exploited in food research. In particular, bacteriocins are used as food preservatives [12] both for dairy products [56] and for meat, fish [57], vegetables and fruits [58], being classified as partially purified bacteriocins, crude-fermented dairy bacteriocins and protective cultures bacteriocins [2].

Bacteriocins are considered natural and safe food additives after being ingested by the gastrointestinal tract [59]. They have the interesting properties of stability, antimicrobial effects, potency, and no flavor alteration [59].

There are different commercially available bacteriocins such as nisin (named Nisaplin) or Pediocin PA-1 against the growth of *Listeria monocytogenes* in meat products [60]. Other bacteriocins, such as those produced by Enterococci, seem to reduce the contamination of cheese due to animal feces [61], while Enterocin AS-48, Enterocin CCM4231 and EJ97 are used to protect both fermented and unfermented vegetables [60]. Bacteriocins can be added to food through the direct inoculation of the producer-strains as a concentrated fermented product [60] or as a gradual-release preparation. They have antimicrobial activity against gram-negative bacteria that infect foods, and this property could be empowered by combining bacteriocins with other compounds (e.g., organic acids, phenolic compounds). Other antimicrobial bacteriocins involved in food protection belong to the class I and II bacteriocins of Bacillus subtilis GAS101 and act against some gram-positive bacterial species such as *Staphylococcus Epidermidis* [62]. Bacteriocins are overall able to reduce the costs of food treatments and at the same time increase the product shelf-life.

Similarly, bacteriophages are used against *Salmonella*, *Campylobacter* and *Enterococcus* on food [28]. The efficacy of bacteriophages is reduced by their spectrum of action, which is oriented against specific serotypes, species or strains of bacteria [28]. However, their narrow spectrum could be more advantageous than antibiotics and may have a lower impact on the other components of the gut microbiota [33].

Bacteriophages can also control the production of some pathogenic toxins such as Cholera, Shiga and Pertussis, and interfere with mechanisms of antibiotic resistance [48]. In the past, they have been used to control the epidemic of bloody diarrhea in Germany caused by *E. coli* strain 0104:H4 through the production of Shiga toxins [63].

Finally, an alteration of gut virome composition could also be found in recurrent *Clostridium Difficile* infection [64]. Interestingly, the presence of a complex of bacteriophages in fecal mass used for therapeutic fecal microbiota transplantation (FMT) has been demonstrated to improve clinical outcomes of this treatment [65].

5. Role of Bacteriophages and Bacteriocins in Extra-Intestinal Diseases

Bacteriophage therapy has strong potential as a treatment for many extra-intestinal diseases, and in particular in those correlated to bacterial infections [66]. Indeed, in chronic bacterial rhino-sinusitis, after twenty days of topical application, a bacteriophage cocktail (P68, K710) is able to control a broad range of *Staphylococcus Aureus* (*S. aureus*) strains, including the methicillin-resistant strain (MRSA) [66]. A common manifestation of invasive *S. aureus* infection is osteomyelitis. *S. aureus* triggers many profound alterations in bone remodeling. Bacteriophage therapy has been applied with promising results, but more data are needed to confirm these findings [67].

In animal models, it has been reported that bacteriophages are able to control *Pseudomonas* lung infections [46]. In fact, two bacteriophages, φMR299-2 and φNH-4, have been proven to induce the formation of a biofilm on lung cells useful in controlling these infections. Hypothetically, they could have beneficial effects in patients with cystic fibrosis who are mostly exposed to this microorganism [68].

Bacteriophage therapy has been also used successfully for acne treatment. Acne has a multifactorial etiology and the inflammatory follicular response caused by the gram-positive skin bacterium *Propionibacterium Acnes* seems to play a primary role. The most common first line treatment is based on topical antimicrobial agents or oral antibiotics. Recent data suggest an alternative treatment, both for acne and for others bacterial skin infections, based on the use of a lytic bacteriophage preparation able to kill specific bacterial cells [69].

Further advantages of bacteriophage treatment have been demonstrated for diabetic foot ulcer healing. A commercial topical preparation of staphylococcal bacteriophage Sb-1 is effective when antibiotic treatment is unsuccessful [70].

On the contrary, bacteriocins such as pyocin were unable to control *Pseudomonas* lung infections in patients with cystic fibrosis. In fact, despite initial positive laboratory experiments, subsequent studies have underlined no evidence of beneficial effects for this bacteriocin [71].

Another frequent infection is provoked by *Streptococcus Pneumoniae*, which is responsible for pneumonia, bacteremia and meningitis, in particular in children. Pneumococcal disease benefit from vaccine and antibiotic treatment, but resistance is increasing. *S. Pneumoniae* is common in the nasopharynx of children, and it produces a circular bacteriocin, known as pneumocyclicin, to attack other bacteria and to protect itself against the immune system. This bacteriocin is similar to the other circular bacteriocins produced by gram-positive bacteria, and it could represent an important target thanks to its correlation to antibiotic resistance mechanisms [72].

Overall, bacteriophage therapy could be very beneficial thanks to its action against all types of pathogens, including those that are multi-drug resistant. A positive aspect of their narrow spectrum is the possibility of preserving the existing microbiome. Bacteriophages also have lower side effects, a wide distribution after their administration, and a possible inhibitory effect on the inflammatory response. They are cost effective and some studies underline their efficacy in comparison with antibiotics [33]. Further, bacteriocins could be very useful in fighting pathogens. They are easier to modify through bioengineering and have targeted activity against specific microorganisms. Numerous studies are trying to prove their use as a natural defense and as an alternative to antibiotics [12] in peculiar cases such as pregnant women and in individuals with contraindications to antibiotic use [73].

6. Bacteriocins, Bacteriophages and Cancer

Bacteriocins and bacteriophages are gaining great importance in the medical oncology field. Both are able to induce an immune modulatory response against T and B cells [74], which are involved in the control of cancerous pathways [75]. In addition, they can stimulate cytokine secretion [76] and modify the tumor microenvironment to make anticancer treatment more effective.

Bacteriophages display a huge genetic flexibility and consequently a variety of surface modifications that can be used as a basis for phage display methodology. These manipulations could potentially lead to the targeted delivery of therapeutic genes. Furthermore, their strong safety profile allows their potential application as cancer gene therapy platforms. The combination of phage display with combinatorial technology has produced the organization of phage libraries, transforming phage display into a high throughput technology. Indeed, random peptide libraries are one of the most important phage libraries, as they offer a huge source of clinically useful peptide ligands [77]. Peptides represent promising pharmaceutical tools in the oncologic field with significant advantages, including the low costs of synthesis, efficient membrane penetration and the absence of immunogenicity. Phage peptide libraries can be interrogated against several oncologic targets such as cancer-homing ligands, and they serve as gene therapy vectors towards malignant cells [77]. Thanks to this method, a large number of peptide ligands can be produced through the addition of specific genetic fragments into genes encoding phage capsid proteins [76]. In this scenario, a filamentous phage is used to vector a functionally active green fluorescent protein into mammalian cells by exerting a mechanism commonly used by fibroblast growth factor for cell internalization [78]. Another group was able to inhibit vascular endothelial growth factor activity and thus angiogenesis through the use of a phage display library [79]. Moreover, these peptides can diminish tumor metastasis and block specific enzymes necessary for tumor progression [76]. In fact, the affinity of the phage T4 (wt4) and its substrain HAP1 with melanoma cells was used efficiently to inhibit lung metastasis in mice [80].

Bacteriocins share similar anticancer properties. In particular, Colicin A and Colicin E1 revealed inhibitory activity against the growth of eleven different tumor-cell lines [81]. Similarly, colicin D and colicin E2 showed an inhibitory effect against murine leukemia cells P388 and colicin E3 suppressed the malignant transformation of a chicken monoblast line [59]. Further, other colicins produced by *E. coli* strains were able to act against human colorectal carcinoma cells [59].

Finally, in mice, nisin was effective in controlling head and neck squamous cell carcinoma and oral cancer. The effects of this treatment resulted in the reduction of tumor volumes and was correlated with an increased cellular apoptosis mediated by CHAC1 expression, a cation transport regulator and apoptosis mediator [82].

7. Conclusions

In summary, bacteriophages and bacteriocins share significant potentially beneficial effects on human health (Table 1). In particular, bacteriocins could fill a gap in medical and food industry applications by playing a role as a "natural" and "safe" antimicrobial agent in the near future. They can regulate competitive interactions in the microbial community. Their narrow-target activity, surprising specificity, high stability and low toxicity make them an alternative or complement to current antibiotics. They could play a key role in antibiotic resistance and could become a useful approach in the treatment of infectious diseases. Moreover, thanks to their non-immunogenicity and ability to modulate cancer cell proliferation, they could act as potential synergistic agents with current conventional cancer treatments. Likewise, bacteriophages could share similar properties of effectiveness and safety in various medical fields (e.g., the modulation of chronic inflammation, antibiotic and cancer therapy, food safety). For this reason, in the world of nanotechnology and nanomaterials, they are emerging as valuable rising stars for modulating the gut barrier and restoring the overall homeostasis of the gut community.

Table 1. An overview of bacteriocins, bacteriophages and antibiotics properties.

	Bacteriocins	Bacteriophages	Antibiotics
Classes	Class I (lanthionine-containing bacteriocins) Class II (non-lanthionine-containing bacteriocins): - IIa - IIb - IIc - IId - IIe Class III Class IV* (also containing lipid or carbohydrate and not only proteins)	Four classes based on the genetic composition: dsDNA ssRNA dsRNA ssDNA	β-Lactams Aminoglycosides Chloramphenicol Glycopeptides Ansamycins Streptogramins Sulfonamides Tetracyclines Macrolides Oxazolidinones Quinolones Lipopeptides
Inhibitory mechanism (mechanisms of action)	-Inhibit the pathogens' growth, acting as pore-forming agents, membrane perturbers. -Dissipate the transmembrane electrical potential, leading to cell death. -Interfere with cellular division processes.	-Infect and use bacterial cells resources through: • lytic cycle • lysogenic cycle or • pseudo-lysogenic cycle • cryptic life cycle • chronic infection -Inhibitory activity against pathogens' growth through their combined action on both gut microflora species and immune system cells. -Interfere with bacterial cellular replication and transcriptional processes.	-Inhibit the biosynthesis of bacteria cell walls. -Inhibit the synthesis of proteins. -Inhibit the synthesis of RNA. -Interfere with bacterial DNA replication and transcription. -Disrupt multiple bacteria cell membrane functions.
Target cells (spectrum of action)	Mainly narrow spectrum on: -Bacterial cells-Viral cells -B and T Lymphocytes	Mainly narrow spectrum on: -Bacterial cells -Archaea	Narrow or broad spectrum on: -Bacterial cells -Parasites
Size	Small or large peptides (from less than 5kDa to 90 kDa)	Short or Long (from 24 to 200 nm)	
Morphology (shape)	Linear Globular Circular	Filamentous Icosahedral, polyhedral Pleomorphic Spiral Isometric With or without tails (contractile or non-contractile) With or without an envelope With or without a capsid	Heterogeneous
Administration	Mainly oral; intravenous, intranasal, intraperitoneal, subcutaneous (studies on animal models)	Intramuscular, intravenous, topical (studies on animal models)	Oral, intramuscular, intravenous, topical
Application	Food preservatives, treatment of intestinal and extraintestinal infections	Models for studying viral transformation, vehicles for vaccine delivery, synthesis of novel polypeptides, control of environmental and dangerous bacterial cell growth	Treatment or prevention of bacterial infections and in specific cases of protozoan infections.
Side effects	More studies are needed to test this		Allergic reactions, hypersensitivity, diarrhea, fever, nausea are the most common.
Resistance	Potential application to fight antibiotic resistance and act against the current multi-drug resistant pathogens		Very common

Author Contributions: This work was contributed to by all authors. The paper was discussed and designed by all authors with the main text being written by L.R.L., M.E.G., A.S. and G.C. All authors then reviewed and contributed further to the review.

Int. J. Mol. Sci. **2019**, *20*, 183

Funding: This research received no external funding.

Acknowledgments: The authors acknowledge continued support from the Crohn's & Colitis Foundation of America Research Fellowship Award (to L.R.L.) and Società Italiana di Medicina Interna Premio di Ricerca (to L.R.L.).

Conflicts of Interest: The authors declare no conflict of interest.

Abbreviations

IBD   Inflammatory Bowel Diseases
CD   Crohn's Disease
UC   Ulcerative Colitis
MRSA   Methicillin-Resistant *S. aureus*

References

1. Klaenhammer, T.R. Bacteriocins of lactic acid bacteria. *Biochimie* **1988**, *70*, 337–349. [CrossRef]
2. Chikindas, M.L.; Weeks, R.; Drider, D.; Chistyakov, V.A.; Dicks, L.M. Functions and emerging applications of bacteriocins. *Curr. Opin. Biotechnol.* **2017**, *49*, 23–28. [CrossRef] [PubMed]
3. Hegarty, J.W.; Guinane, C.M.; Ross, R.P.; Hill, C.; Cotter, P.D. Bacteriocin production: A relatively unharnessed probiotic trait? *F1000Res* **2016**, *5*, 2587. [CrossRef] [PubMed]
4. Zheng, J.; Ganzle, M.G.; Lin, X.B.; Ruan, L.; Sun, M. Diversity and dynamics of bacteriocins from human microbiome. *Environ. Microbiol.* **2015**, *17*, 2133–2143. [CrossRef] [PubMed]
5. Guinane, C.M.; Piper, C.; Draper, L.A.; O'Connor, P.M.; Hill, C.; Ross, R.P.; Cotter, P.D. Impact of Environmental Factors on Bacteriocin Promoter Activity in Gut-Derived Lactobacillus salivarius. *Appl. Environ. Microbiol.* **2015**, *81*, 7851–7859. [CrossRef] [PubMed]
6. Turgis, M.; Vu, K.D.; Millette, M.; Dupont, C.; Lacroix, M. Influence of Environmental Factors on Bacteriocin Production by Human Isolates of Lactococcus lactis MM19 and Pediococcus acidilactici MM33. *Probiotics Antimicrob. Proteins* **2016**, *8*, 53–59. [CrossRef] [PubMed]
7. Tap, J.; Mondot, S.; Levenez, F.; Pelletier, E.; Caron, C.; Furet, J.P.; Ugarte, E.; Munoz-Tamayo, R.; Paslier, D.L.; Nalin, R.; et al. Towards the human intestinal microbiota phylogenetic core. *Environ. Microbiol.* **2009**, *11*, 2574–2584. [CrossRef]
8. Ley, R.E.; Hamady, M.; Lozupone, C.; Turnbaugh, P.J.; Ramey, R.R.; Bircher, J.S.; Schlegel, M.L.; Tucker, T.A.; Schrenzel, M.D.; Knight, R.; et al. Evolution of mammals and their gut microbes. *Science* **2008**, *320*, 1647–1651. [CrossRef]
9. Dethlefsen, L.; McFall-Ngai, M.; Relman, D.A. An ecological and evolutionary perspective on human-microbe mutualism and disease. *Nature* **2007**, *449*, 811–818. [CrossRef]
10. Douillard, F.P.; de Vos, W.M. Functional genomics of lactic acid bacteria: From food to health. *Microb. Cell Fact.* **2014**, *13* (Suppl. 1), S8. [CrossRef]
11. Cotter, P.D.; Hill, C.; Ross, R.P. Bacteriocins: Developing innate immunity for food. *Nat. Rev. Microbiol.* **2005**, *3*, 777–788. [CrossRef]
12. Oldak, A.; Zielinska, D. Bacteriocins from lactic acid bacteria as an alternative to antibiotics. *Postepy Hig. Med. Dosw. (Online)* **2017**, *71*, 328–338. [CrossRef] [PubMed]
13. Umu, O.C.; Bauerl, C.; Oostindjer, M.; Pope, P.B.; Hernandez, P.E.; Perez-Martinez, G.; Diep, D.B. The Potential of Class II Bacteriocins to Modify Gut Microbiota to Improve Host Health. *PLoS ONE* **2016**, *11*, e0164036. [CrossRef]
14. Umu, O.C.O.; Rudi, K.; Diep, D.B. Modulation of the gut microbiota by prebiotic fibres and bacteriocins. *Microb. Ecol. Health Dis.* **2017**, *28*, 1348886. [CrossRef]
15. De Vuyst, L.; Leroy, F. Bacteriocins from lactic acid bacteria: Production, purification, and food applications. *J. Mol. Microbiol. Biotechnol.* **2007**, *13*, 194–199. [CrossRef] [PubMed]
16. Eijsink, V.G.; Skeie, M.; Middelhoven, P.H.; Brurberg, M.B.; Nes, I.F. Comparative studies of class IIa bacteriocins of lactic acid bacteria. *Appl. Environ. Microbiol.* **1998**, *64*, 3275–3281. [PubMed]
17. Anderssen, E.L.; Diep, D.B.; Nes, I.F.; Eijsink, V.G.; Nissen-Meyer, J. Antagonistic activity of Lactobacillus plantarum C11: Two new two-peptide bacteriocins, plantaricins EF and JK, and the induction factor plantaricin A. *Appl. Environ. Microbiol.* **1998**, *64*, 2269–2272. [PubMed]

18. Nissen-Meyer, J.; Rogne, P.; Oppegard, C.; Haugen, H.S.; Kristiansen, P.E. Structure-function relationships of the non-lanthionine-containing peptide (class II) bacteriocins produced by gram-positive bacteria. *Curr. Pharm. Biotechnol.* **2009**, *10*, 19–37. [CrossRef]

19. Criado, R.; Diep, D.B.; Aakra, A.; Gutierrez, J.; Nes, I.F.; Hernandez, P.E.; Cintas, L.M. Complete sequence of the enterocin Q-encoding plasmid pCIZ2 from the multiple bacteriocin producer Enterococcus faecium L50 and genetic characterization of enterocin Q production and immunity. *Appl. Environ. Microbiol.* **2006**, *72*, 6653–6666. [CrossRef]

20. Etayash, H.; Azmi, S.; Dangeti, R.; Kaur, K. Peptide Bacteriocins–Structure Activity Relationships. *Curr. Top. Med. Chem.* **2015**, *16*, 220–241. [CrossRef]

21. Kaur, S.; Kaur, S. Bacteriocins as Potential Anticancer Agents. *Front. Pharmacol.* **2015**, *6*, 272. [CrossRef] [PubMed]

22. Weinstock, G.M. A Glimpse of Microbial Power in Preventive Medicine. *JAMA Pediatr.* **2016**, *170*, 11. [CrossRef] [PubMed]

23. Manrique, P.; Dills, M.; Young, M.J. The Human Gut Phage Community and Its Implications for Health and Disease. *Viruses* **2017**, *9*. [CrossRef] [PubMed]

24. Mills, S.; Ross, R.P.; Hill, C. Bacteriocins and bacteriophage; a narrow-minded approach to food and gut microbiology. *FEMS Microbiol. Rev.* **2017**, *41* (Suppl. 1), S129–S153. [CrossRef] [PubMed]

25. Wang, X.; Wood, T.K. Cryptic prophages as targets for drug development. *Drug Resist. Updates* **2016**, *27*, 30–38. [CrossRef]

26. Drulis-Kawa, Z.; Majkowska-Skrobek, G.; Maciejewska, B.; Delattre, A.S.; Lavigne, R. Learning from bacteriophages—Advantages and limitations of phage and phage-encoded protein applications. *Curr. Protein Pept. Sci.* **2012**, *13*, 699–722. [CrossRef] [PubMed]

27. Lin, D.M.; Koskella, B.; Lin, H.C. Phage therapy: An alternative to antibiotics in the age of multi-drug resistance. *World J. Gastrointest. Pharmacol. Ther.* **2017**, *8*, 162–173. [CrossRef] [PubMed]

28. Wernicki, A.; Nowaczek, A.; Urban-Chmiel, R. Bacteriophage therapy to combat bacterial infections in poultry. *Virol. J.* **2017**, *14*, 179. [CrossRef]

29. Scanlan, P.D. Bacteria-Bacteriophage Coevolution in the Human Gut: Implications for Microbial Diversity and Functionality. *Trends Microbiol.* **2017**, *25*, 614–623. [CrossRef]

30. Abedon, S.T. Phage evolution and ecology. *Adv. Appl. Microbiol.* **2009**, *67*, 1–45.

31. Babickova, J.; Gardlik, R. Pathological and therapeutic interactions between bacteriophages, microbes and the host in inflammatory bowel disease. *World J. Gastroenterol.* **2015**, *21*, 11321–11330. [CrossRef] [PubMed]

32. Rohwer, F.; Edwards, R. The Phage Proteomic Tree: A genome-based taxonomy for phage. *J. Bacteriol.* **2002**, *184*, 4529–4535. [CrossRef] [PubMed]

33. Wittebole, X.; De Roock, S.; Opal, S.M. A historical overview of bacteriophage therapy as an alternative to antibiotics for the treatment of bacterial pathogens. *Virulence* **2014**, *5*, 226–235. [CrossRef] [PubMed]

34. Diaz-Munoz, S.L.; Koskella, B. Bacteria-phage interactions in natural environments. *Adv. Appl. Microbiol.* **2014**, *89*, 135–183.

35. Yu, P.; Mathieu, J.; Li, M.; Dai, Z.; Alvarez, P.J. Isolation of Polyvalent Bacteriophages by Sequential Multiple-Host Approaches. *Appl. Environ. Microbiol.* **2015**, *82*, 808–815. [CrossRef]

36. Lepage, P.; Colombet, J.; Marteau, P.; Sime-Ngando, T.; Dore, J.; Leclerc, M. Dysbiosis in inflammatory bowel disease: A role for bacteriophages? *Gut* **2008**, *57*, 424–425. [CrossRef] [PubMed]

37. Mills, S.; Shanahan, F.; Stanton, C.; Hill, C.; Coffey, A.; Ross, R.P. Movers and shakers: Influence of bacteriophages in shaping the mammalian gut microbiota. *Gut Microbes* **2013**, *4*, 4–16. [CrossRef]

38. Lusiak-Szelachowska, M.; Weber-Dabrowska, B.; Jonczyk-Matysiak, E.; Wojciechowska, R.; Gorski, A. Bacteriophages in the gastrointestinal tract and their implications. *Gut Pathog.* **2017**, *9*, 44. [CrossRef]

39. Wang, J.; Hu, B.; Xu, M.; Yan, Q.; Liu, S.; Zhu, X.; Sun, Z.; Reed, E.; Ding, L.; Gong, J.; et al. Use of bacteriophage in the treatment of experimental animal bacteremia from imipenem-resistant Pseudomonas aeruginosa. *Int. J. Mol. Med.* **2006**, *17*, 309–317. [CrossRef]

40. Matsuzaki, S.; Yasuda, M.; Nishikawa, H.; Kuroda, M.; Ujihara, T.; Shuin, T.; Shen, Y.; Jin, Z.; Fujimoto, S.; Nasimuzzaman, M.D.; et al. Experimental protection of mice against lethal Staphylococcus aureus infection by novel bacteriophage phi MR11. *J. Infect. Dis.* **2003**, *187*, 613–624. [CrossRef]

41. Barr, J.J.; Auro, R.; Furlan, M.; Whiteson, K.L.; Erb, M.L.; Pogliano, J.; Stotland, A.; Wolkowicz, R.; Cutting, A.S.; Doran, K.S.; et al. Bacteriophage adhering to mucus provide a non-host-derived immunity. *Proc. Natl. Acad. Sci. USA* **2013**, *110*, 10771–10776. [CrossRef] [PubMed]

42. Brown-Jaque, M.; Muniesa, M.; Navarro, F. Bacteriophages in clinical samples can interfere with microbiological diagnostic tools. *Sci. Rep.* **2016**, *6*, 33000. [CrossRef]

43. Thannesberger, J.; Hellinger, H.J.; Klymiuk, I.; Kastner, M.T.; Rieder, F.J.J.; Schneider, M.; Fister, S.; Lion, T.; Kosulin, K.; Laengle, J.; et al. Viruses comprise an extensive pool of mobile genetic elements in eukaryote cell cultures and human clinical samples. *FASEB J.* **2017**, *31*, 1987–2000. [CrossRef] [PubMed]

44. Kommineni, S.; Bretl, D.J.; Lam, V.; Chakraborty, R.; Hayward, M.; Simpson, P.; Cao, Y.; Bousounis, P.; Kristich, C.J.; Salzman, N.H. Bacteriocin production augments niche competition by enterococci in the mammalian gastrointestinal tract. *Nature* **2015**, *526*, 719–722. [CrossRef]

45. O'Toole, P.W.; Cooney, J.C. Probiotic bacteria influence the composition and function of the intestinal microbiota. *Interdiscip. Perspect. Infect. Dis.* **2008**, *2008*, 175285. [CrossRef] [PubMed]

46. Rea, M.C.; Alemayehu, D.; Ross, R.P.; Hill, C. Gut solutions to a gut problem: Bacteriocins, probiotics and bacteriophage for control of Clostridium difficile infection. *J. Med. Microbiol.* **2013**, *62 Pt 9*, 1369–1378. [CrossRef]

47. Lopetuso, L.R.; Ianiro, G.; Scaldaferri, F.; Cammarota, G.; Gasbarrini, A. Gut Virome and Inflammatory Bowel Disease. *Inflamm. Bowel Dis.* **2016**, *22*, 1708–1712. [CrossRef]

48. Norman, J.M.; Handley, S.A.; Baldridge, M.T.; Droit, L.; Liu, C.Y.; Keller, B.C.; Kambal, A.; Monaco, C.L.; Zhao, G.; Fleshner, P.; et al. Disease-specific alterations in the enteric virome in inflammatory bowel disease. *Cell* **2015**, *160*, 447–460. [CrossRef]

49. Reyes, A.; Semenkovich, N.P.; Whiteson, K.; Rohwer, F.; Gordon, J.I. Going viral: Next-generation sequencing applied to phage populations in the human gut. *Nat. Rev. Microbiol.* **2012**, *10*, 607–617. [CrossRef]

50. Yu, L.; Wang, S.; Guo, Z.; Liu, H.; Sun, D.; Yan, G.; Hu, D.; Du, C.; Feng, X.; Han, W.; et al. A guard-killer phage cocktail effectively lyses the host and inhibits the development of phage-resistant strains of Escherichia coli. *Appl. Microbiol. Biotechnol.* **2018**, *102*, 971–983. [CrossRef]

51. Vahedi, A.; Dallal, M.M.S.; Douraghi, M.; Nikkhahi, F.; Rajabi, Z.; Yousefi, M.; Mousavi, M. Isolation and identification of specific bacteriophage against enteropathogenic Escherichia coli (EPEC) and in vitro and in vivo characterization of bacteriophage. *FEMS Microbiol. Lett.* **2018**, *365*, fny136. [CrossRef] [PubMed]

52. Galtier, M.; De Sordi, L.; Sivignon, A.; de Vallee, A.; Maura, D.; Neut, C.; Rahmouni, O.; Wannerberger, K.; Darfeuille-Michaud, A.; Desreumaux, P.; et al. Bacteriophages Targeting Adherent Invasive Escherichia coli Strains as a Promising New Treatment for Crohn's Disease. *J. Crohn's Colitis* **2017**, *11*, 840–847. [CrossRef] [PubMed]

53. Sartor, R.B.; Wu, G.D. Roles for Intestinal Bacteria, Viruses, and Fungi in Pathogenesis of Inflammatory Bowel Diseases and Therapeutic Approaches. *Gastroenterology* **2017**, *152*, 327e4–339e4. [CrossRef] [PubMed]

54. Sarker, S.A.; Sultana, S.; Reuteler, G.; Moine, D.; Descombes, P.; Charton, F.; Bourdin, G.; McCallin, S.; Ngom-Bru, C.; Neville, T.; et al. Oral Phage Therapy of Acute Bacterial Diarrhea With Two Coliphage Preparations: A Randomized Trial in Children From Bangladesh. *EBioMedicine* **2016**, *4*, 124–137. [CrossRef] [PubMed]

55. Lepage, P. [The human gut microbiota: Interactions with the host and dysfunctions]. *Rev. Mal. Respir* **2017**, *34*, 1085–1090. [CrossRef] [PubMed]

56. Linares, D.M.; Gomez, C.; Renes, E.; Fresno, J.M.; Tornadijo, M.E.; Ross, R.P.; Stanton, C. Lactic Acid Bacteria and Bifidobacteria with Potential to Design Natural Biofunctional Health-Promoting Dairy Foods. *Front. Microbiol.* **2017**, *8*, 846. [CrossRef]

57. Francoise, L. Occurrence and role of lactic acid bacteria in seafood products. *Food Microbiol.* **2010**, *27*, 698–709. [CrossRef]

58. Di Cagno, R.; Coda, R.; De Angelis, M.; Gobbetti, M. Exploitation of vegetables and fruits through lactic acid fermentation. *Food Microbiol.* **2013**, *33*, 1–10. [CrossRef]

59. Yang, S.C.; Lin, C.H.; Sung, C.T.; Fang, J.Y. Antibacterial activities of bacteriocins: Application in foods and pharmaceuticals. *Front. Microbiol.* **2014**, *5*, 241.

60. Settanni, L.; Corsetti, A. Application of bacteriocins in vegetable food biopreservation. *Int. J. Food Microbiol.* **2008**, *121*, 123–138. [CrossRef]

61. Foulquie Moreno, M.R.; Sarantinopoulos, P.; Tsakalidou, E.; De Vuyst, L. The role and application of enterococci in food and health. *Int. J. Food Microbiol.* **2006**, *106*, 1–24. [CrossRef] [PubMed]
62. Sharma, G.; Dang, S.; Gupta, S.; Gabrani, R. Antibacterial Activity, Cytotoxicity, and the Mechanism of Action of Bacteriocin from Bacillus subtilis GAS101. *Med. Princ. Pract.* **2018**, *27*, 186–192. [CrossRef] [PubMed]
63. Merabishvili, M.; De Vos, D.; Verbeken, G.; Kropinski, A.M.; Vandenheuvel, D.; Lavigne, R.; Wattiau, P.; Mast, J.; Ragimbeau, C.; Mossong, J.; et al. Selection and characterization of a candidate therapeutic bacteriophage that lyses the Escherichia coli O104:H4 strain from the 2011 outbreak in Germany. *PLoS ONE* **2012**, *7*, e52709. [CrossRef] [PubMed]
64. Broecker, F.; Russo, G.; Klumpp, J.; Moelling, K. Stable core virome despite variable microbiome after fecal transfer. *Gut Microbes* **2017**, *8*, 214–220. [CrossRef] [PubMed]
65. Ott, S.J.; Waetzig, G.H.; Rehman, A.; Moltzau-Anderson, J.; Bharti, R.; Grasis, J.A.; Cassidy, L.; Tholey, A.; Fickenscher, H.; Seegert, D.; et al. Efficacy of Sterile Fecal Filtrate Transfer for Treating Patients With Clostridium difficile Infection. *Gastroenterology* **2017**, *152*, 799e7–811e7. [CrossRef] [PubMed]
66. Drilling, A.J.; Ooi, M.L.; Miljkovic, D.; James, C.; Speck, P.; Vreugde, S.; Clark, J.; Wormald, P.J. Long-Term Safety of Topical Bacteriophage Application to the Frontal Sinus Region. *Front. Cell. Infect. Microbiol.* **2017**, *7*, 49. [CrossRef] [PubMed]
67. Abedon, S.T. Commentary: Phage Therapy of Staphylococcal Chronic Osteomyelitis in Experimental Animal Model. *Front. Microbiol.* **2016**, *7*, 1251. [CrossRef]
68. Alemayehu, D.; Casey, P.G.; McAuliffe, O.; Guinane, C.M.; Martin, J.G.; Shanahan, F.; Coffey, A.; Ross, R.P.; Hill, C. Bacteriophages phiMR299-2 and phiNH-4 can eliminate Pseudomonas aeruginosa in the murine lung and on cystic fibrosis lung airway cells. *MBio* **2012**, *3*, e00029-12. [CrossRef]
69. Brown, T.L.; Petrovski, S.; Dyson, Z.A.; Seviour, R.; Tucci, J. The Formulation of Bacteriophage in a Semi Solid Preparation for Control of Propionibacterium acnes Growth. *PLoS ONE* **2016**, *11*, e0151184. [CrossRef]
70. Fish, R.; Kutter, E.; Wheat, G.; Blasdel, B.; Kutateladze, M.; Kuhl, S. Compassionate Use of Bacteriophage Therapy for Foot Ulcer Treatment as an Effective Step for Moving Toward Clinical Trials. *Methods Mol. Biol.* **2018**, *1693*, 159–170.
71. Ghoul, M.; West, S.A.; Johansen, H.K.; Molin, S.; Harrison, O.B.; Maiden, M.C.; Jelsbak, L.; Bruce, J.B.; Griffin, A.S. Bacteriocin-mediated competition in cystic fibrosis lung infections. *Proc. Biol. Sci.* **2015**, *282*. [CrossRef] [PubMed]
72. Bogaardt, C.; van Tonder, A.J.; Brueggemann, A.B. Genomic analyses of pneumococci reveal a wide diversity of bacteriocins—Including pneumocyclicin, a novel circular bacteriocin. *BMC Genom.* **2015**, *16*, 554. [CrossRef] [PubMed]
73. Hammami, R.; Fernandez, B.; Lacroix, C.; Fliss, I. Anti-infective properties of bacteriocins: An update. *Cell. Mol. Life Sci.* **2013**, *70*, 2947–2967. [CrossRef] [PubMed]
74. Gorski, A.; Miedzybrodzki, R.; Borysowski, J.; Dabrowska, K.; Wierzbicki, P.; Ohams, M.; Korczak-Kowalska, G.; Olszowska-Zaremba, N.; Lusiak-Szelachowska, M.; Klak, M.; et al. Phage as a modulator of immune responses: Practical implications for phage therapy. *Adv. Virus Res.* **2012**, *83*, 41–71.
75. Gorski, A.; Miedzybrodzki, R.; Weber-Dabrowska, B.; Fortuna, W.; Letkiewicz, S.; Rogoz, P.; Jonczyk-Matysiak, E.; Dabrowska, K.; Majewska, J.; Borysowski, J. Phage Therapy: Combating Infections with Potential for Evolving from Merely a Treatment for Complications to Targeting Diseases. *Front. Microbiol.* **2016**, *7*, 1515. [CrossRef] [PubMed]
76. Budynek, P.; Dabrowska, K.; Skaradzinski, G.; Gorski, A. Bacteriophages and cancer. *Arch. Microbiol.* **2010**, *192*, 315–320. [CrossRef] [PubMed]
77. Bakhshinejad, B.; Karimi, M.; Sadeghizadeh, M. Bacteriophages and medical oncology: Targeted gene therapy of cancer. *Med. Oncol.* **2014**, *31*, 110. [CrossRef] [PubMed]
78. Larocca, D.; Kassner, P.D.; Witte, A.; Ladner, R.C.; Pierce, G.F.; Baird, A. Gene transfer to mammalian cells using genetically targeted filamentous bacteriophage. *FASEB J.* **1999**, *13*, 727–734. [CrossRef]
79. Lei, H.; An, P.; Song, S.; Liu, X.; He, L.; Wu, J.; Meng, L.; Liu, M.; Yang, J.; Shou, C. A novel peptide isolated from a phage display library inhibits tumor growth and metastasis by blocking the binding of vascular endothelial growth factor to its kinase domain receptor. *J. Biol. Chem.* **2002**, *277*, 43137–43142.

80. Dabrowska, K.; Opolski, A.; Wietrzyk, J.; Switala-Jelen, K.; Boratynski, J.; Nasulewicz, A.; Lipinska, L.; Chybicka, A.; Kujawa, M.; Zabel, M.; et al. Antitumor activity of bacteriophages in murine experimental cancer models caused possibly by inhibition of beta3 integrin signaling pathway. *Acta Virol.* **2004**, *48*, 241–248.

81. Chumchalova, J.; Smarda, J. Human tumor cells are selectively inhibited by colicins. *Folia Microbiol. (Praha)* **2003**, *48*, 111–115. [CrossRef] [PubMed]

82. Joo, N.E.; Ritchie, K.; Kamarajan, P.; Miao, D.; Kapila, Y.L. Nisin, an apoptogenic bacteriocin and food preservative, attenuates HNSCC tumorigenesis via CHAC1. *Cancer Med.* **2012**, *1*, 295–305. [CrossRef] [PubMed]

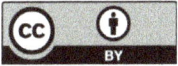

International Journal of
Molecular Sciences

MDPI

Article

A Small Aromatic Compound Has Antifungal Properties and Potential Anti-Inflammatory Effects against Intestinal Inflammation

Clovis Bortolus [1,2,3], Muriel Billamboz [2,4], Rogatien Charlet [1,2,3], Karine Lecointe [1,2,3], Boualem Sendid [1,2,3], Alina Ghinet [2,4,5] and Samir Jawhara [1,2,3,*]

[1] Institut National de la Santé et de la Recherche Médicale, U995/Team2, F-59000 Lille, France; clovis.bortolus@univ-lille.fr (C.B.); charlet-rogatien@hotmail.fr (R.C.); lecointe.karine@gmail.com (K.L.); boualem.sendid@univ-lille.fr (B.S.)
[2] Lille Inflammation Research International Center, University Lille, U995-LIRIC, F-59000 Lille, France; muriel.billamboz@yncrea.fr (M.B.); alina.ghinet@yncrea.fr (A.G.)
[3] Service de Parasitologie Mycologie, Pôle de Biologie Pathologie Génétique, CHU Lille, F-59000 Lille, France
[4] Laboratoire de Chimie Durable et Santé, Ecole des Hautes Etudes d'Ingénieur (HEI), Yncréa Hauts-de-France, 13 Rue de Toul, F-59046 Lille, France
[5] Faculty of Chemistry, Al. I. Cuza' University of Iasi, B-dul Carol 1 nr. 11, 700506 Iasi, Romania
* Correspondence: samir.jawhara@inserm.fr; Tel.: +33-(0)3-20-62-35-46; Fax: +33-(0)3-20-62-34-16

Received: 7 December 2018; Accepted: 4 January 2019; Published: 14 January 2019

Abstract: Resistance of the opportunistic pathogen *Candida albicans* to antifungal drugs has increased significantly in recent years. After screening 55 potential antifungal compounds from a chemical library, 2,3-dihydroxy-4-methoxybenzaldehyde (DHMB) was identified as having potential antifungal activity. The properties of DHMB were then assessed in vitro and in vivo against *C. albicans* overgrowth and intestinal inflammation. Substitution on the aromatic ring of DHMB led to a strong decrease in its biological activity against *C. albicans*. The MIC of DHMB was highly effective at eliminating *C. albicans* when compared to that of caspofungin or fluconazole. Additionally, DHMB was also effective against clinically isolated fluconazole- or caspofungin-resistant *C. albicans* strains. DHMB was administered to animals at high doses. This compound was not cytotoxic and was well-tolerated. In experimental dextran sodium sulphate (DSS)-induced colitis in mice, DHMB reduced the clinical and histological score of inflammation and promoted the elimination of *C. albicans* from the gut. This finding was supported by a decrease in aerobic bacteria while anaerobic bacteria populations were re-established in mice treated with DHMB. DHMB is a small organic molecule with antifungal properties and anti-inflammatory activity by exerting protective effects on intestinal epithelial cells.

Keywords: *Candida albicans*; 2,3-dihydroxy-4-methoxyBenzaldehyde; melanin; colitis; anaerobic bacteria; aerobic bacteria

1. Introduction

Inflammatory bowel diseases (IBDs), comprising Crohn's disease (CD) and ulcerative colitis, have a multifactorial aetiology with complex interactions between genetic susceptibility, the immune system, environment and the microbiota [1]. The biodiversity of the gut microbiota is frequently decreased in IBD patients, in particular a reduction in Firmicutes and an increase in Proteobacteria are often observed [2]. *Escherichia coli* is part of the Proteobacteria phylum and is increased greatly while *Lactobacillus* species belonging to the Firmicutes phylum are reduced in IBD patients [3,4]. Other observations supporting a role for the gut microbiota in IBD include an abundance of fungi in the inflamed mucosa and faeces [5,6].

Colonisation with *Candida albicans*, an opportunistic human fungal pathogen, is consistently increased in CD patients [7]. In addition, abundance of this fungus is correlated with serological markers of CD, namely anti-*Saccharomyces cerevisiae* antibodies (ASCA) [5,8]. Recently, in an experimental murine model of dextran sodium sulphate (DSS)-induced colitis, the population of aerobic bacteria, in particular *E. coli* and *Enterococcus faecalis*, increased, whereas the population of anaerobic bacteria such as *Lactobacillus johnsonii* and *Bifidobacterium* species decreased. These microbiota modifications were associated with overgrowth of fungi suggesting that dysbiosis could play a crucial role in IBD [9].

Different anti-inflammatory compounds including 5-aminosalicylic acid (5-ASA) or anti-TNFα antibodies have been used to treat IBD patients, but no compounds have a dual effect of antifungal and anti-inflammatory activity [10]. Some of the anti-inflammatory drugs are not effective at treating active CD or preventing disease relapse; they only treat the symptoms and are sometimes only effective for a few years [11]. In parallel, an increase in antifungal resistance is considered a major problem to clinicians and leads to high morbidity and mortality rates in patients with invasive mycoses [12]. The increase of new fungal species that are resistant to different classes of available antifungal drugs constitutes an urgent need for developing new antifungal compounds [13].

In the current study, we assessed the in vitro and in vivo antifungal properties of a novel compound, 2,3-dihydroxy-4-methoxybenzaldehyde (DHMB), against *C. albicans* colonisation and intestinal inflammation.

2. Results

2.1. Structure and Characterisation of DHMB

A series of 55 compounds from the private chemical library of the laboratory was screened for antifungal and antibacterial activities, revealing that DHMB was a highly effective molecule against *C. albicans*. The DHMB MIC, at which *C. albicans* growth was fully inhibited, was 8 µg/mL. From a chemical point of view, DHMB is a small organic molecule (M.W. = 168.15 g/mol) bearing a highly reactive aromatic aldehyde moiety and two free phenol groups (Figure 1). We then evaluated some derivatives of DHMB for their antifungal activity; the structure and activities of these derivatives are summarised in Table 1. The biological activity of these compounds against *C. albicans* was evaluated at 4 × MIC (32 µg/mL). The aldehyde group in position 1 was modified with little or no change in positions 2–5 on the aromatic moiety (Table 1, entries 1–6). Deletion of the aldehyde substituent led to a total loss of activity (Compound 1, Table 1, entry 2). Compounds 2 and 3, in which the carbonyl group in position 1 is still present but included in a phenylethanone moiety, exhibited weak inhibition at 32 µg/mL (13% and 27%, respectively). Moreover, as exemplified by compounds 4 and 5, modification of the phenolic hydroxyl groups in positions 2 and 3 led to a loss of activity (Table 1, entries 5–6). Rigidification of the system and introduction of a lactone ring (compound 6) significantly decreased the biological activity (Table 1, entry 7).

From these data, the aldehyde group in position 1 seems to be essential for activity against *C. albicans*. The importance of the catechol and methoxy groups on the aromatic ring was also studied. Unexpectedly, replacement of the 4-methoxy substituent by a hydroxyl one led to a complete loss of activity (Table 1, entry 8). This shows that this *para*-methoxy group plays an essential role in the biological activity, possibly due to its hydrophobicity compared with the hydroxyl moiety. Modification of position 6 was then undertaken whilst retaining the 2,3-dihydroxy-4-methoxy- sequence on the aromatic ring. A carboxylic acid was introduced in that position (3,4-dihydroxy-5-methoxybenzoic acid, compound 8), but no activity against *C. albicans* was detected, and modifications of the hydrophilicity/hydrophobicity of benzoic acid derivatives did not result in a gain in activity (compounds 9 and 10, Table 1). Passing from benzoic acid to benzylic acid did not improve the activity (compare compounds 9 and 11, Table 1, entries 10 and 12). A similar conclusion can be drawn on replacement of the carboxylic acid by an ethoxy substituent at position 6 (compound 12). In the same way, replacing the carboxylic acid by an aldehyde, an acetate or a hydrogen group did not improve the activity (comparison of compound 10 with compounds 13–15).

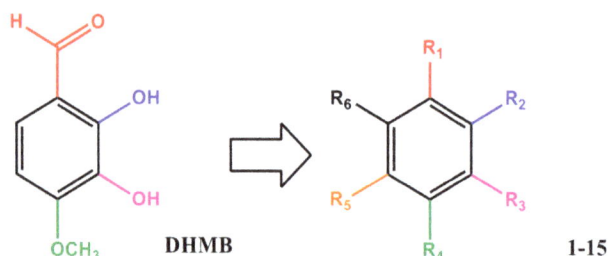

Figure 1. Chemical structure of DHMB and related investigated compounds.

Table 1. Chemical modifications of DHMB and their impact on activity.

Entry	Compound	R_1	R_2	R_3	R_4	R_5	R_6	% Inhibition at 32 µg/mL [a]
1	DHMB	CHO	OH	OH	OCH_3	H	H	100
2	1	H	OH	OH	OCH_3	H	H	3
3	2		OH	OCH_3	OCH_3	H	H	13
4	3		OH	OH	OCH_3	H	H	27
5	4		OH	$OCOCH_2Cl$	OCH_3	H	H	6
6	5		$OCOCH_2Cl$	$OCOCH_2Cl$	OCH_3	H	H	4
7	6						H	2
8	7	CHO	OH	OH	OH	H	H	4
9	8	H	OH	OH	OCH_3	H	COOH	2
10	9	H	OCH_3	OCH_3	OCH_3	H	COOH	2
11	10	H	OCH_3	OH	OCH_3	H	COOH	0
12	11	H	OCH_3	OCH_3	OCH_3	H	CH_2-COOH	1
13	12	H	OCH_3	OCH_3	OCH_3	H	CH_2-OH	2
14	13	H	OCH_3	OH	OCH_3	H	CHO	1
15	14	H	OCH_3	OH	OCH_3	H	$COCH_3$	4
16	15	H	OCH_3	OH	OCH_3	H	H	0

[a] Screening carried out on *C. albicans* ATCC 90028.

2.2. In Vitro Antifungal Activity of DHMB against C. albicans

The antifungal activity of DHMB against *C. albicans* was compared with that of caspofungin and fluconazole. The viability of *C. albicans* cells was tracked in real time using a fungal bioluminescent strain challenged with either DHMB, caspofungin or fluconazole at their MICs (8 µg/mL), 2 × MICs (16 µg/mL) or 4 × MICs (32 µg/mL) utilising different exposure times: 0, 15, 30 and 60 min (Figure 2). DHMB led to a significant reduction in bioluminescence as well as in the number of fungal colonies indicating rapid fungicidal activity after incubation with *C. albicans*. This fungicidal activity of DHMB was similar to that of caspofungin while fluconazole exhibited a fungistatic effect. The antifungal activity of DHMB was assessed on drug-resistant *C. albicans* clinical isolates (Figure 2E,F). The viability of drug-resistant *C. albicans* clinical isolates was significantly reduced after treatment with DHMB at 10 × MIC in terms of viable colony counts using fungal culture media (Figure 3). To assess whether DHMB has an impact on modulation of the glycan cell wall, flow cytometry analysis and confocal microscopic observations were performed. Confocal microscopy revealed that, in contrast to fluconazole and DHMB, caspofungin challenge for 1 h produced a damaged polysaccharide cell wall; in particular, the β-glucan and chitin layers were mainly affected by this antifungal treatment (Figure 3A). Similarly, flow cytometry analysis showed that treatment with either fluconazole or DHMB did not affect the fungal cell wall when compared to untreated *C. albicans* while *C. albicans* challenged with caspofungin exhibited a significant increase in chitin levels when compared to unchallenged *C. albicans*. No changes in mannan levels were observed in *C. albicans* challenged with either fluconazole, caspofungin or DHMB (Figure 3B,C). To determine whether DHMB has an impact on the melanisation, which is involved in the virulence of *C. albicans*, in particular resistance to antifungal agents and protection against oxidative stresses, microscopic observations were realised. A remarkable reduction in the melanin production was observed in *C. albicans* treated with DHMB when compared to that treated with caspofungin (Figure 3D).

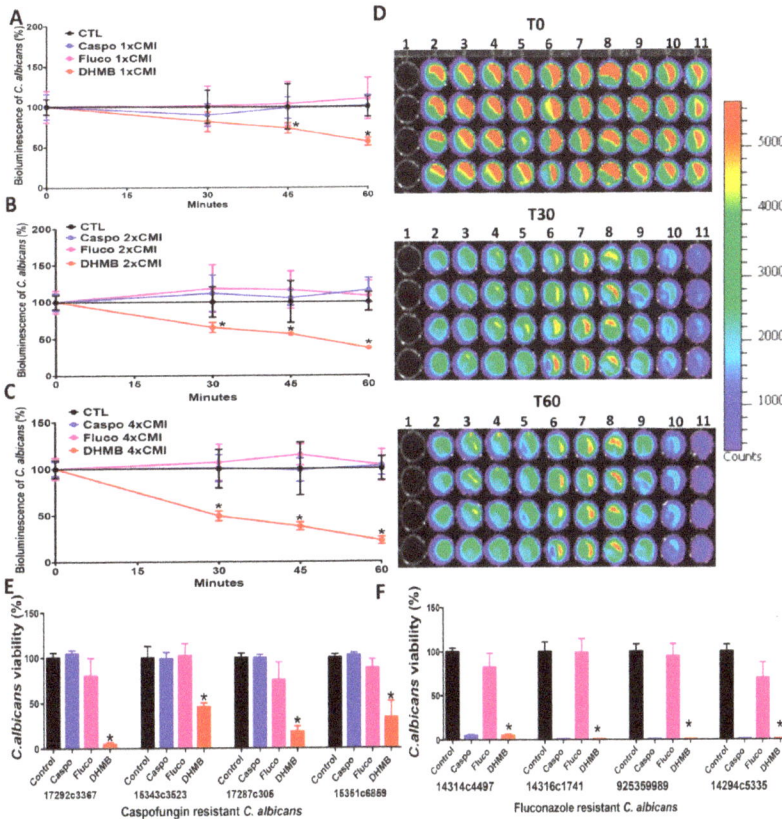

Figure 2. Impact of DHMB on *C. albicans* viability. (**A–C**) Bioluminescent *C. albicans* strain was treated with either DHMB, flucanoazole or caspofungin at their MICs, 2 × MICs or 4 × MICs and monitored at 0, 15, 30 and 60 min. Control corresponds to *C. albicans* alone without antifungal treatment; (**D**) Visualisation of DHMB effect on bioluminescent *C. albicans* strain in real time. Bioluminescent *C. albicans* strain was treated with either DHMB, fluconazole or caspofungin at their MICs, 2 × MICs or 4 × MICs and monitored at 0, 15, 30 and 60 min. Line 1, PBS without yeasts; Line 2, *C. albicans* alone; Lines 3–5, *C. albicans* treated with caspofungin at 1 × MIC, 2 × MIC and 4 × MIC, respectively; Lines 6–8, *C. albicans* challenged with fluconazole at 1 × MIC, 2 × MIC and 4 × MIC, respectively; Lines 9–11, *C. albicans* + DHMB at 1 x MIC, 2 × MIC and 4 × MIC, respectively. * $p < 0.0001$; (**E,F**) Effect of DHMB on drug-resistant *C. albicans* clinical isolates. Control represents *C. albicans* clinical isolate. Caspo (caspofungin), Fluco (fluconazole) or DHMB (2,3-dihydroxy-4-methoxybenzaldehyde) were added to *C. albicans* strains at 10 × MIC.

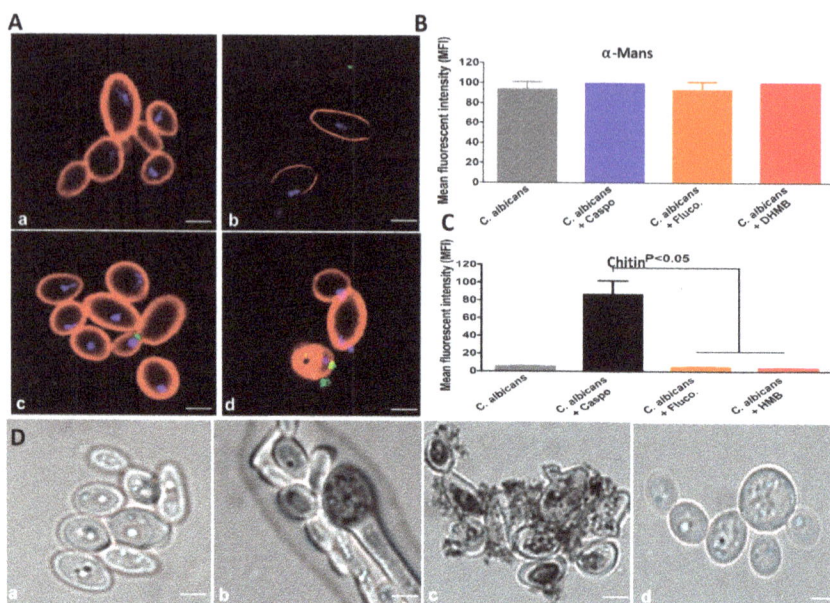

Figure 3. Effect of DHMB on modulation of chitin and α-mannan expression. (**A**) Confocal microscopic observation after antifungal challenge. *C. albicans* was treated with PBS (**a**) caspofungin (**b**), fluconazole (**c**) or DHMB (**d**) at a final concentration of 100 µM for 1 h and the fungal cell wall was analysed by confocal microscopy and flow cytometry; (**B**) Percentage of viable *C. albicans* cells labelled with concanavalin A. α-Mannans were labelled with concanavalin A-rhodamine; (**C**) Percentage of viable *C. albicans* cells labelled with WGA-IFTC. Chitin was labelled with wheat germ agglutinin-fluorescein isothiocyanate (WGA-IFTC); (**D**) Microscopic observation of the melanin pigments in *C. albicans* after DHMB treatment. (**a**) *C. albicans* cells grown without DOPA; (**b**) *C. albicans* grown with 1 mM DOPA; (**c**) *C. albicans* cells grown with DOPA and treated with caspofungin; (**d**), *C. albicans* cells were incubated with DOPA and challenged with DHMB. Bars 10 nm.

2.3. Effect of DHMB on C. albicans Colonisation and Intestinal Inflammation in DSS-Induced Colitis Model

To assess whether DHMB can be tolerated in mice, a high dose of DHMB (100 mg/kg) was injected intraperitoneally in mice. No mortality was observed following DHMB challenge (data not shown). Body weight remained stable and no clinical signs were observed over two weeks.

The efficacy of DHMB at eliminating *C. albicans* was assessed in a DSS-induced colitis model. After *C. albicans* challenge, DHMB was administered for five days (10 mg/kg) to assess the therapeutic properties of this compound. As the DHMB compound has fungicidal activity against *C. albicans*, its effectiveness was compared to that of caspofungin in terms of *C. albicans* elimination from the gut. No sign of inflammation was observed in mice receiving water (CTL), *C. albicans* only (Ca) or DHMB (Figure 4). Following DSS treatment alone (D) or *C. albicans* challenge with DSS treatment (CaD), mice showed a gradual reduction in body mass over two weeks, whereas CaD mice receiving DHMB showed less severe weight loss than those untreated or treated with caspofungin (CaDCaspo) (Figure 4A). The clinical score for inflammation, including diarrhoea and rectal bleeding, decreased significantly in CaD mice treated with DHMB while caspofungin treatment did not significantly decrease these clinical symptoms (Figure 4B). Histological analysis of colon samples showed that DHMB treatment significantly reduced disease severity in CaD mice when compared to those treated with caspofungin (Figure 4C).

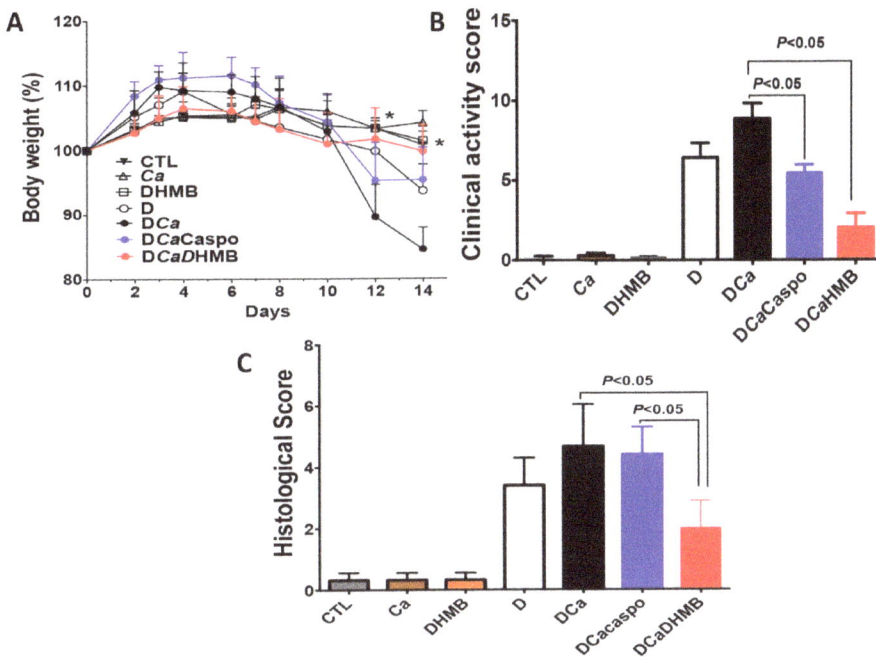

Figure 4. Determination of inflammatory parameters after DHMB treatment in a DSS-induced colitis model. (**A**) Body weight loss during colitis development. CTL refers to the control group receiving water. Ca corresponds to mice receiving *C. albicans* alone. DHMB refers to mice treated with DHMB only. D corresponds to mice receiving DSS only. DCa corresponds to mice receiving DSS and challenged with *C. albicans*. DCaCaspo and DCaDHMB refers to mice receiving DSS and challenged with *C. albicans* and treated with either caspofungin or DHMB (* $p < 0.05$); (**B**) Clinical score for inflammation; (**C**) Histological score for inflammation. Data are the mean ± SD of 10 mice per group from two independent experiments.

In contrast to CaD or CaDCaspo, colon sections from the CaDDHMB group showed low levels of leukocyte infiltrates, oedema and cryptic abscesses, and the surface epithelia structures remained intact (Figure 5).

The number of *C. albicans* colony-forming units (CFUs) and microbiota changes were assessed in freshly collected stool samples from each tagged mouse. A high number of *C. albicans* CFUs was recovered from stools from all groups on Day 1 (Figure 6). In the absence of DSS, *C. albicans* was dramatically decreased in mice. DSS treatment promoted a significant increase in *C. albicans* CFUs starting on Day 12 while DHMB administration favoured *C. albicans* elimination in DSS treated mice. The number of *C. albicans* CFUs was assessed in the stomach, caecum and colon (Figure 6). Treatment with either caspofungin or DHMB promoted *C. albicans* elimination from the mouse gut. For the gut microbiota, high numbers of *E. coli* and *E. faecalis* populations were observed following DSS treatment. Overgrowth of these two populations occurred regardless of *C. albicans* colonisation (Figure 7). DHMB treatment significantly maintained low levels of *E. coli* and *E. faecalis* populations while caspofungin treatment failed to reduce them. In terms of anaerobic bacteria, the number of *L. johnsonii* colonies was significantly reduced in both DSS and *C. albicans* mice, while DHMB treatment significantly restored *L. johnsonii* population in colitic mice challenged with *C. albicans*. In contrast, *L. reuteri* population showed unpredictable changes (Figure 7). The expression levels of pro-inflammatory cytokine IL-1β and anti-inflammatory cytokine IL-10 were assessed in the colons (Figure 8A,B). Expression of IL-1β was significantly lower in the colons of CaD mice treated with DHMB than in CaD or DSS mice

(Figure 8A,B). In contrast, expression of IL-10 was significantly higher in colons of CaD mice challenged with DHMB when compared to that of CaD or DSS mice. Additionally, the expression levels of TLR-4 and TLR-8 were determined. TLR-4 and TLR-8 expression increased significantly in response to both *C. albicans* overgrowth and colitis while treatment with DHMB decreased the expression of these receptors in the colons (Figure 8A,B).

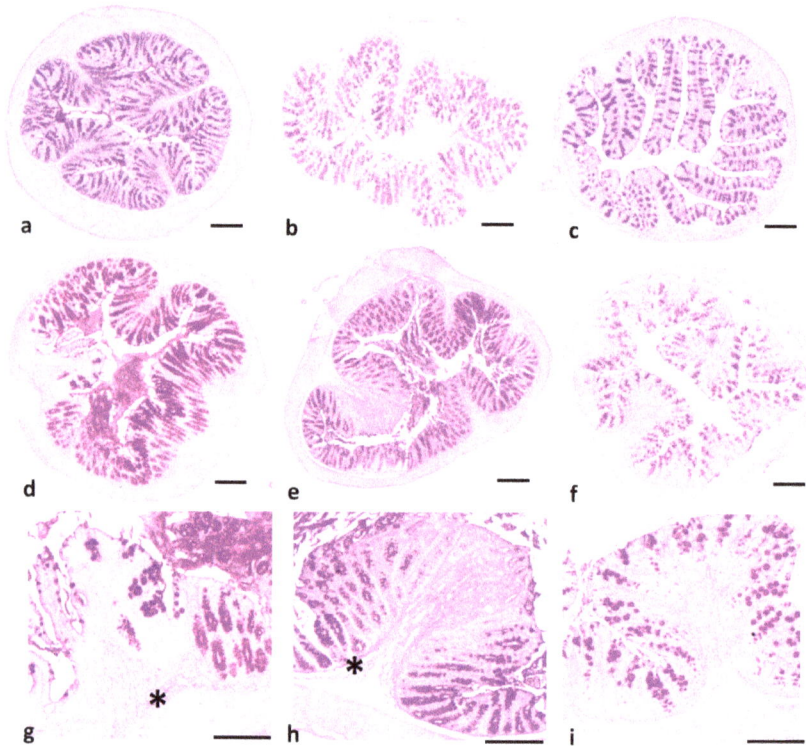

Figure 5. Analysis of histological colon sections from DSS-induced colitis: (**a–c**) colon sections from mice receiving water (control), *C. albicans* alone and DHMB, respectively; (**d**) colon sections from mice receiving DSS; (**e**) colon sections from mice receiving *C. albicans* and DSS; and (**f**) colon sections from CaD mice treated with DHMB; (**g–i**) colon sections from either DSS mice or CaD show tissue destruction, an important inflammatory cell infiltrate and oedema in the mucosa and submucosa of colon wall structures (*). Scale bars represent 50 μm (**a–f**) and 10 μm (**g–i**).

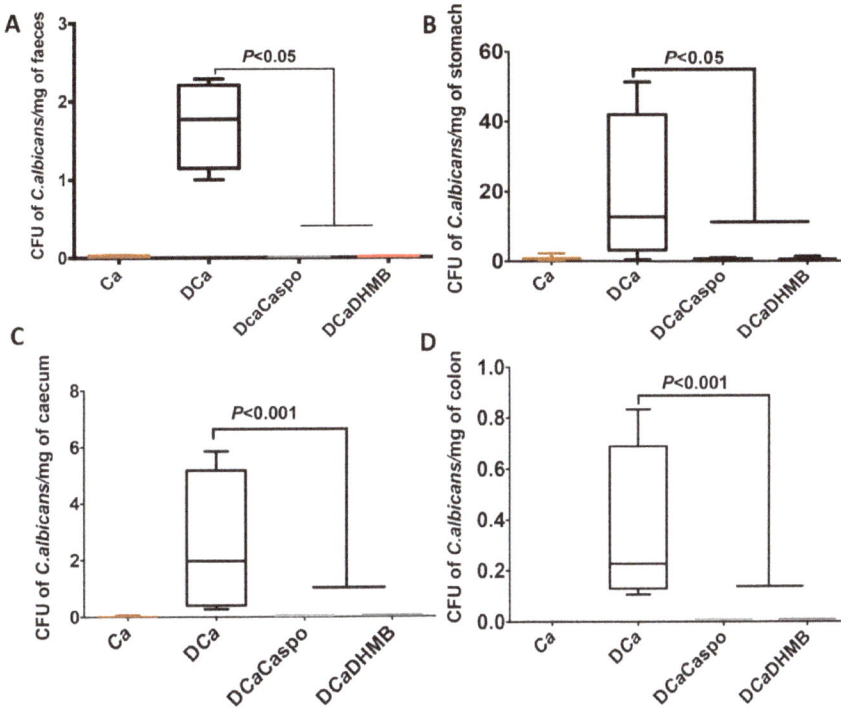

Figure 6. Effect of DHMB on *C. albicans* elimination from the gut. (**A–D**) Number of *C. albicans* colonies recovered from the stools, stomach, cecum and colon. Data are the mean ± SD of 10 mice per group from two independent experiments (*p* < 0.001).

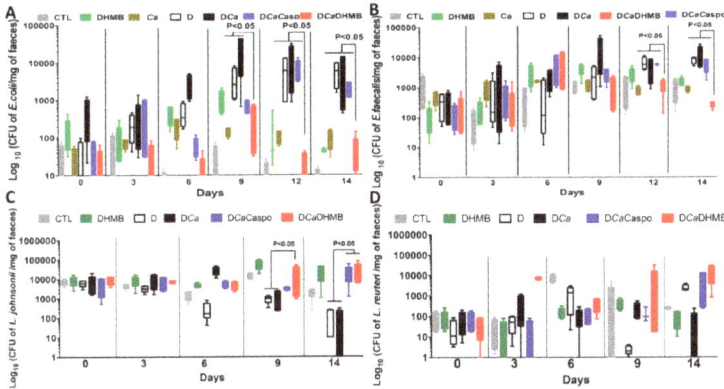

Figure 7. Determination of viable faecal aerobic and anaerobic bacteria in mice with colitis treated with DHMB. For all experiments, stool bacteria were collected from mice on Day 0 before *C. albicans* challenge and DSS treatment. (**A–D**) Number of *E. coli*, *E. faecalis*, *L. johnsonii* and *L. reuteri* colonies recovered from stools. Data are the mean ± SD of 10 mice per group from two independent experiments.

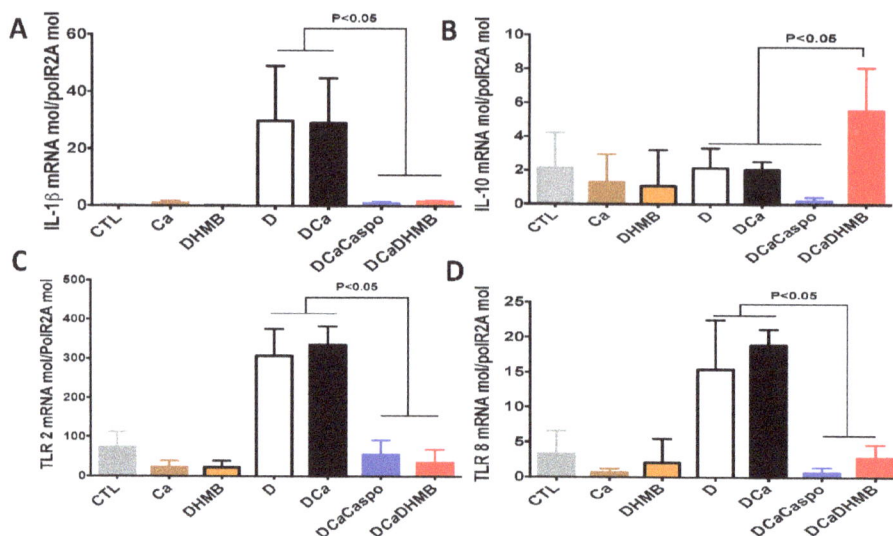

Figure 8. Cytokine and receptor expression after DHMB treatment. (**A–D**) Relative expression levels of IL-1b, IL-10, TLR-2 and TLR-8 mRNA in mouse colons. Data are the mean ± SD of 10 mice per group from two independent experiments.

3. Discussion

The resistance of opportunistic yeast pathogens to antifungal drugs has increased significantly over the past decade and this led us to screen 55 molecules from our chemical library for antifungal activity. DHMB was found to be a promising molecule in terms of MIC value and solubility. In addition, DHMB was not cytotoxic in vitro against a human embryonic kidney cell line (HEK293) at high concentrations (data not shown).

DHMB is often used as a key intermediate in the synthesis of different natural compounds such as the antibacterial agents (±)-isoperbergin and perbergin [14], the antineoplastic agent combretastatin A-1 [15], the allergy-inducing benzofuranoquinone acamelin [16], natural coumarins such as fraxetin and fraxidin [17], or the photoreactive compound pimpinellin [18], but the role of this molecule alone in inflammation and fungal elimination has not yet been studied. An hydroxy-deleted related compound, 2-hydroxy-4-methoxybenzaldehyde (HMB), the principal component of root bark essential oil of *Periploca sepium* Bunge, which is a woody climbing vine [19], exhibits some interesting biological activities. The dried root bark of this plant is traditionally used in the treatment of autoimmune diseases, in particular rheumatoid arthritis [20]. It also appears to have insecticidal activity against several insect species [21].

In the present study, DHMB was highly effective against clinically isolated fluconazole- or caspofungin-resistant *C. albicans* strains indicating that this compound could potentially be used to fight drug-resistant fungi. Some antifungal drugs can induce changes in the cell wall structure after *C. albicans* challenge. In contrast to caspofungin, which induces important cell wall changes in terms of chitin levels, DHMB did not induce any important changes in the cell wall. DHMB was also involved in the inhibition of the melanin production. It has been shown that melanisation is a virulence factor in *C. albicans* while inhibition of melanin biosynthesis by anti-melanin antibodies leads to a decrease in fungal virulence [22,23].

In experimental animals, we observed that the DHMB compound that we administered to animals at high doses was not cytotoxic and was well-tolerated. The animals were still alive and healthy two weeks after the end of the experiment. Furthermore, the efficiency of DHMB was assessed in vivo in the DSS colitis model. This compound reduced the clinical and histological scores for inflammation and promoted elimination of *C. albicans* from the gut. This finding is supported by a decrease in aerobic bacteria while anaerobic bacterial populations were re-established in mice treated with DHMB indicating that DHMB was not only able to reduce *C. albicans* colonisation but also, unexpectedly, to diminish intestinal inflammation. It has been shown that neutrophils and macrophages are recruited to the damaged colonic mucosa during DSS-induced colitis [24]. IL-1β expression, which is predominantly produced by these leukocytes, reduced in mice treated with DHMB. Recently, we observed after colitis development and *C. glabrata* challenge a high production of IL-6 and IL-1β, which are highly important in the recruitment of neutrophils and macrophages into the inflammatory site [9].

It has been shown that melanin concentrate hormone is highly expressed in the colonic mucosa of colitic mice and in patients with IBD suggesting that inhibition of melanin expression by DHMB can potentially reduce the pathogenesis of intestinal inflammation [25].

In conclusion, DHMB is a small organic molecule and any modification or substitution on the aromatic ring led to a strong decrease in the antifungal activity of the molecule, indicating that each group on the ring plays a specific and crucial role in its activity. This compound had antifungal properties against *C. albicans*, was safe and well-tolerated in different culture cell types and animals, and was effective at eliminating drug-resistant fungi, as well as had an anti-tyrosinase effect through the inhibition of the melanisation process in *C. albicans*. In DSS induced colitis model, DHMB had antifungal properties through the elimination of *C. albicans* from the gut and anti-inflammatory activity by re-establishing the anaerobic bacteria. This finding was also supported by a decrease of pro-inflammatory cytokine IL-1β in mice treaded with DHMB. Therefore, this aromatic small molecule holds great potential as an antifungal agent and anti-inflammatory properties.

4. Materials and Methods

4.1. C. albicans Strains and Growth Conditions

The *C. albicans* strains used in the current study are shown in Table 2. Fungal culture was carried out in YPD medium (yeast extract 1%, peptone 1%, dextrose 1%), on a rotary shaker for 18 h at 37 °C. The fungal culture obtained was then centrifuged at 2500 rpm for 5 min and washed twice in PBS (phosphate buffered saline).

Table 2. Antifungal activity of DHMB vs. caspofungin and fluconazole.

Strains	Description	MIC Caspofungin (μg/mL)	MIC Fluconazole (μg/mL)	MIC DHMB (μg/mL)	Ref.
C. albicans ATCC 90028	Wild-type	0.03	0.5	8	This study
Bioluminescent *C. albicans*	*C. albicans* strain CAI4 (ura3::imm434/ura3::imm434)	0.03	0.5	8	[26]
C. albicans 14314c4497	Anal, fluconazole resistant	0.06	128	80	This study
C. albicans 14316c1746	Bronchoalveolar lavage, fluconazole resistant	0.03	128	80	This study
C. albicans 92535989	Tracheal secretion, fluconazole resistant	0.06	64	80	This study
C. albicans 14294c5335	Stools, fluconazole resistant	0.06	5	80	This study
C. albicans 17292c3367	Venous catheter, caspofungin resistant	8	0.5	80	This study
C. albicans 15343c3523	Blood, caspofungin resistant	2	0.5	80	This study
C. albicans 17287c305	Blood, caspofungin resistant	8	0.5	80	This study
C. albicans 15351c6859	Venous catheter, caspofungin resistant	4	1	80	This study

4.2. Antifungal Compounds

The molecule 2,3-dihydroxy-4-methoxybenzaldehyde (DHMB) was synthesised and provided by Hautes Etudes d'Ingénieur (HEI), Lille, France. DHMB was used at a final concentration of 100 μg/mL, diluted in PBS during the various in vitro experiments. Commercially available caspofungin (Merck, Semoy, France) and fluconazole (Fresenius, Sèvres, France) were used as positive controls.

4.3. Fungal Viability Assays

Minimum inhibitory concentrations (MICs) were measured using the broth microdilution method following Clinical Laboratory Standards Institute (CLSI) procedures. After drug inoculation, the plates were incubated at 37 °C for 24 h and MICs were measured as the lowest concentration of drug below growth levels [27]. For antifungal assays on *C. albicans* ATCC 90028, this screening was carried out by CO-ADD (Community for Antimicrobial Drug Discovery) and the University of Queensland (Santa Lucia, Australia). *C. albicans* ATCC 90028 was cultured for 3 days on YPD agar at 30 °C. A yeast suspension of 1×10^6 to 5×10^6 CFU/mL was prepared and the suspension was subsequently diluted and added to each well of the compound-containing plates giving a final cell density of fungi of 2.5×10^3 CFU/mL in a total volume of 50 μL. All plates were covered and incubated at 35 °C for 36 h without shaking. Growth inhibition of *C. albicans* ATCC 90028 was determined by measuring absorbance at 630 nm (OD630), after the addition of resazurin (0.001% final concentration) and incubation at 35 °C for 2 h. The absorbance was measured using a Biotek Multiflo Synergy HTX plate reader. The percentage growth inhibition was calculated for each well, using the negative control (media only) and positive control (fungi without inhibitor) on the same plate. The MIC was determined as the lowest concentration at which growth was fully inhibited, defined by an inhibition of $\geq$80% for *C. albicans* (total inhibition in the case of DHMB at 8 μg/mL concentration).

For the viability assays, the bioluminescent *C. albicans* strain was suspended in PBS at a volume of 10^6 cells/well (96-well black plates, Chimney well). DHMB, caspofungin or fluconazole were then added at their final MIC concentrations (Table 1). Coelenterazine was then added to the wells at a concentration of 2 μM. Bioluminescence kinetics were then measured (at 0, 30 and 60 min) and analysed with a FLUOstar Omega Fluorometer (BMG Labtech, Champigny sur Marne, France). The positive control consisted of *C. albicans* strain alone. The kinetics were also measured with the Xenogen device. For fungal CFU/mL counting, serial dilutions were performed by incubation of 10^5 *C. albicans* cells for 1 h with antifungal at the MIC concentration and an aliquot of 100 μL of each dilution was plated on Sabouraud dextrose agar and incubated for 48 h.

For the melanin production, *C. albicans* yeast cells at 2×10^6 cells/mL were incubated in a minimal medium (15 mM glucose, 10 mM MgSO4, 29.4 mM KH2PO4, 13 mM glycine, 3 mM vitamin B1, pH 5.5) with or without 5 mM L-3,4-dihydroxyphenylalanine (DOPA, Sigma, St. Quentin Fallavier, France) at 37 °C in the dark. After 3 days, *C. albicans* cells grown with DOPA were treated with either DHMB (8 μg/mL) or caspofungin (0.0128 μg/mL). After one day of antifungal incubation, the production of melanin was examined using a Zeiss Axioplan microscope (Axioplan2, Jena, Germany).

4.4. Flow Cytometry and Confocal Microscopy

C. albicans was suspended in PBS at a volume of 10^6 cells/well. DHMB, caspofungin or fluconazole were then added to each well at a final concentration of 100 μM. The expression of chitin or α-Mans was assessed using wheat germ agglutinin-fluorescein isothiocyanate and concanavalin A-rhodamine. The obtained data were analysed using Kaluza software. In parallel, a negative control without addition of lectin marker was prepared under the same conditions as those described previously for the samples. To examine the *C. albicans* cell wall by confocal microscopy after antifungal treatment, *C. albicans* cells were stained with wheat germ agglutinin-fluorescein isothiocyanate, concanavalin A-rhodamine and DAPI. Specific slides (well 6.7 mm; Thermo Scientific, Montigny le Bretonne, France) were used in this experiment and the coverslips were examined by confocal microscopy (Zeiss LSM710, Jena, Germany).

4.5. Animals

The animals used were wild female C57BL/6 mice aged 3–4 months, certified free from infection and purchased from Janvier Laboratories, Le Genest-Saint-Isle, France. The mice were housed at the pet store of the Faculty of Medicine, Lille, France. The temperature of the room was maintained at 21 °C and the mice had free access to water and food with exposure to light 12 h/day. Water bottles and food were daily examined in each cage before the evaluation of the clinical score for each tagged mouse. The studies were carried out in accordance with the decrees relating to the ethics of animal experimentation (Decree 86/609/EC, 8/2/2016).

4.6. C. albicans Challenge and Induction of Colitis

Each mouse was administered with 300 µL of PBS containing 10^7 live *C. albicans* cells by oral gavage on Day 1. For antifungal treatment, mice were injected intraperitoneally for 5 days with 300 µL containing 10 mg/kg/day of DHMB or caspofungin. The DSS model is a reflection of how intestinal inflammation can promote *C. albicans* overgrowth in patients with CD. Mice received 2% DSS (M.W. 36−50 kDa; MP Biomedicals, LLC, Eschwege, Germany) in drinking water from Day 1 to Day 14 to promote colitis development and *C. albicans* intestinal colonisation [28]. The presence of *C. albicans* in the gut was assessed daily by measuring the number of CFUs in stools (approximately 0.1 g/sample). Stools were collected every 2 days from each tagged mouse. Faecal samples were suspended in 1 mL PBS, homogenised with a glass tissue homogeniser and plated onto Candi-Select medium (Bio-Rad Laboratories, Marnes la Coquette, France) [29]. The presence of *C. albicans* was assessed in the stomach, caecum and colon. The tissues were cut longitudinally and washed several times in PBS to avoid surface contamination from organisms present in the lumen. Serial dilutions of gut homogenates were prepared. The results were noted as *C. albicans* CFU/mg of tissue.

For the isolation of aerobic bacteria, the faecal samples were plated onto MacConkey agar (Sigma-Aldrich, Saint Louis, MO, USA) and bile esculin azide agar (BEA, HongKong, China; Sigma-Aldrich, Saint Louis, MO, USA) plates. Serial dilutions of these samples were performed. For the isolation of anaerobic bacteria, Columbia agar (Sigma-Aldrich, Saint Louis, MO, USA) were used. MALDI-TOF MS (Microflex-Bruker Daltonics) was used to identify the bacteria [9].

4.7. Determination of Clinical and Histological Scores of Inflammation

The clinical score was evaluated daily in each tagged mouse based on the presence of blood in the stools, rectal bleeding and stool consistency [5]. These three clinical markers of inflammation were recorded to give a score between 0 (healthy mouse) and 12 (maximum inflammation of the colon reflecting the severity of the inflammation).

Colon samples were fixed in 4% paraformaldehyde-acid and embedded in paraffin for histological analysis. Histological scores were assessed by two independent, blinded investigators who observed two sections per mouse at magnifications of X10 and X100. The histological score was analysed according to two sub-scores: (i) a score for the presence of inflammatory cells; and (ii) a score for epithelial damage. The histological score ranged from 0 (no changes) to 6 (extensive cell infiltration and tissue damage) [5].

4.8. Real-Time mRNA Quantification of Pro-Inflammatory Cytokines and Innate Immune Receptors

RNA extraction was performed with a NucleoSpin RNA® kit (Macherey-Nagel, Hoerdt, France). RNA was quantified by spectrophotometry (Nanodrop; Nyxor Biotech, Paris, France). cDNA synthesis was performed according to the High Capacity DNA Reverse Transcription (RT) protocol, using Master Mix (Applied Biosystems, Foster, CA, USA). Fast SYBR green (Applied Biosystems) was used to amplify the cDNA by PCR using the one-step system (Applied Biosystems). SYBR green dye intensity was assessed using one-step software. All results were normalised to the reference gene, POLR2A.

5. Statistical Analysis

All data are presented as the mean ± standard deviation (SD) of individual experimental groups. Statistical analyses were performed using the Mann–Whitney U test to compare pairs of groups. Differences were considered significant when the p value was as follows: $p < 0.05$; $p < 0.01$; $p < 0.001$. Prism 4.0 from GraphPad and XLSTAT were used for the statistical analyses.

Int. J. Mol. Sci. **2019**, *20*, 321

Author Contributions: C.B., M.B., R.C., K.L., and S.J. performed the experiments. C.B., M.B., R.C., and S.J. analysed the data. C.B., M.B., R.C., K.L., A.G., B.S. and S.J. interpreted the results of the experiments. M.B., A.G., and B.S. contributed reagents/materials/analysis tools. S.J. designed the experiments and drafted the manuscript.

Funding: This work was partially funded by Agence Nationale de la Recherche (ANR) in the setting the project "InnateFun", promotional reference ANR-16-IFEC-0003-05, in the "Infect-ERA" program.

Acknowledgments: The authors thank Nadine François and Antonino Bongiovanni for their excellent technical assistance. The authors would like to thank the Community for Antimicrobial Drug Discovery (CO-ADD), funded by the Welcome Trust (UK), and the University of Queensland (Australia) for performing the DHMB antimicrobial screening.

Conflicts of Interest: The authors declare no conflict of interest.

References

1. Baumgart, D.C.; Sandborn, W.J. Inflammatory bowel disease: Clinical aspects and established and evolving therapies. *Lancet* **2007**, *369*, 1641–1657. [CrossRef]
2. Oyri, S.F.; Muzes, G.; Sipos, F. Dysbiotic gut microbiome: A key element of Crohn's disease. *Comp. Immunol. Microbiol. Infect. Dis.* **2015**, *43*, 36–49. [CrossRef] [PubMed]
3. Gevers, D.; Kugathasan, S.; Denson, L.A.; Vazquez-Baeza, Y.; Van Treuren, W.; Ren, B.; Schwager, E.; Knights, D.; Song, S.J.; Yassour, M.; et al. The treatment-naive microbiome in new-onset Crohn's disease. *Cell Host Microbe* **2014**, *15*, 382–392. [CrossRef] [PubMed]
4. Darfeuille-Michaud, A.; Neut, C.; Barnich, N.; Lederman, E.; Di Martino, P.; Desreumaux, P.; Gambiez, L.; Joly, B.; Cortot, A.; Colombel, J.F. Presence of adherent Escherichia coli strains in ileal mucosa of patients with Crohn's disease. *Gastroenterology* **1998**, *115*, 1405–1413. [CrossRef]
5. Jawhara, S.; Thuru, X.; Standaert-Vitse, A.; Jouault, T.; Mordon, S.; Sendid, B.; Desreumaux, P.; Poulain, D. Colonization of mice by Candida albicans is promoted by chemically induced colitis and augments inflammatory responses through galectin-3. *J. Infect. Dis.* **2008**, *197*, 972–980. [CrossRef] [PubMed]
6. Jawhara, S.; Poulain, D. Saccharomyces boulardii decreases inflammation and intestinal colonization by Candida albicans in a mouse model of chemically-induced colitis. *Med. Mycol.* **2007**, *45*, 691–700. [CrossRef] [PubMed]
7. Standaert-Vitse, A.; Sendid, B.; Joossens, M.; Francois, N.; Vandewalle-El Khoury, P.; Branche, J.; Van Kruiningen, H.; Jouault, T.; Rutgeerts, P.; Gower-Rousseau, C.; et al. Candida albicans colonization and ASCA in familial Crohn's disease. *Am. J. Gastroenterol.* **2009**, *104*, 1745–1753. [CrossRef]
8. Poulain, D.; Sendid, B.; Standaert-Vitse, A.; Fradin, C.; Jouault, T.; Jawhara, S.; Colombel, J.F. Yeasts: Neglected pathogens. *Dig. Dis.* **2009**, *27* (Suppl. 1), 104–110. [CrossRef]
9. Charlet, R.; Pruvost, Y.; Tumba, G.; Istel, F.; Poulain, D.; Kuchler, K.; Sendid, B.; Jawhara, S. Remodeling of the Candida glabrata cell wall in the gastrointestinal tract affects the gut microbiota and the immune response. *Sci. Rep.* **2018**, *8*, 3316. [CrossRef]
10. Ardizzone, S.; Cassinotti, A.; Manes, G.; Porro, G.B. Immunomodulators for all patients with inflammatory bowel disease? *Ther. Adv. Gastroenterol.* **2010**, *3*, 31–42. [CrossRef]
11. Campieri, M. New steroids and new salicylates in inflammatory bowel disease: A critical appraisal. *Gut* **2002**, *50* (Suppl. 3), III43–III46. [CrossRef] [PubMed]
12. Wiederhold, N.P. Antifungal resistance: Current trends and future strategies to combat. *Infect. Drug Resist.* **2017**, *10*, 249–259. [CrossRef] [PubMed]
13. Ostrosky-Zeichner, L.; Casadevall, A.; Galgiani, J.N.; Odds, F.C.; Rex, J.H. An insight into the antifungal pipeline: Selected new molecules and beyond. *Nat. Rev. Drug Discov.* **2010**, *9*, 719–727. [CrossRef] [PubMed]
14. Almabruk, K.H.; Chang, J.H.; Mahmud, T. Total Synthesis of (+/−)-Isoperbergins and Correction of the Chemical Structure of Perbergin. *J. Nat. Prod.* **2016**, *79*, 2391–2396. [CrossRef] [PubMed]
15. Pettit, G.R.; Singh, S.B.; Niven, M.L.; Hamel, E.; Schmidt, J.M. Isolation, structure, and synthesis of combretastatins A-1 and B-1, potent new inhibitors of microtubule assembly, derived from Combretum caffrum. *J. Nat. Prod.* **1987**, *50*, 119–131. [CrossRef]
16. McKittrick, B.A.; Stevenson, R. A simple synthesis of the natural benzofuranoquinone, acamelin. *J. Chem. Soc. Perkin Trans. 1* **1983**, *10*, 2423–2424. [CrossRef]
17. Spath, E.; Dobrovolny, E. Natural coumarins. XLII. Synthesis of fraxetin, fraxidin and isofraxidin. *Berichte der Deutschen Chemischen Gesellschaft* **1938**, *71B*, 1831–1836. [CrossRef]

18. Cervi, A.; Aillard, P.; Hazeri, N.; Petit, L.; Chai, C.L.; Willis, A.C.; Banwell, M.G. Total syntheses of the coumarin-containing natural products pimpinellin and fraxetin using Au(I)-catalyzed intramolecular hydroarylation (IMHA) chemistry. *J. Org. Chem.* **2013**, *78*, 9876–9882. [CrossRef]

19. Wang, L.; Yin, Z.Q.; Zhang, L.H.; Ye, W.C.; Zhang, X.Q.; Shen, W.B.; Zhao, S.X. Chemical constituents from root barks of Periploca sepium. *China J. Chin. Mater. Med.* **2007**, *32*, 1300–1302.

20. Tokiwa, T.; Harada, K.; Matsumura, T.; Tukiyama, T. Oriental medicinal herb, Periploca sepium, extract inhibits growth and IL-6 production of human synovial fibroblast-like cells. *Biol. Pharm. Bull.* **2004**, *27*, 1691–1693. [CrossRef]

21. Chu, S.S.; Jiang, G.H.; Liu, W.L.; Liu, Z.L. Insecticidal activity of the root bark essential oil of Periploca sepium Bunge and its main component. *Nat. Prod. Res.* **2012**, *26*, 926–932. [CrossRef] [PubMed]

22. Morris-Jones, R.; Gomez, B.L.; Diez, S.; Uran, M.; Morris-Jones, S.D.; Casadevall, A.; Nosanchuk, J.D.; Hamilton, A.J. Synthesis of melanin pigment by Candida albicans in vitro and during infection. *Infect. Immun.* **2005**, *73*, 6147–6150. [CrossRef] [PubMed]

23. Eisenman, H.C.; Duong, R.; Chan, H.; Tsue, R.; McClelland, E.E. Reduced virulence of melanized Cryptococcus neoformans in Galleria mellonella. *Virulence* **2014**, *5*, 611–618. [CrossRef] [PubMed]

24. Qualls, J.E.; Kaplan, A.M.; van Rooijen, N.; Cohen, D.A. Suppression of experimental colitis by intestinal mononuclear phagocytes. *J. Leukoc. Biol.* **2006**, *80*, 802–815. [CrossRef]

25. Kokkotou, E.; Moss, A.C.; Torres, D.; Karagiannides, I.; Cheifetz, A.; Liu, S.; O'Brien, M.; Maratos-Flier, E.; Pothoulakis, C. Melanin-concentrating hormone as a mediator of intestinal inflammation. *Proc. Natl. Acad. Sci. USA* **2008**, *105*, 10613–10618. [CrossRef]

26. Doyle, T.C.; Nawotka, K.A.; Kawahara, C.B.; Francis, K.P.; Contag, P.R. Visualizing fungal infections in living mice using bioluminescent pathogenic Candida albicans strains transformed with the firefly luciferase gene. *Microb. Pathog.* **2006**, *40*, 82–90. [CrossRef] [PubMed]

27. Bustamante, B.; Martins, M.A.; Bonfietti, L.X.; Szeszs, M.W.; Jacobs, J.; Garcia, C.; Melhem, M.S. Species distribution and antifungal susceptibility profile of Candida isolates from bloodstream infections in Lima, Peru. *J. Med. Microbiol.* **2014**, *63 Pt 6*, 855–860. [CrossRef]

28. Choteau, L.; Parny, M.; Francois, N.; Bertin, B.; Fumery, M.; Dubuquoy, L.; Takahashi, K.; Colombel, J.F.; Jouault, T.; Poulain, D.; et al. Role of mannose-binding lectin in intestinal homeostasis and fungal elimination. *Mucosal Immunol.* **2016**, *9*, 767–776. [CrossRef]

29. Sendid, B.; Francois, N.; Standaert, A.; Dehecq, E.; Zerimech, F.; Camus, D.; Poulain, D. Prospective evaluation of the new chromogenic medium CandiSelect 4 for differentiation and presumptive identification of the major pathogenic Candida species. *J. Med. Microbiol.* **2007**, *56 Pt 4*, 495–499. [CrossRef]

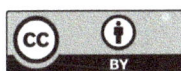

International Journal of
Molecular Sciences

MDPI

Article

Intravenous Immunoglobulin Therapy Eliminates *Candida albicans* and Maintains Intestinal Homeostasis in a Murine Model of Dextran Sulfate Sodium-Induced Colitis

Rogatien Charlet [1,2,3], Boualem Sendid [1,2,3], Srini V. Kaveri [4], Daniel Poulain [1,2,3], Jagadeesh Bayry [4,*] and Samir Jawhara [1,2,3,*]

[1] Inserm, U995/Team2, Université Lille, 1 place Verdun, F-59000 Lille, France; charlet-rogatien@hotmail.fr (R.C.); boualem.sendid@univ-lille.fr (B.S.); daniel.poulain@univ-lille.fr (D.P.)

[2] University Lille2, U995-LIRIC, Lille Inflammation Research International Centre, F-59000 Lille, France

[3] CHU Lille, Service de Parasitologie Mycologie, Pôle de Biologie Pathologie Génétique, F-59000 Lille, France

[4] Inserm Centre de Recherche des Cordeliers, Equipe-Immunopathologie et Immuno-intervention Thérapeutique, Sorbonne Universités, Université Paris Descartes, Sorbonne Paris Cité, F-75006 Paris, France; srini.kaveri@crc.jussieu.fr

* Correspondence: jagadesh.bayry@crc.jussieu.fr (J.B.); samir.jawhara@univ-lille.fr (S.J.); Tel.: +33-(0)320-6235-46 (J.B.); Fax: +33-(0)3-20-6234-16 (S.J.)

Received: 13 February 2019; Accepted: 21 March 2019; Published: 23 March 2019

Abstract: Intravenous immunoglobulin (IVIg) therapy has diverse anti-inflammatory and immunomodulatory effects and has been employed successfully in autoimmune and inflammatory diseases. The role of IVIg therapy in the modulation of intestinal inflammation and fungal elimination has not been yet investigated. We studied IVIg therapy in a murine model of dextran sulfate sodium (DSS)-induced colitis. Mice received a single oral inoculum of *Candida albicans* and were exposed to DSS treatment for 2 weeks to induce colitis. All mice received daily IVIg therapy starting on day 1 for 7 days. IVIg therapy not only prevented a loss of body weight caused by the development of colitis but also reduced the severity of intestinal inflammation, as determined by clinical and histological scores. IVIg treatment significantly reduced the *Escherichia coli*, *Enterococcus faecalis*, and *C. albicans* populations in mice. The beneficial effects of IVIg were associated with the suppression of inflammatory cytokine interleukin (IL)-6 and enhancement of IL-10 in the gut. IVIg therapy also led to an increased expression of peroxisome proliferator-activated receptor gamma (PPARγ), while toll-like receptor 4 (TLR-4) expression was reduced. IVIg treatment reduces intestinal inflammation in mice and eliminates *C. albicans* overgrowth from the gut in association with down-regulation of pro-inflammatory mediators combined with up-regulation of anti-inflammatory cytokines.

Keywords: intravenous immunoglobulin G; colitis; dextran sulfate sodium; mice; inflammation; cytokines; *Candida albicans*; *Escherichia coli*; *Enterococcus faecalis*

1. Introduction

Candida albicans infections continue to be a serious clinical problem in terms of their high morbidity and mortality [1,2]. The interaction between the fungus and its host occurs at the level of the cell wall, which consists mainly of polysaccharides associated with proteins and lipids. Its innermost layers are composed of a dense network of polysaccharides consisting of glucans (β-1,3 and β-1,6 linked glucose) and chitin (a polymer of β-1,4-linked N-acetylglucosamine) [3]. Fungal polysaccharides are shed into the circulation during infection, and their detection enables the early diagnosis of invasive fungal infection [1]. Clinical and experimental studies have shown that *C. albicans* infections can generate anti-glycan antibodies known as ASCA (anti-*Saccharomyces cerevisiae* mannan antibodies) [4]. These anti-fungal glycan antibodies were initially described as serological markers of Crohn's disease (CD), but subsequent studies have established that they can also be generated during *Candida* infection, suggesting a link between CD gut dysbiosis and endogenous opportunistic fungal species [5,6]. CD and ulcerative colitis (UC) are the main forms of inflammatory bowel disease (IBD). CD and UC are distinguishable by the location of the inflammation and by the pattern of histological alterations in the gastrointestinal (GI) tract. Animal models have played a significant role in increasing our understanding of IBD pathogenesis, especially models of murine colitis [7]. Experimental studies have shown that *C. albicans* exacerbates the intestinal inflammation induced by dextran sulfate sodium (DSS) in mice, and, conversely, that DSS colitis promotes fungal colonization [8,9].

Immunotherapy with intravenous immunoglobulin (IVIg) is widely used in the management of various autoimmune and inflammatory diseases [10–12]. Experimental studies and evaluation of patients undergoing IVIg therapy show that the beneficial effects of IVIg in inflammatory and autoimmune diseases involve diverse mechanisms, including inhibition of activation of innate immune cells and release of inflammatory cytokines, reciprocal regulation of effector T-cells (Th1 and Th17) and regulatory T-cells (Tregs), neutralization of autoantibodies and complement, and suppression of autoantibody production [13,14].

Several case studies and open-label trials showed that IVIg could induce significant improvement in aminosalicylate- and steroid-resistant CD [15]. Although the number of patients is small, the data imply that IVIg could induce swift relief from inflammation and significantly improve these patients without causing side-effects. However, the mechanism by which IVIg therapy benefits CD patients is currently unknown.

We investigated the protective effects of IVIg therapy in a murine model of DSS-induced colitis. By using clinical and histological parameters, we reported that IVIg therapy reduced the intestinal inflammation and was associated with the prevention of a loss of body weight. Further, IVIg therapy significantly reduced the burden of *C. albicans* in the intestine and other organs. The beneficial effects of IVIg in DSS-induced colitis were associated with the suppression of inflammatory cytokine interleukin (IL)-6 and enhancement of IL-10 in the gut. IVIg therapy also led to an increased expression of peroxisome proliferator-activated receptor gamma (PPARγ), while toll-like receptor 4 (TLR-4) expression was reduced. These data provide experimental evidence for the therapeutic utility of IVIg in IBD.

2. Results

2.1. IVIg Treatment Reduces the Severity of Intestinal Inflammation in C. albicans Colonized Mice with DSS-Induced Colitis

In order to analyze the efficiency of IVIg in the modulation of intestinal inflammation, mice received 2% DSS for 2 weeks in drinking water to promote the development of colitis. IVIg (Sandoglobulin) was administered via intraperitoneal injection (0.8 g/kg/day for 7 days) to mice treated with DSS and challenged with *C. albicans*. Mice treated with DSS or DSS + *C. albicans* had a mortality rate of approximately 20%, while no mortality was recorded in mice treated with IVIg alone (Figure 1A).

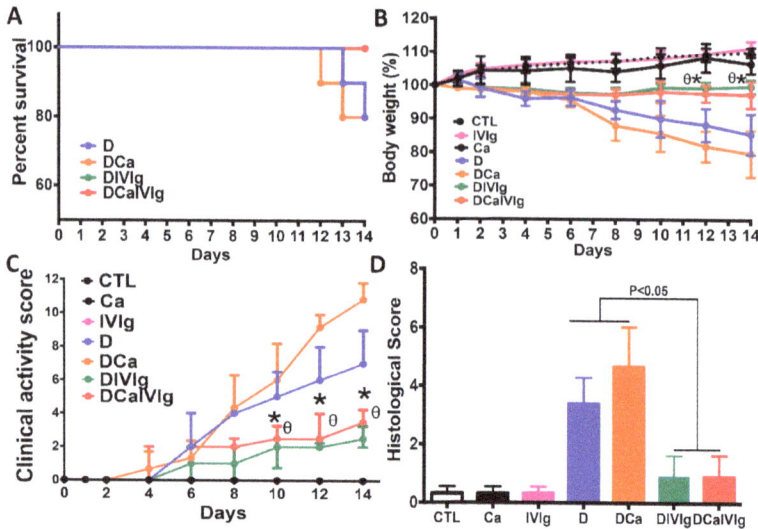

Figure 1. Effect of intravenous immunoglobulin (IVIg) treatment on the survival of mice, body weight, and inflammatory scores in the dextran sulfate sodium (DSS)-induced colitis model. (**A**) Mouse survival. Results are expressed as percent survival from the time of *C. albicans* challenge and DSS treatment. CTL, Ca, IVIg or D correspond to control groups receiving water, *C. albicans*, IVIg treatment or DSS, respectively. DCa corresponds to mice receiving *C. albicans* and treated with DSS. DIVIg corresponds to mice receiving DSS and treated with IVIg. DCaIVIg represents mice receiving *C. albicans* challenged with IVIg and treated with DSS. No mouse mortality was recorded in the Ca or IVIg groups, while DSS treatment induced 20% mouse mortality in groups D and DCa; (**B**) Body weight. Results are expressed as a percent; (**C**) Clinical analysis of DSS-induced colitis in mice after IVIg treatment. Clinical score was determined by assessing weight loss, change in stool consistency, and presence of gross bleeding. The clinical score ranged from 0 to 12 (each value corresponds to the mean value over 14 days per group). * $p < 0.05$ for DCaIVIg mice vs. DCa and D mice; (**D**) Histological scores. Scores range from 0 (no changes) to six (extensive cell infiltration and tissue damage). Data are the mean ± SD of 14 mice per group.

DSS treatment led to a 15% loss of body weight of mice at 2 weeks (Figure 1B). Although *C. albicans* did not alter the body weight of mice in the absence of DSS-induced colonic inflammation, *C. albicans* triggered a further loss of body weight (nearly 20%) in DSS-induced colitis, while mice treated with DSS solely displayed 15% of body weight loss. In both groups of mice, the clinical scores increased significantly from day 7 onwards (Figure 1C). However, IVIg therapy not only rescued the mice from body weight loss but also significantly reduced the severity of intestinal inflammation, as determined by clinical and histological scores in DIVIg or DCaIVIg mice.

Histological analysis of the colon revealed that *C. albicans* alone did not induce either epithelial injury or inflammatory cell infiltration in the colon wall (Figure 1D). In DSS-induced colitis, *C. albicans* enhanced inflammatory cell infiltration in the colon wall structures and massive tissue destruction. However, IVIg protected the mice from this severe tissue destruction (Figure 2).

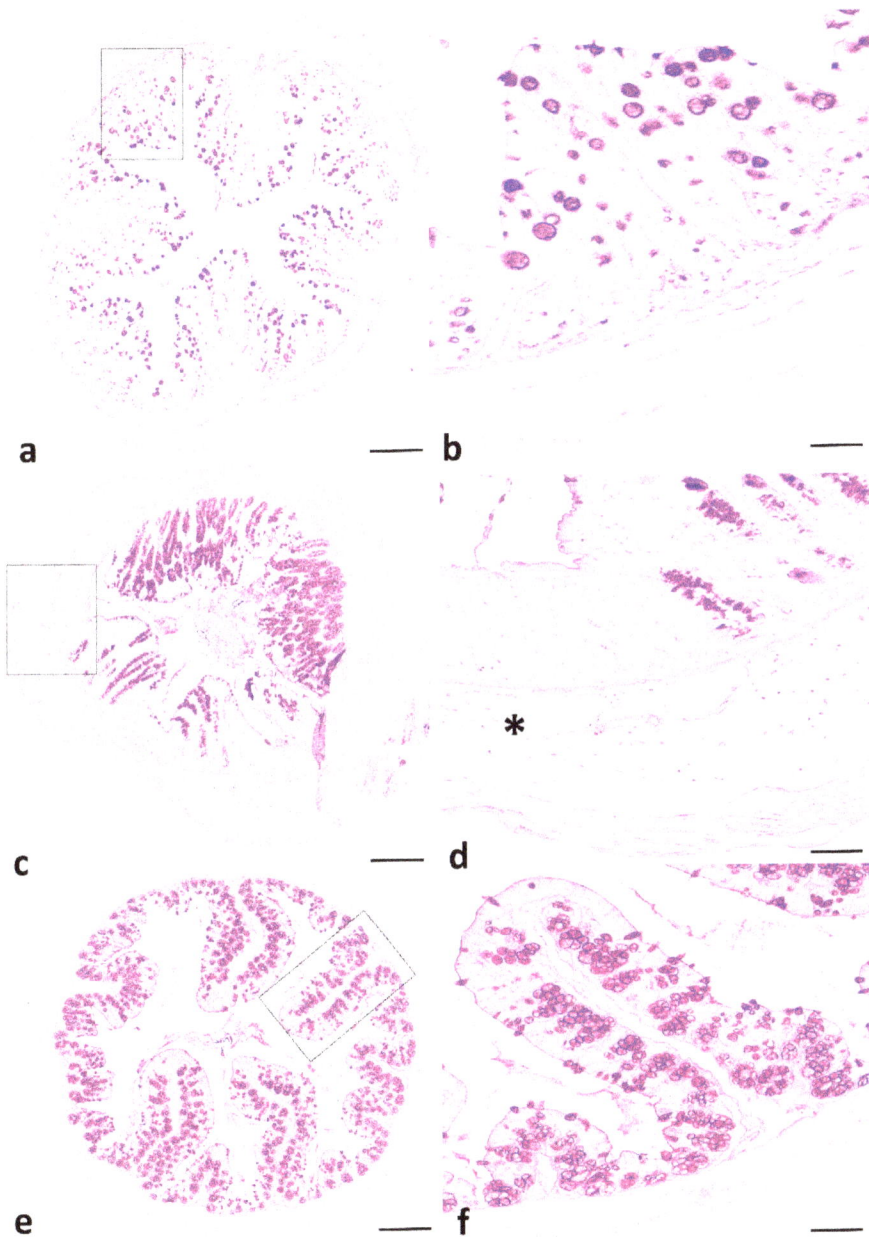

Figure 2. Histological analysis of colons from mice with dextran sulfate sodium (DSS)-induced colitis. Panels (**a,b**) display sections from mice that received *C. albicans;* panels (**c,d**) correspond to *C. albicans* + DSS; and panels (**e,f**) denote colon sections from mice that received *C. albicans* + DSS + intravenous immunoglobulin (IVIg). *C. albicans* alone did not induce any epithelial injury or an inflammatory cell infiltrate in the colon wall structure. Colon sections from DCa mice show an inflammatory cell infiltrate in colon wall structures and massive tissue destruction (asterisk), while colon sections from DCaIVIg mice show minimal tissue damage. The scale bars represent 50 μm (**a,c,e**) and 10 μm (**b,d,f**).

2.2. IVIg Treatment Decreases the Escherichia coli, Enterococcus faecalis, and C. albicans Populations in Mice with DSS-Induced Colitis

To determine the effect of IVIg treatment on the growth of the *E. coli* and *E. faecalis* populations, the colonic luminal contents were analyzed at day 14 in all groups (Figure 3). We found that *C. albicans* alone or IVIg treatment, in the absence of colitis, did not induce any significant changes in the *E. coli* and *E. faecalis* populations, while DSS-induced colitis and *C. albicans* overgrowth promoted an increased *E. coli* and *E. faecalis* populations in mice. In contrast, IVIg treatment significantly reduced *E. coli* and *E. faecalis* in mice treated with DSS solely or DSS + *C. albicans* (Figure 3). The effect of IVIg treatment on *C. albicans* colonization was assessed in stool samples, stomach, and large intestine of mice (Figure 4). DSS promoted C. albicans colonization in the stomach, caecum, and colon. Thus, colonic inflammation induced by DSS promoted the establishment of *C. albicans* colonization. The number of *C. albicans* colony forming units (CFU) gradually increased during colitis development. Interestingly, IVIg treatment significantly reduced the burden of *C. albicans* and CFU of *C. albicans* in various organs (Figure 4).

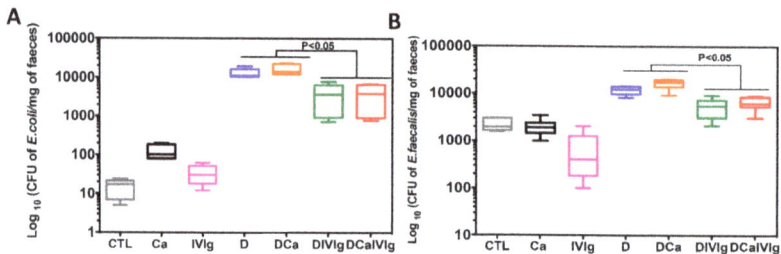

Figure 3. Determination of viable fecal aerobic bacteria in mice with colitis and treated with intravenous immunoglobulin (IVIg) (**A,B**) The number of *E. coli* and *E. faecalis* colonies recovered from colonic luminal contents. Data are expressed as box-and-whiskers plots, with min to the max range as whiskers. CFU: colony forming units.

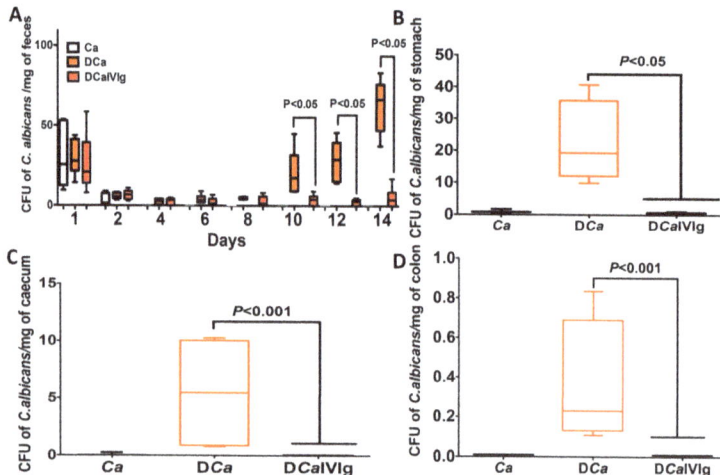

Figure 4. Evaluation of *C. albicans* colonization in various organs following intravenous immunoglobulin (IVIg) treatment of mice with dextran sulfate sodium (DSS)-induced colitis. (**A**) The number of *C. albicans* colony forming units (CFU) recovered from stools. Data are expressed as box-and-whiskers plots, with min to the max range as whiskers. (**B–D**) The number of *C. albicans* CFU recovered from the stomach, cecum, and colon. Data are expressed as box-and-whiskers plots, with min to the max range as whiskers.

2.3. IVIg Treatment Reduces Inflammatory Cytokines and Enhances IL-10 in the Colon

A significant reduction in the severity of intestinal inflammation, as measured by clinical and histological scores, suggests that IVIg treatment altered the inflammatory cytokines in the colon (Figure 5). IVIg significantly reduced IL-6 in the colon and was associated with a reciprocal enhancement of the anti-inflammatory cytokine IL-10. In addition, the transcript levels of PPARγ, a ligand-activated transcription factor that tilts the balance towards the production of anti-inflammatory mediators in innate cells, was significantly increased by IVIg. Interestingly, IVIg also reduced the transcript levels of TLR-4, in line with its role in intestinal inflammation (Figure 5).

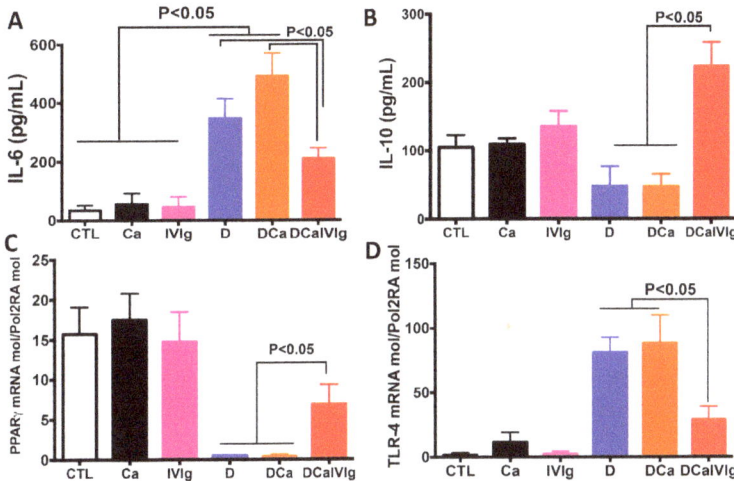

Figure 5. Cytokine and receptor expression after intravenous immunoglobulin (IVIg) treatment of mice with *C. albicans* and dextran sulfate sodium (DSS)-induced colitis. (**A,B**) Protein levels of interleukin (IL)-6 and IL-10 in mouse colons. (**C,D**) Relative expression of peroxisome proliferator-activated receptor gamma (PPARγ) and toll-like receptor 4 (TLR-4) mRNA in mouse colons. Data are the mean ± SD of 14 mice per group.

3. Discussion

IVIg has diverse anti-inflammatory and immunomodulatory effects and has been employed successfully in autoimmune and inflammatory diseases. It is considered non-immunosuppressive and safe. By using the murine model of dextran sulfate sodium-induced colitis, we demonstrate that IVIg therapy not only reduces the intestinal inflammation but also eradicates *C. albicans* overgrowth from the gut. Although we used a mouse model, for the reasons discussed below, we employed human therapeutic normal immunoglobulin preparation rather than murine immunoglobulin for the therapy. IVIg is obtained from the pooled plasma of several thousand healthy donors (typically 3000 to 10,000 donors) with highly variable genetic, epigenetic, and environmental backgrounds. Reproducing these factors and the entire array of human immunoglobulin repertoire is quite impossible in mouse immunoglobulin preparation, and hence mouse immunoglobulin preparation equivalent of human IVIg is not available. As IVIg is infused at 1–2 g/kg body weight, obtaining such big quantities of mouse immunoglobulin is also a daunting task. On the other hand, the use of human IVIg has direct translational value for exploring this therapy in patients.

IVIg has been used in the treatment of CD and has been shown to bring about a rapid and clinically significant improvement in a patient's condition. However, the role of IVIg in the modulation of intestinal inflammation and fungal elimination has not been yet studied. In the present study, low doses of DSS (2%) were administered to mice for 2 weeks to induce colonic inflammation and to promote the establishment of *C. albicans* overgrowth. In a pilot experiment, IVIg was administered to mice intraperitoneally, intravenously or orally. Intraperitoneal injection of IVIg after *C. albicans* challenge was more efficient at reducing inflammatory clinical signs than the other routes of administration (data not shown). This finding is consistent with previous reports showing that intraperitoneal injection is better than other routes in the setting of colitis amelioration [16,17].

IVIg has been used as an anti-infectious agent against viruses or bacteria in both patients and experimental models [18–21]. As IVIg is a pool of IgG from thousands of healthy donors, the exposure of individual donors to vaccinations, endemic infectious diseases, and ubiquitous microorganisms contribute to IgG antibodies against diverse microbes and their products [19,22,23]. These antibodies play an important role in the prevention of infectious episodes in primary immunodeficient patients. However, the beneficial effects of IVIg in infectious diseases go beyond simple neutralization of microbes or their toxins. Anti-inflammatory pathways are also critical for protection against infection [24]. IL-10 was shown to be critical for the protection rendered by IVIg against fatal herpes simplex virus (HSV) encephalitis in mice [25].

Investigations on IVIg therapy in fungal infections is, however, limited despite the fact that several compelling pieces of evidence have shown the protective role of immunoglobulins in the infections and inflammation mediated by several fungal species, including Candida, Aspergillus, Cryptococci, and others [26,27]. Antibodies either in the circulation of an individual that are formed due to natural exposure to fungi species or when used in the form of specific protective monoclonal antibodies could mediate protection against fungal infections by several mutually nonexclusive mechanisms, such as neutralization of fungi species and their pathogen-associated molecular patterns, alteration of expression of fungal transcripts, metabolism and signaling pathways, and suppression of formation of biofilm and liberation of polysaccharides. In addition, antibodies are also shown to enhance opsonization of fungi and promote complement activation and phagocytosis of fungi by innate cells like macrophages and monocytes [26].

Several observational studies have reported that infusion of IVIg reduces the incidence of fungal infections in immunocompromised patients. As IVIg is a pooled IgG purified from the plasma of several thousand healthy donors, these observations highlight the importance of anti-fungal IgG in the circulation to mediate resistance against fungal infections. Thus, prophylaxis IVIg therapy in hepatic allograft individuals receiving oral acyclovir led to a significant decrease in the occurrence of fungal infections [28]. Epidemiologic investigation in soldiers who received IVIg as a prophylactic vaccination reduced the rate of skin fungal infections [29]. Although not used in the form of IVIg, prophylaxis oral administration of bovine anti-Candida antibodies, that are obtained from the bovines immunized with many Candida species, were reported to reduce fungal colonization in the majority of the bone marrow transplant patients [30]. In line with these observations, our recent report demonstrates that IVIg protects from experimental allergic bronchopulmonary aspergillosis in mice [31]. Whether used as prophylaxis or therapy, IVIg in this model significantly reduced the *Aspergillus fumigatus* burden in the lungs. Of interest, this report also provided convincing evidence that beneficial effects of IVIg in fungal infections go beyond neutralization of fungi wherein we found that protective effects of IVIg were associated with reduced Th17 responses and concomitant enhancement of regulatory T cells and IL-10, the mechanisms implicated in the beneficial effects of IVIg in autoimmune conditions [32,33].

In the present study, IVIg promoted the elimination of *C. albicans* from the gut and reduced intestinal inflammation. This finding is also supported by decreased clinical and histological scores of inflammation. Although IVIg is known to contain IgG against *Candida* [34] and may help in the neutralization of *C. albicans*, the anti-inflammatory effects of IVIg appear to be crucial in the DSS-induced colitis model. In terms of the gut bacteria, we focused on *E. coli* and *E. faecalis* populations that are known to be involved in IBD [35,36]. *E. coli* and *E. faecalis* populations increased in mice that developed colitis, while the IVIg treatment reduced these aerobic bacteria. These observations are consistent with clinical and experimental studies, which show an increase in *E. coli* and *E. faecalis* in CD patients [36,37]. The beneficial effects of IVIg were associated with the suppression of inflammatory cytokine IL-6 and enhancement of IL-10 in the gut. Our data, along with previous data from an HSV encephalitis model, suggest that IL-10 plays a central role in mediating protection against the inflammation associated with infection.

In addition to cytokines, IVIg therapy also led to increased expression of PPARγ, a ligand-activated transcription factor that mediates anti-inflammatory functions and resolution of inflammation [38]. Previous studies have shown that IVIg suppresses the activation of monocytes/macrophages and neutrophils [39–43]. Clinically, blocking the pro-inflammatory cytokine stimulates IL-10 production by regulatory macrophages, which are involved in mucosal healing in IBD patients [44]. As PPARγ influences innate immune signaling and the induction of pro-inflammatory cytokines, including IL-6, it is plausible that increased expression of PPARγ might contribute to the anti-inflammatory action of IVIg and cytokine blockers on these innate cells [45].

Because of their role in sensing microbes and mediating the inflammatory response, toll-like receptors (TLR), including TLR-4, occupy a central place in the pathogenesis of IBD. Dysregulated TLR signaling due to mutations or abnormal intestinal microbiota is a common feature of IBD, in particular, *E. coli* and *E. faecalis*. During chronic intestinal inflammation, TLR-4 expression is increased and in addition to promoting inflammation, it also stimulates colon carcinogenesis [46]. In the present study, we observed that TLR-4 expression was correlated with increased *E. coli* population while following the IVIg treatment, the expression of TLR-4 was decreased, concurring with the histological and clinical scores data. Altogether, IVIg treatment reduces intestinal inflammation in mice and eliminates *C. albicans* overgrowth from the gut in association with suppression of inflammatory cytokine IL-6 and enhancement of IL-10. Further work is necessary to identify whether protection is associated with alterations in the adaptive immune compartments and the underlying mechanisms, particularly the relative contribution of Fc versus F(ab')$_2$ fragments in mediating the anti-inflammatory activity.

4. Methods

4.1. Animals

Female C57BL/6 mice (8–10-weeks-old) were purchased from Charles River Laboratories (France). Two complete experimental series were carried out independently. Mice were divided into four control groups, including mice receiving water (CTL), *C. albicans* (Ca), IVIg and DSS (D) alone, and two experimental groups, including *C. albicans* + DSS (DCa) and *C. albicans* + DSS + IVIg (DCaIVIg). All experiments were performed according to protocols approved by the subcommittee for Research Animal Care of the Regional Hospital Centre of Lille, France and the French Ministry of Post-Graduate Education and Research (00550.05, 8/2/2016), and in accordance with European legal and institutional guidelines (86/609/CEE) for the care and use of laboratory animals.

4.2. Yeast Strain, Inoculum Preparation, and Induction of Colitis

C. albicans SC5314 strain was maintained at 4 °C in yeast peptone dextrose broth (YPD; 1% yeast extract, 2% peptone, 2% dextrose). Each mouse was inoculated on day 1 by oral gavage with 200 μL of PBS containing 5×10^7 live *C. albicans* cells. Mice were given 2% DSS (MW 36−50 kDa; MP Biomedicals, LLC, Germany) in drinking water from day 1 to day 14 to induce intestinal inflammation. For IVIg treatment, mice were administered IVIg Sandoglobulin® (CSL Behring SA; Lot No. 4319800016) intraperitoneally on day 1 (0.8 g/kg) for 7 days. Sandoglobulin® contains at least 96% IgG (typically 99%) with the distribution of the IgG subclasses closely resembling that in normal human plasma. In terms of the subclass distribution, Sandoglobulin® contains 64.5% IgG1, 32.4% IgG2, 2.3% IgG3, and 0.8% IgG4. The product also contains traces of immunoglobulin A (IgA) and immunoglobulin M (IgM).

The presence of *C. albicans* in the intestinal tract was monitored daily by measuring the number of colony-forming units (CFUs) in feces (approximately 0.1 g/sample) collected from each animal. Fecal samples were suspended in 1 mL saline, ground in a glass tissue homogenizer, and plated onto

Candi-Select medium (Bio-Rad Laboratories, Marnes la Coquette, France). The CFU of *C. albicans* were counted after 48 h incubation at 37 °C. The results were expressed as CFU/µg of feces. To assess *C. albicans* colonization in the gut, animals were sacrificed, and the GI tract was removed and separated into the stomach, ileum, and colon. The tissues were cut longitudinally. After removal of the intestinal contents, the tissues were washed several times in PBS to minimize surface contamination from organisms present in the lumen. Serial dilutions of homogenates were performed. The results were noted as *C. albicans* CFU/mg of tissue [7,8].

For the isolation of *E. coli* and *E. faecalis* populations, the colonic luminal contents were plated at day 14 onto MacConkey agar (Sigma-Aldrich, St. Quentin Fallavier, France) and Bile esculin azide agar (BEA; Sigma-Aldrich, St. Quentin Fallavier, France). Serial dilutions of these samples were realized. The agar plates were incubated at 37 °C and examined 24 h and 48 h later. Fluconazole (Fresenius Kabi, Louviers, France; 60 mg/L) was added to these two-aerobic media to eliminate the fungal growth cells. For the identification of *E. coli* and *E. faecalis*, a volume of 1.5 µL of matrix solution (α-cyano-4-hydroxycinnamic acid [HCCA]; Bruker Daltonics, Leipzig, Germany) dissolved in 50% acetonitrile, 47.5% water, and 2.5% trifluoroacetic acid was added to each bacterial colony and allowed to dry prior to analysis by MALDI-TOF MS (Microflex-Bruker Daltonics, Bruker Daltonics, Leipzig, Germany).

4.3. Assessment of Clinical and Histological Scores

The body weight of each tagged mouse was recorded daily, and the stool consistency and the presence of blood in the rectum were also assessed [47]. Clinical scores, as described previously, were assessed independently by two investigators blinded to the protocol [7,48]. Two scores (stool consistency and bleeding) were added resulting in a total clinical score ranging from 0 (healthy) to 12 (the maximal activity of colitis). Histological scoring was determined by two independent investigators blinded to the protocols. The two subscores (the infiltration of inflammatory cells and the epithelial damage) were added, with the combined histological scores ranging from 0 (no changes) to 6 (extensive cell infiltration and tissue damage) [47,49].

4.4. Real-Time mRNA Quantification of Innate Immune Receptors

Total RNA was isolated from the colon using a commercial kit (Nucleospin RNA/Protein; Macherey-Nagel, France). Proteins and mRNA are obtained from the same colon sample and not from two portions of the same sample using this kit. RNA quantification was performed by spectrophotometry (Nanodrop; Nyxor Biotech, France). Reverse transcription of mRNA was carried out in a final volume of 20 µL from 1 µg total RNA (high capacity cDNA RT kit; Applied Biosystems, Villebon Sur Yvette, France). cDNA was amplified by PCR using Fast SYBR green (Applied Biosystems) in the one-step system (Applied Biosystems). SYBR green dye intensity was analyzed using one-step software. All results were normalized to the reference gene, *POLR2A* [50,51].

4.5. Quantification of Cytokines

Representative pro-inflammatory (IL-6) and anti-inflammatory (IL-10) cytokine profiles were selected in this study. Cytokine concentrations in the colons were measured using a commercial ELISA kit according to the manufacturer's instructions (eBioscience, San Diego, CA, USA). Briefly, a volume of 100 µL/well of capture antibodies (anti-mouse IL-10 antibody and anti-mouse IL-6 antibody) in coating buffer (diluted in PBS) was added in NUNC 96 well ELISA plate. The plate was then incubated overnight at 4 °C. After several washings, blocking buffer with 200 µL/well was added to the plate. After different washings, the colon mouse samples were added. The plates were subsequently incubated with biotinylated anti-IL-10 and anti-IL-6 (eBioscience, San Diego, CA, USA), respectively. One hundred microliters per well of Avidin-horseradish peroxidase (HRP) was added to each well, and the absorbance of each well was determined by using a microplate reader at 450 nm. The data are expressed as pg/mL.

4.6. Statistical Analysis

All data are expressed as the mean ± standard deviation (SD) of individual experimental groups. Data were analyzed using the Mann-Whitney U test to compare pairs of groups. Differences were considered significant when the p-value was as follows: $p < 0.05$; $p < 0.01$; $p < 0.001$.

All statistical analyses were performed with Prism 4.0 from GraphPad and XLSTAT.

Author Contributions: R.C. and S.J. performed the experiments. R.C., B.S., J.B., and S.J. analyzed the data. R.C., B.S., DP, J.B., and S.J. interpreted the results of the experiments. S.V.K. and J.B. contributed the reagents/materials/analysis tools. S.J. designed the experiments. J.B. and S.J. drafted the manuscript.

Funding: This work was funded by the FP7 Health 260338 "ALLFUN" project "Fungi in the setting of inflammation, allergy, and auto-immune diseases: translating basic science into clinical practices". This work was partially funded by the Agence Nationale de la Recherche (ANR) in the setting of project "InnateFun", promotional reference ANR-16-IFEC-0003-05, in the "Infect-ERA" program.

Acknowledgments: The authors thank Zein Jawhara, Antonino Bongiovanni, and Gaëlle Minet for their excellent technical assistance.

Conflicts of Interest: The authors declare no conflict of interest.

References

1. Poulain, D. Candida albicans, plasticity and pathogenesis. *Crit. Rev. Microbiol.* **2015**, *41*, 208–217. [CrossRef]
2. Kullberg, B.J.; Arendrup, M.C. Invasive candidiasis. *N. Engl. J. Med.* **2015**, *373*, 1445–1456. [CrossRef] [PubMed]
3. Gow, N.A.; van de Veerdonk, F.L.; Brown, A.J.; Netea, M.G. Candida albicans morphogenesis and host defence: Discriminating invasion from colonization. *Nat. Rev. Microbiol.* **2012**, *10*, 112–122. [CrossRef] [PubMed]
4. Sendid, B.; Dotan, N.; Nseir, S.; Savaux, C.; Vandewalle, P.; Standaert, A.; Zerimech, F.; Guery, B.P.; Dukler, A.; Colombel, J.F.; et al. Antibodies against glucan, chitin, and saccharomyces cerevisiae mannan as new biomarkers of candida albicans infection that complement tests based on c. Albicans mannan. *Clin. Vaccine Immunol.* **2008**, *15*, 1868–1877. [CrossRef] [PubMed]
5. Frank, D.N.; St Amand, A.L.; Feldman, R.A.; Boedeker, E.C.; Harpaz, N.; Pace, N.R. Molecular-phylogenetic characterization of microbial community imbalances in human inflammatory bowel diseases. *Proc. Natl. Acad. Sci. USA* **2007**, *104*, 13780–13785. [CrossRef] [PubMed]
6. Standaert-Vitse, A.; Sendid, B.; Joossens, M.; Francois, N.; Vandewalle-El Khoury, P.; Branche, J.; Van Kruiningen, H.; Jouault, T.; Rutgeerts, P.; Gower-Rousseau, C.; et al. Candida albicans colonization and asca in familial crohn's disease. *Am. J. Gastroenterol.* **2009**, *104*, 1745–1753. [CrossRef] [PubMed]
7. Jawhara, S.; Poulain, D. Saccharomyces boulardii decreases inflammation and intestinal colonization by candida albicans in a mouse model of chemically-induced colitis. *Med. Mycol.* **2007**, *45*, 691–700. [CrossRef] [PubMed]
8. Jawhara, S.; Thuru, X.; Standaert-Vitse, A.; Jouault, T.; Mordon, S.; Sendid, B.; Desreumaux, P.; Poulain, D. Colonization of mice by candida albicans is promoted by chemically induced colitis and augments inflammatory responses through galectin-3. *J. Infect. Dis.* **2008**, *197*, 972–980. [CrossRef]
9. Jawhara, S.; Mogensen, E.; Maggiotto, F.; Fradin, C.; Sarazin, A.; Dubuquoy, L.; Maes, E.; Guerardel, Y.; Janbon, G.; Poulain, D. Murine model of dextran sulfate sodium-induced colitis reveals candida glabrata virulence and contribution of beta-mannosyltransferases. *J. Biol. Chem.* **2012**, *287*, 11313–11324. [CrossRef]
10. Perez, E.E.; Orange, J.S.; Bonilla, F.; Chinen, J.; Chinn, I.K.; Dorsey, M.; El-Gamal, Y.; Harville, T.O.; Hossny, E.; Mazer, B.; et al. Update on the use of immunoglobulin in human disease: A review of evidence. *J. Allergy Clin. Immunol.* **2017**, *139*, S1–S46. [CrossRef] [PubMed]
11. Gilardin, L.; Bayry, J.; Kaveri, S.V. Intravenous immunoglobulin as clinical immune-modulating therapy. *CMAJ* **2015**, *187*, 257–264. [CrossRef]
12. Lunemann, J.D.; Nimmerjahn, F.; Dalakas, M.C. Intravenous immunoglobulin in neurology–mode of action and clinical efficacy. *Nat. Rev. Neurol.* **2015**, *11*, 80–89. [CrossRef] [PubMed]
13. Galeotti, C.; Kaveri, S.V.; Bayry, J. Ivig-mediated effector functions in autoimmune and inflammatory diseases. *Int. Immunol.* **2017**, *29*, 491–498. [CrossRef] [PubMed]

14. Bruckner, C.; Lehmann, C.; Dudziak, D.; Nimmerjahn, F. Sweet signs: Igg glycosylation leads the way in ivig-mediated resolution of inflammation. *Int. Immunol.* **2017**, *29*, 499–509. [CrossRef] [PubMed]

15. Rogosnitzky, M.; Danks, R.; Holt, D. Intravenous immunoglobulin for the treatment of crohn's disease. *Autoimmun. Rev.* **2012**, *12*, 275–280. [CrossRef]

16. Wang, M.; Liang, C.; Hu, H.; Zhou, L.; Xu, B.; Wang, X.; Han, Y.; Nie, Y.; Jia, S.; Liang, J.; et al. Intraperitoneal injection (ip), intravenous injection (iv) or anal injection (ai)? Best way for mesenchymal stem cells transplantation for colitis. *Sci. Rep.* **2016**, *6*, 30696. [CrossRef]

17. Castelo-Branco, M.T.; Soares, I.D.; Lopes, D.V.; Buongusto, F.; Martinusso, C.A.; do Rosario, A., Jr.; Souza, S.A.; Gutfilen, B.; Fonseca, L.M.; Elia, C.; et al. Intraperitoneal but not intravenous cryopreserved mesenchymal stromal cells home to the inflamed colon and ameliorate experimental colitis. *PLoS ONE* **2012**, *7*, e33360. [CrossRef]

18. Bayry, J.; Lacroix-Desmazes, S.; Kazatchkine, M.D.; Kaveri, S.V. Intravenous immunoglobulin for infectious diseases: Back to the pre-antibiotic and passive prophylaxis era? *Trends Pharm. Sci.* **2004**, *25*, 306–310. [CrossRef] [PubMed]

19. Diep, B.A.; Le, V.T.; Badiou, C.; Le, H.N.; Pinheiro, M.G.; Duong, A.H.; Wang, X.; Dip, E.C.; Aguiar-Alves, F.; Basuino, L.; et al. Ivig-mediated protection against necrotizing pneumonia caused by mrsa. *Sci. Transl. Med.* **2016**, *8*, 357ra124. [CrossRef] [PubMed]

20. Shopsin, B.; Kaveri, S.V.; Bayry, J. Tackling difficult staphylococcus aureus infections: Antibodies show the way. *Cell Host Microbe* **2016**, *20*, 555–557. [CrossRef]

21. Ben-Nathan, D.; Lustig, S.; Tam, G.; Robinzon, S.; Segal, S.; Rager-Zisman, B. Prophylactic and therapeutic efficacy of human intravenous immunoglobulin in treating west nile virus infection in mice. *J. Infect. Dis.* **2003**, *188*, 5–12. [CrossRef] [PubMed]

22. Gauduchon, V.; Cozon, G.; Vandenesch, F.; Genestier, A.L.; Eyssade, N.; Peyrol, S.; Etienne, J.; Lina, G. Neutralization of staphylococcus aureus panton valentine leukocidin by intravenous immunoglobulin in vitro. *J. Infect. Dis.* **2004**, *189*, 346–353. [CrossRef]

23. Krause, I.; Wu, R.; Sherer, Y.; Patanik, M.; Peter, J.B.; Shoenfeld, Y. In vitro antiviral and antibacterial activity of commercial intravenous immunoglobulin preparations—A potential role for adjuvant intravenous immunoglobulin therapy in infectious diseases. *Transfus Med.* **2002**, *12*, 133–139. [CrossRef]

24. Srivastava, R.; Ramakrishna, C.; Cantin, E. Anti-inflammatory activity of intravenous immunoglobulins protects against west nile virus encephalitis. *J. Gen. Virol.* **2015**, *96*, 1347–1357. [CrossRef]

25. Ramakrishna, C.; Newo, A.N.; Shen, Y.W.; Cantin, E. Passively administered pooled human immunoglobulins exert il-10 dependent anti-inflammatory effects that protect against fatal hsv encephalitis. *PLoS Pathog.* **2011**, *7*, e1002071. [CrossRef]

26. Elluru, S.R.; Kaveri, S.V.; Bayry, J. The protective role of immunoglobulins in fungal infections and inflammation. *Semin Immunopathol.* **2015**, *37*, 187–197. [CrossRef] [PubMed]

27. Casadevall, A.; Pirofski, L.A. Immunoglobulins in defense, pathogenesis, and therapy of fungal diseases. *Cell Host Microbe* **2012**, *11*, 447–456. [CrossRef] [PubMed]

28. Stratta, R.J.; Shaefer, M.S.; Cushing, K.A.; Markin, R.S.; Reed, E.C.; Langnas, A.N.; Pillen, T.J.; Shaw, B.W., Jr. A randomized prospective trial of acyclovir and immune globulin prophylaxis in liver transplant recipients receiving okt3 therapy. *Arch. Surg.* **1992**, *127*, 55–63. [CrossRef] [PubMed]

29. Mimouni, D.; Gdalevich, M.; Mimouni, F.B.; Grotto, I.; Eldad, A.; Shpilberg, O. Does immune serum globulin confer protection against skin diseases? *Int. J. Derm.* **2000**, *39*, 628–631. [CrossRef] [PubMed]

30. Tollemar, J.; Gross, N.; Dolgiras, N.; Jarstrand, C.; Ringden, O.; Hammarstrom, L. Fungal prophylaxis by reduction of fungal colonization by oral administration of bovine anti-candida antibodies in bone marrow transplant recipients. *Bone Marrow Transplant.* **1999**, *23*, 283–290. [CrossRef]

31. Bozza, S.; Kasermann, F.; Kaveri, S.V.; Romani, L.; Bayry, J. Intravenous immunoglobulin protects from experimental allergic bronchopulmonary aspergillosis via a sialylation-dependent mechanism. *Eur. J. Immunol.* **2019**, *49*, 195–198. [CrossRef] [PubMed]

32. Maddur, M.S.; Kaveri, S.V.; Bayry, J. Circulating normal igg as stimulator of regulatory t cells: Lessons from intravenous immunoglobulin. *Trends Immunol.* **2017**, *38*, 789–792. [CrossRef] [PubMed]

33. Othy, S.; Topcu, S.; Saha, C.; Kothapalli, P.; Lacroix-Desmazes, S.; Kasermann, F.; Miescher, S.; Bayry, J.; Kaveri, S.V. Sialylation may be dispensable for reciprocal modulation of helper t cells by intravenous immunoglobulin. *Eur. J. Immunol.* **2014**, *44*, 2059–2063. [CrossRef] [PubMed]

34. Neely, A.N.; Holder, I.A. Effects of immunoglobulin g and low-dose amphotericin b on candida albicans infections in burned mice. *Antimicrob Agents Chemother.* **1992**, *36*, 643–646. [CrossRef]

35. Darfeuille-Michaud, A.; Neut, C.; Barnich, N.; Lederman, E.; Di Martino, P.; Desreumaux, P.; Gambiez, L.; Joly, B.; Cortot, A.; Colombel, J.F. Presence of adherent escherichia coli strains in ileal mucosa of patients with crohn's disease. *Gastroenterology* **1998**, *115*, 1405–1413. [CrossRef]

36. Kim, S.C.; Tonkonogy, S.L.; Karrasch, T.; Jobin, C.; Sartor, R.B. Dual-association of gnotobiotic il-10-/- mice with 2 nonpathogenic commensal bacteria induces aggressive pancolitis. *Inflamm. Bowel Dis.* **2007**, *13*, 1457–1466. [CrossRef]

37. Hoarau, G.; Mukherjee, P.K.; Gower-Rousseau, C.; Hager, C.; Chandra, J.; Retuerto, M.A.; Neut, C.; Vermeire, S.; Clemente, J.; Colombel, J.F.; et al. Bacteriome and mycobiome interactions underscore microbial dysbiosis in familial crohn's disease. *MBio* **2016**, *7*, e01250-16. [CrossRef] [PubMed]

38. Croasdell, A.; Duffney, P.F.; Kim, N.; Lacy, S.H.; Sime, P.J.; Phipps, R.P. Ppargamma and the innate immune system mediate the resolution of inflammation. *Ppar Res.* **2015**, *2015*, 549691. [CrossRef]

39. Ruiz de Souza, V.; Carreno, M.P.; Kaveri, S.V.; Ledur, A.; Sadeghi, H.; Cavaillon, J.M.; Kazatchkine, M.D.; Haeffner-Cavaillon, N. Selective induction of interleukin-1 receptor antagonist and interleukin-8 in human monocytes by normal polyspecific igg (intravenous immunoglobulin). *Eur. J. Immunol.* **1995**, *25*, 1267–1273. [CrossRef] [PubMed]

40. Kozicky, L.K.; Zhao, Z.Y.; Menzies, S.C.; Fidanza, M.; Reid, G.S.; Wilhelmsen, K.; Hellman, J.; Hotte, N.; Madsen, K.L.; Sly, L.M. Intravenous immunoglobulin skews macrophages to an anti-inflammatory, il-10-producing activation state. *J. Leukoc Biol.* **2015**, *98*, 983–994. [CrossRef]

41. Galeotti, C.; Hegde, P.; Das, M.; Stephen-Victor, E.; Canale, F.; Munoz, M.; Sharma, V.K.; Dimitrov, J.D.; Kaveri, S.V.; Bayry, J. Heme oxygenase-1 is dispensable for the anti-inflammatory activity of intravenous immunoglobulin. *Sci. Rep.* **2016**, *6*, 19592. [CrossRef] [PubMed]

42. Casulli, S.; Topcu, S.; Fattoum, L.; von Gunten, S.; Simon, H.U.; Teillaud, J.L.; Bayry, J.; Kaveri, S.V.; Elbim, C. A differential concentration-dependent effect of ivig on neutrophil functions: Relevance for anti-microbial and anti-inflammatory mechanisms. *PLoS ONE* **2011**, *6*, e26469. [CrossRef] [PubMed]

43. Schneider, C.; Wicki, S.; Graeter, S.; Timcheva, T.M.; Keller, C.W.; Quast, I.; Leontyev, D.; Djoumerska-Alexieva, I.K.; Kasermann, F.; Jakob, S.M.; et al. Ivig regulates the survival of human but not mouse neutrophils. *Sci. Rep.* **2017**, *7*, 1296. [CrossRef] [PubMed]

44. Vos, A.C.; Wildenberg, M.E.; Duijvestein, M.; Verhaar, A.P.; van den Brink, G.R.; Hommes, D.W. Anti-tumor necrosis factor-alpha antibodies induce regulatory macrophages in an fc region-dependent manner. *Gastroenterology* **2011**, *140*, 221–230. [CrossRef] [PubMed]

45. Peng, Y.; Liu, H.; Liu, F.; Wang, H.; Liu, Y.; Duan, S. Inhibitory effect of ppar-gamma activator on il-6 and mpges protein expression in pbmc induced by homocysteine. *Hemodial Int.* **2005**, *9* (Suppl. 1), S15–S20. [CrossRef] [PubMed]

46. Fukata, M.; Chen, A.; Vamadevan, A.S.; Cohen, J.; Breglio, K.; Krishnareddy, S.; Hsu, D.; Xu, R.; Harpaz, N.; Dannenberg, A.J.; et al. Toll-like receptor-4 promotes the development of colitis-associated colorectal tumors. *Gastroenterology* **2007**, *133*, 1869–1881. [CrossRef] [PubMed]

47. Charlet, R.; Pruvost, Y.; Tumba, G.; Istel, F.; Poulain, D.; Kuchler, K.; Sendid, B.; Jawhara, S. Remodeling of the candida glabrata cell wall in the gastrointestinal tract affects the gut microbiota and the immune response. *Sci. Rep.* **2018**, *8*, 3316. [CrossRef] [PubMed]

48. Bortolus, C.; Billamboz, M.; Charlet, R.; Lecointe, K.; Sendid, B.; Ghinet, A.; Jawhara, S. A small aromatic compound has antifungal properties and potential anti-inflammatory effects against intestinal inflammation. *Int. J. Mol. Sci.* **2019**, *20*, 321. [CrossRef]

49. Jawhara, S.; Habib, K.; Maggiotto, F.; Pignede, G.; Vandekerckove, P.; Maes, E.; Dubuquoy, L.; Fontaine, T.; Guerardel, Y.; Poulain, D. Modulation of intestinal inflammation by yeasts and cell wall extracts: Strain dependence and unexpected anti-inflammatory role of glucan fractions. *PLoS ONE* **2012**, *7*, e40648. [CrossRef]

50. Choteau, L.; Parny, M.; Francois, N.; Bertin, B.; Fumery, M.; Dubuquoy, L.; Takahashi, K.; Colombel, J.F.; Jouault, T.; Poulain, D.; et al. Role of mannose-binding lectin in intestinal homeostasis and fungal elimination. *Mucosal Immunol.* **2016**, *9*, 767–776. [CrossRef]

51. Charlet, R.; Bortolus, C.; Barbet, M.; Sendid, B.; Jawhara, S. A decrease in anaerobic bacteria promotes candida glabrata overgrowth while beta-glucan treatment restores the gut microbiota and attenuates colitis. *Gut Pathog.* **2018**, *10*, 50. [CrossRef] [PubMed]

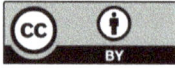

International Journal of
Molecular Sciences

MDPI

Article

Microbial Co-Occurrence Patterns and Keystone Species in the Gut Microbial Community of Mice in Response to Stress and Chondroitin Sulfate Disaccharide

Fang Liu [1], Zhaojie Li [1], Xiong Wang [1], Changhu Xue [1], Qingjuan Tang [1,*] and Robert W. Li [2,*]

[1] College of Food Science and Engineering, Ocean University of China, Qingdao 266003, China; liufang910205@163.com (F.L.); lizhaojie@ouc.edu.cn (Z.L.); wangxiong9202@163.com (X.W.); chxue@ouc.edu.cn (C.X.)

[2] United States Department of Agriculture, Agriculture Research Service (USDA-ARS), Animal Genomics and Improvement Laboratory, Beltsville, MD 20705, USA

* Correspondence: tangqingjuan@ouc.edu.cn (Q.T.); robert.li@ars.usda.gov (R.W.L.); Tel.: +86-532-66782591 (Q.T.); +1-301-504-5185 (R.W.L.)

Received: 15 March 2019; Accepted: 26 April 2019; Published: 30 April 2019

Abstract: Detecting microbial interactions is essential to the understanding of the structure and function of the gut microbiome. In this study, microbial co-occurrence patterns were inferred using a random matrix theory based approach in the gut microbiome of mice in response to chondroitin sulfate disaccharide (CSD) under healthy and stressed conditions. The exercise stress disrupted the network composition and microbial co-occurrence patterns. Thirty-four Operational Taxonomic Units (OTU) were identified as module hubs and connectors, likely acting as generalists in the microbial community. *Mucispirillum schaedleri* acted as a connector in the stressed network in response to CSD supplement and may play a key role in bridging intimate interactions between the host and its microbiome. Several modules correlated with physiological parameters were detected. For example, Modules M02 (under stress) and S05 (stress + CSD) were strongly correlated with blood urea nitrogen levels ($r = 0.90$ and -0.75, respectively). A positive correlation between node connectivity of the OTUs assigned to Proteobacteria with superoxide dismutase activities under stress ($r = 0.57$, $p < 0.05$) provided further evidence that Proteobacteria can be developed as a potential pathological marker. Our findings provided novel insights into gut microbial interactions and may facilitate future endeavor in microbial community engineering.

Keywords: 16S rRNA gene; chondroitin sulfate disaccharide; co-occurrence network; global network; microbial interactions; microbiome; modularity; superoxide dismutase

1. Introduction

Glucosamine (GS) and chondroitin sulfate (CS), a large class of sulfated glycosaminoglycans, are major structural components of joint cartilage and have been widely used as a dietary supplement for maintaining cartilage integrity as well as alleviating osteoarthritis symptoms. CS possesses various biological functions by acting as extracellular signaling molecules/modulators and co-receptors, in addition to their structural role [1]. CS and its component oligosaccharides have different modulatory effects on the structure and function of the gut microbiome [2–5]. Chondroitin sulfate component disaccharide (CSD) can significantly modify the function of gut microbiome and increase intestinal *Bacteroides acidifaciens* populations in a rodent model [2]. Moreover, our previous results show that CSD has the potential to change kidney morphology and repair kidney cortex damaged by exhaustive exercise stress. CSD dietary treatments significantly decrease blood urea nitrogen (BUN) levels ($p < 0.05$) [2]. A randomized human trial demonstrated that glucosamine and chondroitin supplementation lowers systemic inflammation and reduces oxidative stress, as measured by urinary prostaglandin F2α [6]. Malondialdehydes (MDA) are one of the frequently used markers of oxidative stress in response to exercise [7]. Free radicals generated during the stress attack polyunsaturated fatty acids in the cell membrane, leading to a chain of chemical reactions termed lipid peroxidation. Superoxide dismutase (SOD) acts as one of the key enzymatic antioxidant defenses against superoxide radicals [8]. Endurance exercise generally results in an increase in total activities of superoxide dismutase (SOD), which acts as one of the key enzymatic antioxidant defenses against superoxide radicals [8] and leads to enhanced resistance to oxidative stress [9]. In pigs, long-term aerobic exercise increases SOD1 protein concentrations as well as SOD1 enzyme activities, which tends to lower biomolecular indexes of oxidative stress, as reflected by decreased MDA values [10].

While effectiveness of CSD and GS supplements is still debated, several studies have raised questions on their potential renal toxicity [11]. Renal dysfunction and cardiovascular diseases are two of the serious medical concerns. Blood urea nitrogen (BUN) is an important physiological parameter of health; and long-term elevated BUN levels are associated with an increased risk of cardiovascular and renal conditions [12,13]. For example, BUN acts as a significant prognostic factor for the mortality in patients with acute ischemic stroke [14]. Moreover, BUN levels, especially the BUN to creatinine ratio (CR), are correlated with renal health. Recent studies suggest that the intestinal microbiome play critical roles in maintaining renal function [15,16]. The rats treated with *Lactobacillus* probiotics displayed improved BUN values and may ameliorate renal damage [17]. Gut microbiome-derived metabolites, such as trimethylamine-N-oxide and short-chain fatty acids, also play an important role in cardiovascular diseases [18]. As a result, targeting gut microbiota has become a potentially promising therapy for diabetic kidney disease recently [19].

The detection of species interactions and interdependence in a microbial community is beyond the scope of traditional alpha and beta diversity metrics. Network analysis tools enable a better understanding of microbial interactions and potential ecological roles of keystone species in complex microbial communities [20]. However, little is known about biotic interactions among different microbial species in the gut microbial communities in response to CSD and/or GS. Moreover, co-occurrence patterns between various microbial taxa in these microbial communities have not been explored; and microbial taxa that may be significantly correlated with various physiological parameters, such as BUN, SOD, and MDA, have not been identified. In this study, we attempted to understand microbial interactions and identify key microbial taxa that may be strongly correlated with BUN as well as other physiological parameters, such as SOD and MDA, in response to CSD dietary intervention under both healthy and exhaustive exercise-induced stressed conditions using co-occurrence network tools.

2. Results

2.1. Stress from Exhaustive Exercise Induced a Distinctly Different Microbial Co-Occurrence Network in Mice

The mean number of raw reads (2×300 bp paired-end) for the dataset is $227,448 \pm 98,540$ per sample ($n = 30$). After various quality control procedures, including trimming and merging of the pair-ended reads, rarefaction was performed at a depth of 100,000 retained quality sequences. Both closed and open-reference protocols in the QIIME pipeline were used for OTU picking at 97% similarity. A total of 2257 OTU was obtained for the study (Supplementary file). The numbers of OTU in the input datasets used for global network inference were 915 (Group N), 925 (Group M), 854 (Group C), and 844 (Group S), respectively. Global microbial co-occurrence networks were constructed using a Random Matrix Theory (RMT)-based method, as described in the Phylogenetic Molecular Ecological Network pipeline [21,22]. The mean numbers of nodes per module ranged from 7.80 (the S group) to 12.37 in the C group. Topological properties of microbial co-occurrence networks inferred in the four experimental groups were described in Supplementary Materials (Table S1). The numbers of nodes in the global networks inferred from the normal healthy groups (N) and exercise-induced stress group (M) were 539 (788) and 502 (782), respectively. Among them, 340 OTUs (nodes), accounting for 63% and 68% of all nodes in global networks in N and M groups, respectively, were shared by both networks. While the overall network sizes between the two groups appeared to be similar, the network composition and structure were distinctly different. Individual modules differed in the number of nodes (size) and shape (connections) in both groups. Approximately half of all modules, 27 in total, in each network contained only 2 to 3 members. These small modules were generally isolated with no links to the remaining network. There were 20 and 21 modules with six or more members in N and M groups, respectively. The node composition in global networks of each experimental group was substantially different. Many modules in each network was unique. For example, 16 of the 26 members consisting of the module N7 were unique to the N network, while eight of the 13 members in the module N14 was unique. Similarly, six of the seven members in the module M22 were unique to its own network. Very few compositional (or functional) equivalent modules can be paired in the two global networks. One exception may be N2 and M1 modules in N and M global networks. Among 30 and 38 members in N2 and M1 modules, respectively, 21 members were shared between the two networks, suggesting that the two modules may be functional equivalents. The phylogenetic composition of the nodes in each global network appeared relatively stable. For example, the most predominant phylum in each of the four global networks, *Firmicutes*, accounted for approximately 75.5% of all nodes in the networks. However, the percentage of *Proteobacteria* in each of the global networks varied substantially. The stress appeared to increase the percentage of *Proteobacteria* from 5.2% in normal/healthy group (N) to 6.77% in the stressed network (M). Intriguingly, CSD dietary treatments decreased the percentage of nodes assigned to the phylum *Proteobacteria*, from 5.2% to 3.9% under the healthy condition, and 6.8% to 4.1% under the stressed condition.

2.2. Keystone Species and their Possible Ecological Roles

Nodes play different topological roles in the network. Plots generated based on within-module degree z and among-module connectivity p, allow us to identify some key nodes in the network. As shown in Supplementary materials (Figures S1–S4), the majority of the nodes, accounting for >98% of all nodes, in the global networks generated from the 4 experimental groups were peripherals with low Zi and low Pi values. Among them, between 79% to 92% of all nodes had no links with outside of their own modules ($Pi = 0$). Between seven and 11 nodes were identified that may serve as module hubs in the four networks. These nodes represented approximately 1.3% to 2.2% of all nodes in the networks, in a good agreement with the findings in other environmental microbial communities [22]. These nodes were highly connected and tended to link to other nodes within their own module (a high $Zi > 2.5$ and a low $Pi \leq 0.62$) which may be important to the coherence of their own modules. For example, an OTU from the genus *Bacteroides* (GreenGeneID# 1135084) and OTU# (GreengeneID#183321) from *Prevotella*, were module hubs in the network from the C group while an OTU from *Ruminococcus* (GreenGeneID# 339031) and an OTU from *Lactococcus* (#586387) behaved like module hubs only in the healthy group (N). The relative abundance of the majority of the module hubs, six out of the eight OTUs, identified in the C group were significantly changed by CSD (absolute $\log_{10}$ LDA score > 2.0). For example, the abundance of OTU# 1135084 was significantly increased by CSD under both healthy and stressed conditions [2]. Intriguingly, the module hubs were distinctly different in each of the four global networks. Only one node, an OTU (GreenGeneID# 766563), belonging to the genus *Leuconostoc*, acted as a module hub in the networks from both healthy and stressed groups. These findings suggested that the hubs of different global networks and resultant network structure under different stress and dietary conditions were substantially different. Only a few nodes acting as a connector that linked different modules together was identified in scatter plots (Figure 1). Of note, an OTU, GreenGeneID#549991, belonging to the genus *Lactobacillus* acted as a connector species, which links two or more different modules together, under the healthy condition, was identified. The abundance of this OTU was significantly depressed by the exercise stress (LDA score > 2.0). Another OTU (GreenGeneID#1136443), assigned to *Mucispirillum schaedleri*, served as a connector in the global network from the S group.

A network hub, the node with a very high between-module and among-module connectivity value, is likely important to the coherence of the global network and as well as its own module and can be considered keystone species in a microbial community [23]. However, no network hubs were identified in each of the four global networks analyzed in this study.

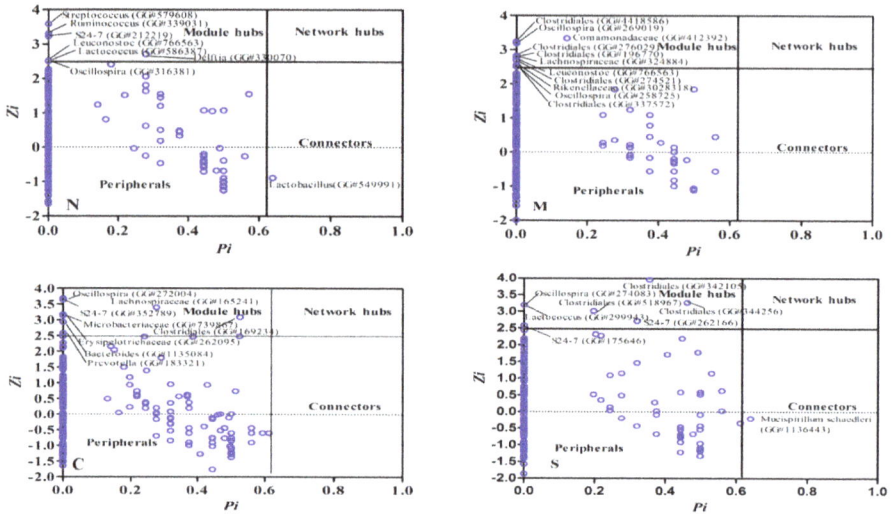

Figure 1. The scatter plot showing the distribution of OTU based on their topological roles in the network. The detailed information for each OTU can be found in Table S3. Each dot represents an OTU. Zi: within-module connectivity. Pi: Among-module connectivity. The network topological role classification was originally proposed by Olesen et al., 2007. N: healthy mice supplemented with phosphate-buffered saline (PBS); C: healthy mice supplemented with a daily dose of 150 mg/kg bodyweight of chondroitin sulfate disaccharide (CSD) for 16 consecutive days; M: mice subjected to exhaustive exercise stress supplemented with PBS; S: the stressed mice supplemented with a daily dose of 150 mg/kg bodyweight of CSD for 16 days.

2.3. The Correlations between Modules and Physiological Parameters

To understand the response of individual modules to physiological parameters, the correlations between module-based eigengenes and the four physiological measurements were calculated (Table 1). Under normal or healthy condition (N), at least 4 modules were positively correlated with three physiological traits. Both the modules N01 and N05 (Figure 2) in the healthy network and Modules C15 and S05 of the groups C and S (Figure 3), respectively, were strongly correlated with the BUN value ($p < 0.05$), while the module N14 was correlated with CR. Several modules in the group M network (Figure 4) also displayed a strong correlation with either BUN (Module M03) or creatinine ratio (CR, Module M13) alone or both (Modules M02 and M21). At least two modules, N09 and M27, had a strong correlation with the kidney concentration of malondialdehyde (MDA), an important lipid peroxidation marker (Figure 5). In the experimental group C, the module C10 (Figure 6) showed a strong negative correlation with SOD ($r = -0.94$; $p = 0.006$), while module C15 was positively correlated with BUN ($r = 0.89$; $p = 0.02$). Among the eight members consisting of the module C10, the OTUs from the phylum *Bacteroidetes* were predominant; and six of the eight members belonged to the order *Bacteroidales*, including at least 2 OTUs assigned to *Bacteroides acidifaciens*. Moreover, the relative abundance of at least 5 OTUs belonging to *Bacteroidetes* were significantly affected by the CSD treatment. In the stressed group (M), the module M02 displayed a strong ($r = 0.90$) and significant positive correlation with both BUN and CR values ($p = 0.002$) (Table 1). Similarly, the module M21 (Figure 4) was positively correlated with both BUN and CR ($r = 0.87$; $p = 0.005$). The module M03 was negatively correlated with the

BUN value ($r = -0.89$; $p = 0.003$). Moreover, the module M01 were positively correlated with the SOD value ($r = 0.71$; $p = 0.05$) while M14 was negatively correlated with SOD (Figure 6). The module M01 contained a total of 38 members, including eight members from the phylum *Bacteroidetes*, 27 members from *Firmicutes*; and two members from *Proteobacteria*. All eight members of the phylum *Bacteroidetes* belong to the family *S24-7*. In the experimental group S, the module S05 was negatively correlated with BUN ($r = -0.75$; $p = 0.05$).

Table 1. The correlations between the eigengene values of select modules and physiological traits. N: healthy mice supplemented with PBS; C: healthy mice supplemented with a daily dose of 150 mg/kg bodyweight of chondroitin sulfate disaccharide (CSD) for 16 consecutive days; M: mice subjected to exhaustive exercise stress supplemented with PBS; S: the stressed mice supplemented with a daily dose of 150 mg/kg bodyweight of CSD for 16 days. BUN: Blood urea nitrogen; CR: creatinine ratio; MDA: malondialdehydes; SOD: superoxide dismutase.

Module	Physiological Parameters	r	p Value	Module Members
Global Network/Group: N				
N01	BUN	0.68	0.040	34
N05	BUN	0.69	0.040	29
N14	CR	0.76	0.002	12
N09	MDA	0.67	0.050	40
Global Network/Group: M				
M02	BUN	0.90	0.002	54
M03	BUN	−0.89	0.003	29
M21	BUN	0.87	0.005	8
M02	CR	0.90	0.002	54
M21	CR	0.87	0.005	8
M13	CR	−0.65	0.080	20
M27	MDA	0.67	0.070	8
M01	SOD	0.71	0.050	38
M14	SOD	−0.72	0.050	22
Global Network/Group: S				
S05	BUN	−0.75	0.050	46
S02	CR	0.68	0.090	32
Global Network/Group: C				
C15	BUN	0.89	0.020	9
C01	CR	0.73	0.100	77
C03	CR	0.75	0.090	42
C04	CR	0.77	0.080	31
C07	SOD	0.76	0.080	20
C10	SOD	−0.94	0.006	8

The relationship of network topology and physiological parameters were also assessed by calculating the correlation between the OTU significance (GS), r^2 (the square of Pearson correlation coefficients) of OTU abundance profiles with traits and node connectivity. Under the normal or healthy condition, the node connectivity of the OTUs assigned to the order *Pseudomonodales* as well as that of the OTUs assigned to the families *Porphyromonadaceae* and *Moraxellaceae* was significantly correlated with GS of the BUN value (Table 2). Under the stressed condition (M), the node connectivity of the phylum *Proteobacteria* was positively correlated with changes in the SOD value ($p < 0.05$). With CSD treatment under both normal and stressed conditions (C and S), the node connectivity of the OTUs belonging to *Pseudomonodales* became positively correlated with CR values, similar to what happened under the normal condition (N). Moreover, the node connectivity of the OTUs in the family *Lactobacillacease* was positively but marginally correlated with both BUN and SOD values ($p < 0.05$ in both cases).

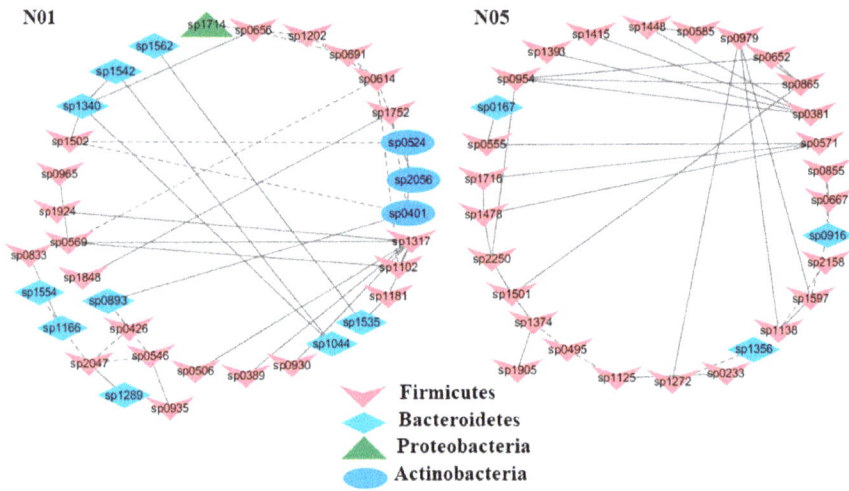

Figure 2. Select modules displaying a strong correlation with blood urea nitrogen contents (BUN) in healthy mice. The interactions among different nodes (OTUs) within a module were shown: solid line: positive correlation; dashed line: negative correlation. The color of each node (OTU) indicated the phylum that this OTU was assigned to. The detailed annotation of each OTU node can be found in Table S3.

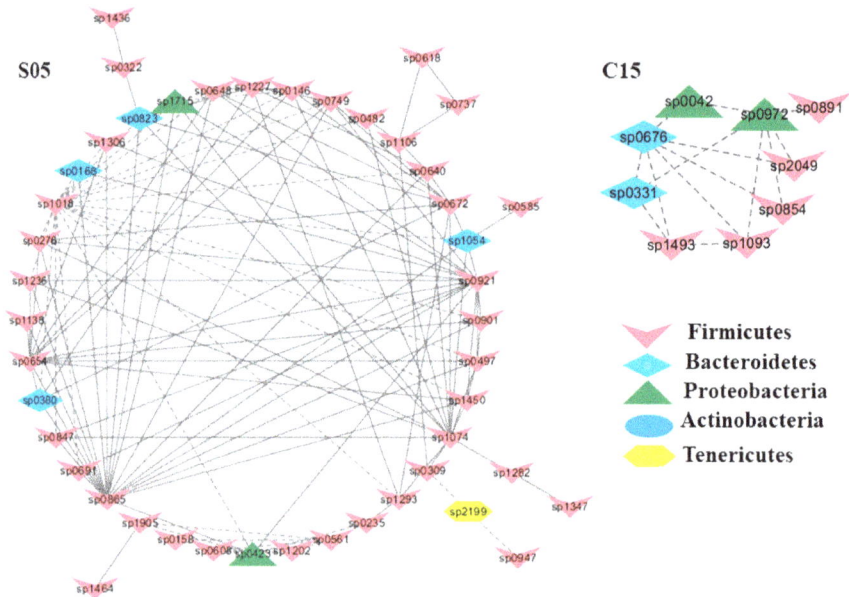

Figure 3. Modules C15 and S05 in the C and S network, respectively, showing a strong correlation with blood urea nitrogen levels (BUN). The detailed annotation of each OTU node can be found in Table S3.

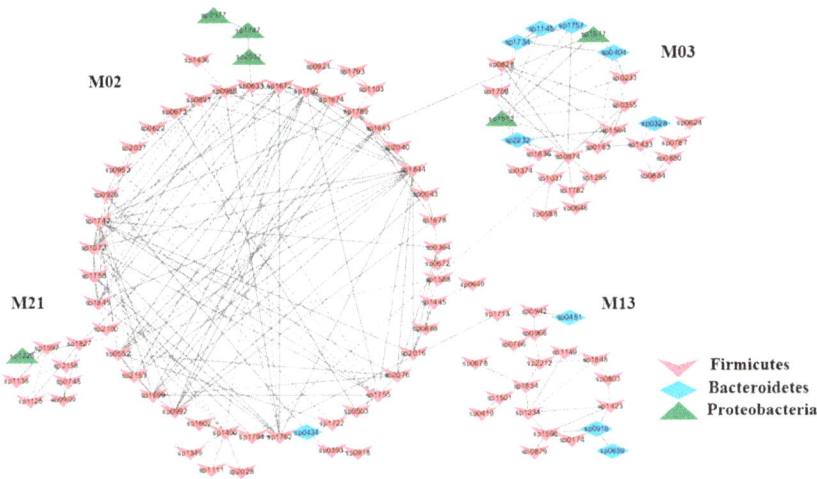

Figure 4. The modules in the mice subjected to exhaustive exercise stress (M) displaying a strong correlation with either blood urea nitrogen contents (BUN) (Module M03) or BUN to creatinine ratio (CR, Module M13) alone or both (Modules M02 and M21). The group N: healthy mice supplemented with PBS. The group M: mice subjected to exhaustive exercise stress supplemented with PBS. The group C: healthy mice supplemented with a daily dose of 150 mg/kg bodyweight of chondroitin sulfate disaccharide for 16 consecutive days. The group S: the stressed mice supplemented with a daily dose of 150 mg/kg bodyweight of CSD for 16 days. The detailed annotation of each OTU node can be found in Table S3.

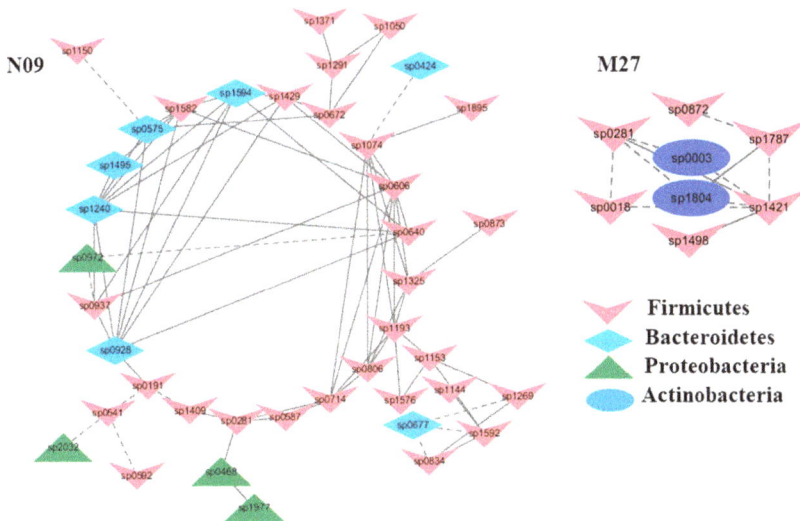

Figure 5. The modules with a strong correlation with kidney malondialdehyde concentrations (MDA), a lipid peroxidation marker. The interactions among different nodes (OTUs) within a module were shown: solid line: positive correlation; dashed line: negative correlation. The color of each node (OTU) indicated the phylum this OTU was assigned. Modules M27 and N09 were identified from the groups M and N, respectively. The group N: healthy mice supplemented with PBS; The group M: mice subjected to exhaustive exercise stress supplemented with PBS. The detailed annotation of each OTU node can be found in Table S3.

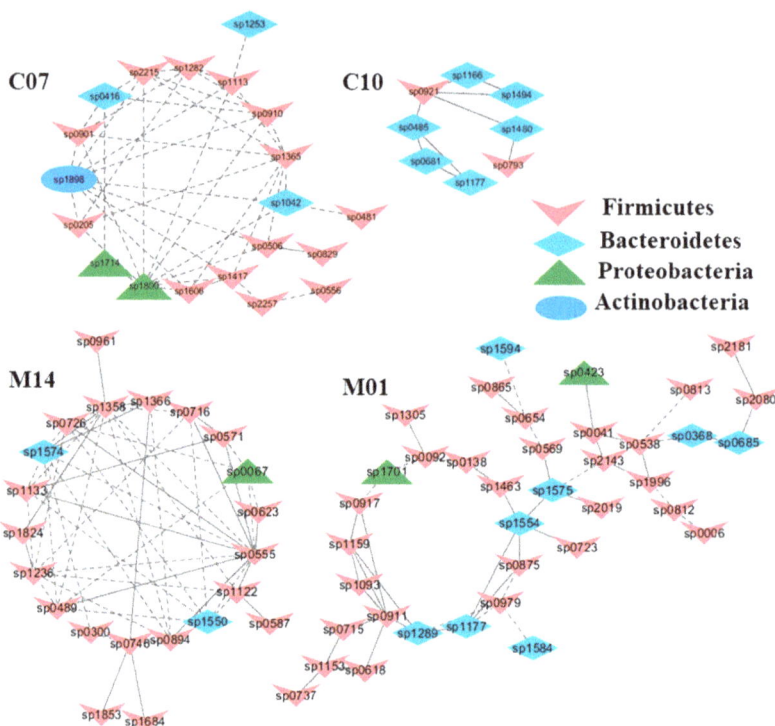

Figure 6. The modules displaying a strong correlation with kidney superoxide dismutase activities (SOD). The interactions among different nodes (OTUs) within a module were shown: solid line: positive correlation; dashed line: negative correlation. The color of each node (OTU) indicated the phylum this OTU was assigned. The modules C07 and C10, identified from the group C (healthy mice supplemented with a daily dose of 150 mg/kg bodyweight of chondroitin sulfate disaccharide for 16 consecutive days); showed a positive (C07) and negative (C10) correlation with SOD ($p < 0.05$), respectively. Similarly, Modules M01 and M14 displayed a positive (M01) and negative (M14) correlation with SOD in the group M, i.e., mice subjected to exhaustive exercise stress supplemented with PBS. The detailed annotation of each OTU node can be found in Table S3.

Table 2. The partial Mantel test revealed the correlation between node connectivity of some taxa and the OTU significance of physiological traits in microbial co-occurrence networks. N: healthy mice supplemented with PBS; C: healthy mice supplemented with a daily dose of 150 mg/kg bodyweight of chondroitin sulfate disaccharide (CSD) for 16 consecutive days; M: mice subjected to exhaustive exercise stress supplemented with PBS; S: the stressed mice supplemented with a daily dose of 150 mg/kg bodyweight of CSD for 16 days. BUN: Blood urea nitrogen; CR: creatinine ratio; SOD: superoxide dismutase.

Treatment Group	Physiological Parameter	Taxon (Level)	*r* (Correlation Coefficient)	Significance (Probability)
N	BUN	Pseudomonodales (Order)	0.8144	0.0020
N	BUN	Porphyromonadaceae (Family)	0.9165	0.0250
N	BUN	Moraxellaceae (Family)	0.7874	0.0040
C	CR	Pseudomonodales (Order)	0.6137	0.0250
C	BUN	Lactobacillaceae (Family)	0.3149	0.0460
C	SOD	Lactobacillaceae (Family)	0.5234	0.0039
M	SOD	Proteobacteria (Phylum)	0.5663	0.0250
S	CR	Pseudomonodales (Order)	0.6167	0.0333

3. Discussion

Over the past few years, various computational algorithms have been developed to infer microbial co-occurrence networks from the microbiome data [24–27]. While different methods, no matter how they measure various features, either Bray-Curtis abundance similarity, Pearson or Spearman correlation coefficients, or Maximal Information coefficients, varied substantially in sensitivity and precision [28], they had common goals to detect robust microbial associations and infer co-occurrence network patterns between microbial entities in a given habitat or environment. The knowledge obtained can provide novel insights into the organization of complex microbial communities and deciphering key microbial populations and their ecological roles. The network approach may allow us to understand functional roles of a closed related group of microbes, especially those unculturable or elusive but ecologically relevant species. In addition, characterization of species interactions or interdependence in a gut microbial community will undoubtedly enrich our understanding of true microbial diversity. In this study, we used a Random matrix theory (RMT) based on method (MENA) to infer microbial co-occurrence networks in fecal microbiome samples of the mice in response to chondroitin sulfate disaccharide dietary treatments under both healthy and stressed conditions. One of the unique features of this RMT method is automatic detection of similarity threshold values by calculating the transition from Gaussian to Poisson distributions [21,22]. This method, while paired with Pearson correlations, significantly improves the precision and tends to generate the fewest false positives [28].

Our previous study demonstrates that exhaustive exercise stress has a profound impact on the structure and function of the murine gut microbiome, resulting in a significant alteration of the fecal microbial community, including a significant change in relative abundance of 4 genera (*Aeromicrobium*, *Anaerostipes*, and *Turicibacter*, and *Anaerotruncus*) and 76 OTUs [2]. Of note, the abundance of at least 10 OTUs in the family *S24-7* was significantly repressed by the stress. In this study, our results suggest that while the overall size and structure of the global networks appeared to be similar, the network composition was distinctly different between healthy and stressed conditions. The networks from each condition had a similar number of modules or subnetworks, especially the large modules with six or more members (20 and 21 larger modules for healthy and stressed conditions, respectively). However, only approximately 60% of all nodes were common components in both networks. Moreover, none of the modules appeared to be paired with similar node compositions, suggesting that the exercise stress significantly disrupted the network structure and composition. Furthermore, compared to the healthy condition, the percentage of the nodes (OTUs) assigned to *Proteobacteria* was much higher in the network from the stressed condition. The increased *Proteobacteria* abundance is a striking feature of an unstable microbial community and associated with inflammation [29,30]. Intriguingly, the percentage of the nodes belonging to *Proteobacteria* in the networks was significantly reduced by the CSD intervention under both conditions. Our previous study identified a significant reduction in the relative abundance of *Proteobacteria* by CSD [2], which may contribute to its anti-inflammatory properties. Together, our findings suggest that CSD supplementation had a potential to reduce both relative abundance and microbial interactions of pro-inflammatory *Proteobacteria*.

Modularity, the extent to which species interaction are organized into modules or subnetworks in a network, may reflect habitat heterogeneity or phylogenetic clustering of closely related species; and modules with closed linked species may represent some key coevolution units [31]. In this study, all four global networks were identified with a very high modularity, ranging from 0.8 to 0.9. In these networks, greater than 98% of the OTUs were peripherals, likely acted as specialists in the microbial community. Collectively, 32 OTUs were identified as module hubs or highly connected species linked to other nodes in their own modules. Only two OTUs were connector species that linked several modules together. Module hubs and connectors can serve as generalists in the microbial community. An OTU belonging to *M. schaedleri* acted as a connector species in the S network. As a member of the core murine gut microbiome, this species is residing in the mucus layer of the gastrointestinal tract. The increased abundance of *M. schaedleri* has been documented in chemically reduced colitis and inflammatory models [32,33]. The species is known to express secretion systems and effector proteins, which can modify the gene expression of host mucosa. Moreover, this species may possess capacity to degrade mucin. Together, these data suggest that *M. schaedleri* undergoes intimate interactions with its host and may play a role in inflammation. Many of the generalists identified in this study acted as module hubs. Moreover, each network had a distinct set of module hubs, which likely reflected habitat heterogeneity or trophic specialization under different experimental conditions. The OTU# 1135084, assigned to the genus *Bacteroides*, which was significantly increased by CSD supplementation under both healthy and stressed conditions [2], acted as a module hub in the module C9 in the C group. Many *Bacteroides* species possess species-specific dynamics responses to CS or CSD availability [34]. For example, *B. thetaiotaomicron*, can rapidly activate the transcription of CS utilization genes after a sudden exposure to CS and then dynamically adjust their transcription in response to the rate at which CS is broken down [35]. *B. acidifaciens* is a predominant member colonized in the murine gut and possesses strong immunomodulating activities. The abundance of several OTU assigned to *B. acidifaciens* was significantly increased by the CSD supplement [2]. The effect of niche disturbances or perturbation likely spreads more slowly in a modular structure [31]. The elimination or a significant reduction of a module hub may cause a modular structure to collapse without a major cascading effect on other modules. Likewise, the expansion of a module hub, such as the one in the genus *Bacteroides*, can have a broad effect on microbial interactions, especially on the species of its own module. As a result, dietary interventions targeting on generalists or super generalists, such as connectors or key module hubs, may have a higher success rate to achieve a desired effect.

The correlation analysis between module-based eigengenes and physiological traits was used to aid the understanding of the responses of individual modules to changes in physiological parameters. For example, numerous published reports support the notion that glucosamine and chondroitin, alone or in combination, possess chondroprotective properties, including a significant reduction of osteoarthritis symptoms with less adverse events [36]. However, several studies suggest a possible link between these supplements and renal dysfunction, manifested in part by elevated levels of BUN and creatinine [37]. In this study, we detected several modules significantly correlated with BUN traits in each of the four networks. Under the healthy condition, Modules N01 and N05 were positively correlated with BUN ($p < 0.05$). The module M02 was strongly positively correlated with BUN ($r = 0.90$, $p < 0.005$) while the module M03 was strongly negatively correlated with BUN ($r = -0.89$, $p < 0.005$) under the stressed condition. Similarly, positive and negative correlations with BUN were detected in the eigengenes of the module C15 ($r = 0.89$, $p < 0.05$) and the module S5 ($r = -0.75$, $p < 0.05$) by the CSD treatment under healthy and stressed conditions, respectively. A close examination of the module membership failed to identify any shared module composition in these networks, even though they were all somehow correlated with BUN. Nevertheless, carefully designed experiments to gain a deep understanding of microbial interactions in these modules may unravel mechanisms of action of chondroitin supplements. In addition, positive and negative correlations were detected between the M01 and M14 eigengenes, respectively, and SOD values under the stressed condition. The Mantel test was used to calculate the correlations between the node connectivity and physiological parameters. Under the stressed condition, the node connectivity of the OTUs assigned to the phylum *Proteobacteria* was positively correlated with SOD ($r = 0.57$, $p < 0.05$). SOD is known to play an important role in inflammation and other diseases. Together, our findings provide further evidence that *Proteobacteria* can be developed as a stress or pathological marker. In addition, the findings suggest that altered network topologies, especially the node connectivity in some key modules, may have important implications on tissue and blood physiological parameters. It is well known that numerous biotic and abiotic factors affect the gut microbial composition and species interdependence in the gut microbial community. It is important to design focused experiments to validate the microbial interactions inferred using network tools. Nevertheless, the microbial co-occurrence network inference approach can provide us with novel insight into the potential functional role of key microbial taxa in not just microbial communities but also the complicated traits or physiological parameters of the host. The knowledge obtained via this approach should facilitate microbial community engineering by targeted elimination and expansion of keystone species in a network and will be of practical significance in modeling the effect of a successful dietary intervention.

4. Materials and Methods

4.1. Animals Experiment

The animal experiment was previously described [2]. Briefly, 30 Balb/c mice were housed in the same room and fed the same basal diet. The mice were randomly assigned to 4 groups: Healthy control mice + Phosphate-buffered saline or PBS (the group N; $n = 9$), Exhaustive exercise stressed mice + PBS (the group M; $n = 8$), Healthy mice supplemented with CSD at a daily dose of 150 mg/kg body weight for 16 consecutive days (the group C; $n = 6$); and Exhaustive exercise stressed mice supplemented with CSD at a daily dose of 150 mg/kg body weight for 16 days (the group S; $n = 7$). Animals in both M and S groups were subjected to a forced exercise wheel-track treadmill. After an initial resting period to collect baseline data, exercise commenced at 20 rpm running speed for 3 h each day for 2 days. A recovery and resting period of 5 days was allowed after the 2-day exercise. The entire experiment lasted for 16 days, including 6 days in which exhaustive exercise was endured. The CSD dietary supplement was initiated at the same time as the exercise stress commenced and lasted for 16 days. The animal protocol (Project# SCXK-Jing-2007-0001G) was approved by the Committee on the Ethics of Animal Experiments of Ocean University of China (approval date: 27 December 2007); and the experiment was conducted by strictly following the Institutional Animal Care and Use Committee guideline (IACUC).

4.2. Physiological Parameters

All assay kits were purchased from Nanjing Jiancheng Bioengineering Institute (NJBI, Nanjing, China). Blood creatinine kinase (CK) activities and BUN values were measured as previously reported [2]. All physiological parameter data can be found in the Supplementary Material (Table S2).

SOD activities and MDA concentrations in the renal tissue were measured using assay kits purchased from NJBI. Total SOD activities were measured based on a WST1 [2-(4-iodophenyl)-3-(4-nitrophenyl)-5-(2,4-disulfo-phenyl)-2H-tetrazolium, monosodium salt] SOD inhibition assay using a colorimetric microplate reader. Briefly, renal tissue samples were weighed and homogenized in a microfuge tube immersed in an ice slurry. The homogenate was then incubated at 4 °C for 30 min. After a 5-min centrifugation at 12,000× g (4 °C) to pellet tissue debris, the supernatant was transferred to a new tube for assay analysis. The SOD activity was defined as units per mg protein.

4.3. 16S rRNA Gene Sequencing and Data Analysis

Feces were collected at necropsy and stored at −80 °C until total DNA was extracted. Total DNA was extracted using a bead-beating method as described [2,38]. The quality of the total DNA was verified using a BioAnalyzer 2100 (Agilent, Palo Alto, CA, USA). DNA concentration was first measured using a Nanodrop instrument and then verified by a Quantus fluorometer (Promega, Madison, WI, USA). The hypervariable V1-V3 regions of the 16S rRNA gene were directly amplified from 20 ng of fecal total DNA with Polyacrylamide Gel Electrophoresis (PAGE)-purified Illumina platform-compatible adaptors that contain features such as sequencing primers, sample-specific barcodes, and 16S PCR primers (forward primer, 9F, GAGTTTGATCMTGGCTCAG; reverse primer, 515R: CCGCGGCKGCTGGCAC). The PCR reaction included 2.5 units of AccuPrime Taq DNA Polymerase High Fidelity (Invitrogen, Carlsbad, CA, USA) in a 50 µL reaction buffer containing 200 nM primers, 200 nM dNTP, 60 mM Tris-SO$_4$, 18 mM (NH4)$_2$SO$_4$, 2.0 mM MgSO$_4$, 1% glycerol, and 100 ng/uL bovine serum albumin (New England BioLabs, Ipswich, MA, USA). PCR was performed using the following cycling profile: initial denaturing at 95 °C for 2 min followed by 20 cycles of 95 °C 30 s, 60 °C 30 s, and 72 °C 60 s. Amplicons were purified using Agencourt AMPure XP beads (Beckman Coulter Genomics, Danvers,

MA, USA), quantified using a BioAnalyzer high-sensitivity DNA chip, and pooled at equal molar ratios. The pool was then sequenced using an Illumina MiSeq sequencer, as described previously [38]. The raw sequences have been deposited to the NCBI Sequence Read Archive (*SRA*) database and are freely accessible (SRA accession# SRP137092)

4.4. Network Construction and Visualization

The quality control, preprocessing, and OTU picking steps were conducted using the Quantitative Insights Into Microbial Ecology (QIIME) pipeline (v1.9.1) [39]. Both "closed reference" and "open-reference" protocols in the pipeline were used for OTU picking. The global networks were constructed for each of the 4 experimental groups using a Random-Matrix theory (RMT) based pipeline described [21,22] (http://ieg4.rccc.ou.edu/mena/). The input datasets used for the network construction were the OTU abundance table derived using the "closed reference" protocol in the QIIME pipeline. Because the OTU sparsity has a drastic effect on the precision and sensitivity of network inference [28], the rare OTU, that is, those OTU detected in <50% of all samples, were excluded. While this practice may have a negative effect on network structure, it improves the false positive rate of interaction detection. A similarity matrix, which measures the degree of concordance between the abundance profiles of individual OTUs across different samples [21], was then obtained by using Pearson correlation analysis of the abundance data. A threshold was automatically determined by calculating the transition from Gaussian orthogonal ensemble to Poisson distribution of the nearest-neighbor spacing distribution of eigenvalues, in the pipeline and then applied to generate an adjacent matrix for network inference [22]. In this study, the stringent threshold with significance >0.05 was selected to control the false positive rate. The threshold values used in this study were 0.87 for the N group, 0.92 for M, 0.98 for C, and 0.94 for S, respectively. The fast-greedy modularity optimization procedure was used for module separation. The within-module degree (Zi) and among-module connectivity (Pi) were then calculated and plotted to generate a scatter plot for each network to gain insights into topological roles of individual nodes in the network. The Olesen classification approach was used to define node topological roles [31]. A partial Mantel test was performed to measure the relationship of the network topology and physiological traits by calculating OTU significance and node connectivity, as described [21]. Finally, the networks were visualized using Cytoscape v3.6.1 [40].

5. Conclusions

Global network analysis allows a better understanding of microbial interactions and potential ecological roles of keystone species in complex microbial communities in the gut. Under healthy condition, CSD alters the abundance of the majority of module hubs or connector species, such as those from *Bacteroides* and *Prevotella* while *Mucispirillum schaedleri*, a mucin-utilizing bacterium, acts as a connector in the network stressed by exercise. One of mechanisms by which CSD exerts its potential therapeutic effects is via modulation of network composition and microbial co-occurrence patterns significantly disrupted by exercise stress. The study highlights the importance of microbial community engineering based approaches in expanding the therapeutic potential of CSD to diseases and pathophysiological conditions with abnormal blood urea nitrogen levels and superoxide dismutase activities.

Supplementary Materials: Supplementary materials can be found at http://www.mdpi.com/1422-0067/20/9/2130/s1. Table S1: Topological properties of the global network inferred using a Random-Matrix theory (RMT) based network pipeline under various experimental conditions. Table S2: Physiological parameters measured in mice. Table S3: OTU tables and network parameters. Figure S1: Visualization of global networks with modules identified using the fast greedy modularity optimization method under the four experimental conditions in healthy mice supplemented with PBS. Figure S2: Visualization of global networks with modules identified using the fast greedy modularity optimization method under the four experimental conditions in healthy mice supplemented with a daily dose of 150 mg/kg bodyweight of chondroitin sulfate disaccharide (CSD) for 16 consecutive days. Figure S3: Visualization of global networks with modules identified using the fast greedy modularity optimization method under the four experimental conditions in mice subjected to exhaustive exercise stress supplemented with PBS. Figure S4: Visualization of global networks with modules identified using the fast greedy modularity optimization

Int. J. Mol. Sci. **2019**, *20*, 2130

method under the four experimental conditions in the stressed mice supplemented with a daily dose of 150 mg/kg bodyweight of CSD for 16 days.

Author Contributions: Conceived and designed the experiment: F.L., Q.T., R.W.L. Performed the experiment: F.L., Z.L., X.W., C.X., and Q.T. Analyzed the data: F.L. and R.W.L. Wrote the manuscript: F.L. All authors reviewed and approved the manuscript.

Funding: This research was partially fundede by National Natural Science Foundation of China (No. U1606403 to C.X.).

Acknowledgments: Names or commercial products in this publication is solely for the purpose of providing specific information and does not imply recommendation or endorsement by USDA. The USDA is an equal opportunity provider and employer.

Conflicts of Interest: The authors declare that they have no conflict of interest.

References

1. Mikami, T.; Kitagawa, H. Biosynthesis and function of chondroitin sulfate. *Biochim. Biophys. Acta* **2013**, *1830*, 4719–4733. [CrossRef] [PubMed]

2. Liu, F.; Zhang, N.; Li, Z.; Wang, X.; Shi, H.; Xue, C.; Li, R.W.; Tang, Q. Chondroitin sulfate disaccharides modified the structure and function of the murine gut microbiome under healthy and stressed conditions. *Sci. Rep.* **2017**, *7*, 6783. [CrossRef]

3. Wang, Q.; Huang, S.Q.; Li, C.Q.; Xu, Q.; Zeng, Q.P. Akkermansia muciniphila May Determine Chondroitin Sulfate Ameliorating or Aggravating Osteoarthritis. *Front. Microbiol.* **2017**, *8*, 1955. [CrossRef]

4. Shang, Q.; Shi, J.; Song, G.; Zhang, M.; Cai, C.; Hao, J.; Li, G.; Yu, G. Structural modulation of gut microbiota by chondroitin sulfate and its oligosaccharide. *Int. J. Biol. Macromol.* **2016**, *89*, 489–498. [CrossRef]

5. Shang, Q.; Yin, Y.; Zhu, L.; Li, G.; Yu, G.; Wang, X. Degradation of chondroitin sulfate by the gut microbiota of Chinese individuals. *Int. J. Biol. Macromol.* **2016**, *86*, 112–118. [CrossRef] [PubMed]

6. Navarro, S.L.; White, E.; Kantor, E.D.; Zhang, Y.; Rho, J.; Song, X.; Milne, G.L.; Lampe, P.D.; Lampe, J.W. Randomized trial of glucosamine and chondroitin supplementation on inflammation and oxidative stress biomarkers and plasma proteomics profiles in healthy humans. *PLoS ONE* **2015**, *10*, e0117534. [CrossRef] [PubMed]

7. Urso, M.L.; Clarkson, P.M. Oxidative stress, exercise, and antioxidant supplementation. *Toxicology* **2003**, *189*, 41–54. [CrossRef]

8. Powers, S.K.; Lennon, S.L. Analysis of cellular responses to free radicals: Focus on exercise and skeletal muscle. *Proc. Nutr. Soc.* **1999**, *58*, 1025–1033. [CrossRef]

9. Fielding, R.A.; Meydani, M. Exercise, free radical generation, and aging. *Aging (Milano)* **1997**, *9*, 12–18. [CrossRef] [PubMed]

10. Rush, J.W.; Turk, J.R.; Laughlin, M.H. Exercise training regulates SOD-1 and oxidative stress in porcine aortic endothelium. *Am. J. Physiol. Heart Circ. Physiol.* **2003**, *284*, H1378–H1387. [CrossRef]

11. Danao-Camara, T. Potential side effects of treatment with glucosamine and chondroitin. *Arthritis. Rheum.* **2000**, *43*, 2853. [CrossRef]

12. Jujo, K.; Minami, Y.; Haruki, S.; Matsue, Y.; Shimazaki, K.; Kadowaki, H.; Ishida, I.; Kambayashi, K.; Arashi, H.; Sekiguchi, H.; et al. Persistent high blood urea nitrogen level is associated with increased risk of cardiovascular events in patients with acute heart failure. *ESC Heart Fail.* **2017**, *4*, 545–553. [CrossRef]

13. Kajimoto, K.; Minami, Y.; Sato, N.; Takano, T.; Investigators of the Acute Decompensated Heart Failure Syndromes (ATTEND) registry. Serum sodium concentration, blood urea nitrogen, and outcomes in patients hospitalized for acute decompensated heart failure. *Int. J. Cardiol.* **2016**, *222*, 195–201. [CrossRef]

14. You, S.; Zheng, D.; Zhong, C.; Wang, X.; Tang, W.; Sheng, L.; Zheng, C.; Cao, Y.; Liu, C.F. Prognostic Significance of Blood Urea Nitrogen in Acute Ischemic Stroke. *Circ J.* **2018**, *82*, 572–578. [CrossRef]

15. Anders, H.J.; Andersen, K.; Stecher, B. The intestinal microbiota, a leaky gut, and abnormal immunity in kidney disease. *Kidney Int.* **2013**, *83*, 1010–1016. [CrossRef]

16. Ramezani, A.; Raj, D.S. The gut microbiome, kidney disease, and targeted interventions. *J. Am. Soc. Nephrol.* **2014**, *25*, 657–670. [CrossRef]

17. Yoshifuji, A.; Wakino, S.; Irie, J.; Tajima, T.; Hasegawa, K.; Kanda, T.; Tokuyama, H.; Hayashi, K.; Itoh, H. Gut Lactobacillus protects against the progression of renal damage by modulating the gut environment in rats. *Nephrol. Dial. Transplant.* **2016**, *31*, 401–412. [CrossRef]

18. Tang, W.H.; Hazen, S.L. The Gut Microbiome and Its Role in Cardiovascular Diseases. *Circulation* **2017**, *135*, 1008–1010. [CrossRef]

19. Chen, Z.; Zhu, S.; Xu, G. Targeting gut microbiota: A potential promising therapy for diabetic kidney disease. *Am. J. Transl. Res.* **2016**, *8*, 4009–4016.

20. Williams, R.J.; Howe, A.; Hofmockel, K.S. Demonstrating microbial co-occurrence pattern analyses within and between ecosystems. *Front. Microbiol.* **2014**, *5*, 358. [CrossRef]

21. Zhou, J.; Deng, Y.; Luo, F.; He, Z.; Yang, Y. Phylogenetic molecular ecological network of soil microbial communities in response to elevated CO_2. *MBio* **2011**, *2*, e00122-11. [CrossRef]

22. Deng, Y.; Jiang, Y.H.; Yang, Y.; He, Z.; Luo, F.; Zhou, J. Molecular ecological network analyses. *BMC Bioinform.* **2012**, *13*, 113. [CrossRef]

23. Layeghifard, M.; Hwang, D.M.; Guttman, D.S. Disentangling Interactions in the Microbiome: A Network Perspective. *Trends Microbiol.* **2017**, *25*, 217–228. [CrossRef]

24. Ruan, Q.; Dutta, D.; Schwalbach, M.S.; Steele, J.A.; Fuhrman, J.A.; Sun, F. Local similarity analysis reveals unique associations among marine bacterioplankton species and environmental factors. *Bioinformatics* **2006**, *22*, 2532–2538. [CrossRef]

25. Faust, K.; Raes, J. Microbial interactions: From networks to models. *Nat. Rev. Microbiol.* **2012**, *10*, 538–550. [CrossRef]

26. Friedman, J.; Alm, E.J. Inferring correlation networks from genomic survey data. *PLoS Comput. Biol.* **2012**, *8*, e1002687. [CrossRef]

27. Xia, L.C.; Ai, D.; Cram, J.; Fuhrman, J.A.; Sun, F. Efficient statistical significance approximation for local similarity analysis of high-throughput time series data. *Bioinformatics* **2013**, *29*, 230–237. [CrossRef]

28. Weiss, S.; Van Treuren, W.; Lozupone, C.; Faust, K.; Friedman, J.; Deng, Y.; Xia, L.C.; Xu, Z.Z.; Ursell, L.; Alm, E.J.; et al. Correlation detection strategies in microbial data sets vary widely in sensitivity and precision. *ISME J.* **2016**, *10*, 1669–1681. [CrossRef]

29. Carvalho, F.A.; Koren, O.; Goodrich, J.K.; Johansson, M.E.; Nalbantoglu, I.; Aitken, J.D.; Su, Y.; Chassaing, B.; Walters, W.A.; Gonzalez, A.; et al. Transient inability to manage proteobacteria promotes chronic gut inflammation in TLR5-deficient mice. *Cell Host Microbe* **2012**, *12*, 139–152. [CrossRef]

30. Shin, N.R.; Whon, T.W.; Bae, J.W. Proteobacteria: Microbial signature of dysbiosis in gut microbiota. *Trends Biotechnol.* **2015**, *33*, 496–503. [CrossRef]

31. Olesen, J.M.; Bascompte, J.; Dupont, Y.L.; Jordano, P. The modularity of pollination networks. *Proc. Natl. Acad. Sci. USA* **2007**, *104*, 19891–19896. [CrossRef] [PubMed]

32. Berry, D.; Schwab, C.; Milinovich, G.; Reichert, J.; Ben Mahfoudh, K.; Decker, T.; Engel, M.; Hai, B.; Hainzl, E.; Heider, S.; et al. Phylotype-level 16S rRNA analysis reveals new bacterial indicators of health state in acute murine colitis. *ISME J.* **2012**, *6*, 2091–2106. [CrossRef]

33. Loy, A.; Pfann, C.; Steinberger, M.; Hanson, B.; Herp, S.; Brugiroux, S.; Gomes Neto, J.C.; Boekschoten, M.V.; Schwab, C.; Urich, T.; et al. Lifestyle and Horizontal Gene Transfer-Mediated Evolution of Mucispirillum schaedleri, a Core Member of the Murine Gut Microbiota. *mSystems* **2017**, *2*, e00171-16. [CrossRef]

34. Raghavan, V.; Groisman, E.A. Species-specific dynamic responses of gut bacteria to a mammalian glycan. *J. Bacteriol.* **2015**, *197*, 1538–1548. [CrossRef] [PubMed]

35. Raghavan, V.; Lowe, E.C.; Townsend, G.E., 2nd; Bolam, D.N.; Groisman, E.A. Tuning transcription of nutrient utilization genes to catabolic rate promotes growth in a gut bacterium. *Mol. Microbiol.* **2014**, *93*, 1010–1025. [CrossRef] [PubMed]

36. Shmagel, A.; Demmer, R.; Knights, D.; Butler, M.; Langsetmo, L.; Lane, N.E.; Ensrud, K. The Effects of Glucosamine and Chondroitin Sulfate on Gut Microbial Composition: A Systematic Review of Evidence from Animal and Human Studies. *Nutrients* **2019**, *11*, 294. [CrossRef] [PubMed]

37. Guillaume, M.P.; Peretz, A. Possible association between glucosamine treatment and renal toxicity: Comment on the letter by Danao-Camara. *Arthritis. Rheum.* **2001**, *44*, 2943–2944. [CrossRef]

38. Li, R.W.; Li, W.; Sun, J.; Yu, P.; Baldwin, R.L.; Urban, J.F. The effect of helminth infection on the microbial composition and structure of the caprine abomasal microbiome. *Sci. Rep.* **2016**, *6*, 20606. [CrossRef]

39. Caporaso, J.G.; Kuczynski, J.; Stombaugh, J.; Bittinger, K.; Bushman, F.D.; Costello, E.K.; Fierer, N.; Pena, A.G.; Goodrich, J.K.; Gordon, J.I.; et al. QIIME allows analysis of high-throughput community sequencing data. *Nat. Methods* **2010**, *7*, 335–336. [CrossRef]

40. Shannon, P.; Markiel, A.; Ozier, O.; Baliga, N.S.; Wang, J.T.; Ramage, D.; Amin, N.; Schwikowski, B.; Ideker, T. Cytoscape: A software environment for integrated models of biomolecular interaction networks. *Genome Res.* **2003**, *13*, 2498–2504. [CrossRef]

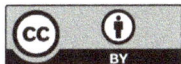

International Journal of
Molecular Sciences

MDPI

Review

Interplay among Vaginal Microbiome, Immune Response and Sexually Transmitted Viral Infections

Maria Gabriella Torcia

Department of Clinical and Experimental Medicine, University of Firenze, 50139 Firenze, Italy;
maria.torcia@unifi.it; Tel.: +39-0552758227

Received: 6 December 2018; Accepted: 8 January 2019; Published: 11 January 2019

Abstract: The vaginal ecosystem is important for women's health and for a successful reproductive life, and an optimal host-microbial interaction is required for the maintenance of eubiosis. The vaginal microbiota is dominated by *Lactobacillus* species in the majority of women. Loss of *Lactobacillus* dominance promotes the colonization by anaerobic bacterial species with an increase in microbial diversity. Vaginal dysbiosis is a very frequent condition which affects the immune homeostasis, inducing a rupture in the epithelial barrier and favoring infection by sexually transmitted pathogens. In this review, we describe the known interactions among immune cells and microbial commensals which govern health or disease status. Particular attention is given to microbiota compositions which, through interplay with immune cells, facilitate the establishment of viral infections, such as Human Immunodeficiency Virus (HIV), Human Papilloma Virus (HPV), Herpes Simplex Virus 2 (HSV2).

Keywords: vaginal microbiota; HIV; HPV; HSV2; cytokines; chemokines; innate immunity; adaptive immunity

1. The Vaginal Ecosystem

The vaginal mucosal ecosystem is comprised of a stratified squamous epithelium covered by a mucosal layer continuously lubricated by cervicovaginal fluid (CVF), which contains products of epithelial cells, such as mucins and antimicrobial molecules B-Defensin, Lipocalin, Elafine and secretory leukocyte protease inhibitor (SLPI) [1,2], IgA and IgG antibodies produced by mucosal plasma cells. CVF continuously lubricates epithelium, maintains the fluidity of the ecosystem and represents the first line of defense against exogenous pathogen colonization through the activity of mucins which entrap microbes and facilitate their binding to antibodies [3].

Cervicovaginal fluid also helps to contain the vaginal microbiota, microbial communities which exist in a mutualistic relationship with the host. The vaginal microbiota is unique in that, in many women, it is most often dominated by *Lactobacillus* species [4,5]. The latter produce lactic acid and bacteriocins, which contribute to prevent bacterial growth and, by maintaining a low vaginal pH (3.0–4.5), eventually favor *Lactobacillus* dominance. Moreover, *Lactobacillus* species adhere to epithelial surfaces, preventing the adhesion of bacteria able to infect epithelial cells, promote the autophagy of cells infected by viruses, bacteria or protozoa, facilitating their elimination [6], and modulate any inflammatory process that could have negative consequences, especially during pregnancy [7].

These activities are also necessary to prevent immune reactions against sperm. It is believed that the human behavior with sexual activities at any time during the menstrual cycle, as well as during gestation, may have contributed to select *Lactobacillus* species in the vaginal microbiota.

The detailed composition of vaginal microbiota and the relative abundance of the bacterial species has recently been defined through high-throughput 16s rRNA gene sequencing. At least five microbial communities, here referred as Community State Type (CST) were identified. Four CSTs are dominated by *Lactobacillus* (*L.*) species highly adapted to the vaginal environment [4,5]. In particular CST-I is dominated by *Lactobacillus crispatus*; CST-II by *Lactobacillus gasseri*; CST-III by *Lactobacillus iners*; CST-V by *Lactobacillus jensenii*. The CST-IV is comprised by polymicrobial communities, with prevalence of strictly anaerobic species of the order *Gardnerella, Atopobium, Mobiluncus, Megasphoera Prevotella, Streptococcus, Mycoplasma, Ureaplasma, Dialister, Bacteroides*, etc. [4,8,9]. The latter CST is very common in black and Hispanic women, ranging from 10% in United States [4] to 60% in South Africa [10]. The factors driving racial and geographic differences in cervicovaginal communities are not known yet, but could include changes in sexual behavior, hygienic practices, rectal colonization or even host genetics [11].

In many cases, a low vaginal pH may be maintained by microbes of CST-IV through the production of lactic acid [9], in this case, the presence of CST-IV is completely asymptomatic. However, loss of *Lactobacillus* dominance facilitates Bacterial Vaginosis (BV), the most common vaginal infection in reproductive-aged women [12,13], characterized by vaginal discharge, irritation, fishy odor and a vaginal pH often >4.5. Hormonal changes strongly affect the composition of vaginal microbiota during a woman's life, in particular at menopausal age, when reduced estrogen levels decrease the glycogen availability with the consequent depletion in *Lactobacillus* species [14].

In addition to epithelial cells and microbiota, the vaginal ecosystem comprises also cells of innate and adaptive immunity as neutrophils, macrophages, classic dendritic cells, Langerhans cells, NK cells, T and B lymphocytes. [15]. CD3+ T lymphocytes, predominantly CD8+ lymphocytes, are distributed in the lamina propria of the cervix and vagina. In particular, in ectocervical mucosa they have an effector/memory (CD27− CD45RA−) or effector phenotype (CD27−CD45RA+); B cells are found as aggregates or follicular-like structures surrounded by T lymphocytes. Plasma cells, as well as a small number of macrophages CD68+ and dendritic cells, are distributed throughout the lamina propria. Dendritic cells and monocyte/macrophagic CD14+ cells represent the most prevalent antigen-presenting cells in the vaginal ecosystem. Immune cell trafficking and activation throughout the reproductive tract is tightly mediated by the expression of pattern recognition receptors (PRR) [16,17] and is regulated by endocrine signaling [18].

2. Interplay between Host and Vaginal Microbiota in Health and Disease

Interplay between the cervicovaginal microbiota and the cells of immune system is determinant to prevent infections by external pathogens and to maintain an immuno-tolerant environment, particularly during pregnancy. Sex hormones are key regulators of this interplay: they regulate the production of antimicrobial peptides (beta-defensin, alpha Defensin, SLPI) and of pro-inflammatory cytokines (IL-6, IL-8) by the vaginal epithelial cells to ensure, when necessary, survival of sperm and to prevent ascending infections [19]; estrogens in particular also contribute to select microbial populations. At prepuberal age, vaginal microbiota is dominated by anaerobic species of the *Enterobacteriacee* and/or *Staphylococcacee* family. At puberty, the increased concentrations of estrogens promote the accumulation of glycogen by mature epithelial cells. Maltotriose and alpha-dextrins, derived from alpha-amylase-mediated glycogen digestion are selective food for *Lactobacillus* species that use these products for the synthesis of lactic acid. The low pH, the maintenance of mucous viscosity and the prevention of bacterial binding on epithelial surfaces are all factors that favor *Lactobacillus* dominance [20].

When *Lactobacillus* dominance is lost and microbial diversity increases, changes in immune and epithelial homeostasis often appear, induced through multiple mechanisms, as: (a) production of pro-inflammatory cytokines and chemokines, (b) recruitment of immune cells (c) reduction in the viscosity of the CVF, due to the production of mucin-degrading enzymes (including sialidase, α-fucosidase, α-and β-galactosidase, N-acetyl-glucosaminidase, and glycine and arginine aminopeptidases [21,22]. Physical/chemical changes in vaginal ecosystem ultimately affect the barrier properties of both CVF and the genital epithelium and increase the risk of infection with sexually transmitted pathogens. In fact, vaginal dysbiosis was associated with increased risk of acquisition of Sexual Transmitted Infections (STI) such as *Neisseria gonorrhoeae, Chlamydia trachomatis, Trichomonas vaginalis*, Herpes Simplex Virus (HSV), Human Papilloma Virus (HPV), and Human Immunodeficiency Virus (HIV) [12,13]. Even in the absence of clinical symptomatology, women harboring CST-IV in vaginal microbiota may be at high risk of STI or of early pregnancy loss and pre-term delivery [20].

STI impose major health and economic burdens globally, in particular in low- and middle-income countries (LMICs) [23]. It is estimated that about 18.9 million people, of whom 48% aged 15 to 24 years, acquired a new STI every year [24]. This is likely an underestimation of the real incidence of STI, as they are often asymptomatic.

Sexually transmitted viral infections, the subject of this review, also represent a serious health problem globally. A total of 34 million people were living with HIV at the end of 2011. Worldwide prevalence of genital HPV infection is estimated at 440 million persons, causing 510,000 cases of cervical cancer and approximately 288,000 deaths [25]. An estimated 417 million people aged 15–49 (11%) worldwide have Herpes Simplex Virus type 2 (HSV-2) infection, and HSV-2 incidence was 23.6 million new cases per year [26]. Prevalence of HSV-2 infection was estimated to be highest in Africa (31.5%), followed by the Americas (14.4%). It increases with age, though the highest numbers of people newly-infected were adolescents [27].

Risk factors commonly associated with acquisition of STI include biological and behavioral factors, number of sexual partners, lack of information about transmission modalities, difficulty to access to prevention services and, as reported above, selected compositions of the vaginal microbiota [28]. Moreover, the epidemiology of these infections is extremely complicated by the fact that each of them increases the risk of contracting other STI.

Metagenomic studies largely contributed to define the microbial communities most frequently associated with these infections. The assessment of the interplay among microbial communities, immune cells reactivity and epithelial homeostasis has contributed to define the environment in which infections are established and, in particular for HPV infection, also the one that facilitates persistence of the pathogen. This information will be helpful for the development of new diagnostic assays as well as new therapeutic strategies based on the replacement of harmful microbial communities. The following sections describe in greater detail current knowledge on the interplay between vaginal microbiota, immune system and epithelial cells in the most prevalent sexually transmitted viral infections: HIV, HPV, HSV-2.

3. The Vaginal Microbiota and HIV Infection

The importance of understanding how bacterial communities modulate female genital health has come strongly into focus, in particular with the evolving knowledge about the influence of cervicovaginal microbiota on HIV acquisition. As known, the highest incidence of HIV infections, with an extraordinarily high number of infected women in reproductive age, is in the African continent and, particularly in the sub-Saharan regions.

Socio-economic factors largely contribute to such high incidence. The prevalence of CST-IV in the vaginal microbiota of African women, however, also suggested that this CST may affect the susceptibility to HIV infection. The molecular mechanisms that have been suggested are:

(A) A decrease in D-lactate concentrations and the lowering of virions trapping. In fact, D-lactate, the main metabolic product of numerous *Lactobacillus* species, including *L. crispatus*, contributes to trap virions by favoring hydrogen bridges between HIV surface proteins and carboxylic groups of mucins [29].

(B) CST-IV microbes produce enzymes that degrade the mucus included sialidase, α-fucosidase, α-and β-galactosidase, N-acetyl-glucosaminidase, and glycine and arginine aminopeptidases [21,22,30].

(C) Antigen-presenting cells activated by bacterial products, in particular LPS, produce cytokines and chemokines which increase the recruitment of activated CD4+ lymphocytes [10].

The first observations on the associations between defined microbial communities and HIV susceptibility were obtained in cross-sectional studies. These studies have a serious limitation since the recruited people were at "high risk" of infection (e.g., sex workers) and left the doubt that changes in the microbiome may be a consequence of HIV infection rather than a contributing cause [10,31–33]. Recently, however, these doubts have been resolved: a prospective study on a cohort of healthy HIV-uninfected black South African women who were monitored for incident HIV infection clearly showed that none of the women who acquired HIV had a *L. crispatus* dominant community [34]; in contrast, women belonging to CST-IV experienced up to four-fold greater rates of HIV acquisition during follow-up compared to women of the CST-I, dominated by *L. crispatus* [34]. In particular, a subgroup of CST-IV dominated by *Prevotella bivia*, *Prevotella melaninogenica*, *Veillonella montpellierensis*, *Mycoplasma* species, and *Sneathia sanguinegens* was identified as the cervicotype with significantly higher risk of HIV acquisition [34]. Recent observations expanded the number of bacterial taxa associated with increased risk of HIV acquisition: in addition to *Prevotella* species, *Parvimonas* species type 1 and type 2, *Gemella asaccharolytica*, *Eggerthella* species type 1 and vaginal *Megasphaera* species were significantly associated with HIV acquisition [35].

The mechanisms underlying the increased HIV susceptibility likely reside in the ability of the bacterial taxa to induce a strong inflammation in the cervicovaginal environment with elevated concentrations of IL-17, IL-23 and IL-1β and high recruitment of CCR5$^+$ CD4 T cells, the primary target of HIV infection. These cells also show an activated phenotype (HLA-DR+CD38$^+$) and thus they are highly permissive for viral replication [34]. High numbers of activated $\gamma\delta$ CD4 T lymphocytes expressing the Vδ2 chain, which potentially are targets of HIV and permissive for its replication, were also found increased in women with vaginal microbiota not dominated by *Lactobacillus* species [36], thus defining a framework where selected microbial communities are closely linked with immune activation and HIV infection.

Such knowledge also suggests that, in addition to vaccines, strategies to prevent HIV infection may include the stable colonization of vaginal microbiota with non-dangerous bacterial taxa to limit inflammation and T-cell recruitment. Since vaginal dysbiosis may undermine the efficacy of locally administered antiviral drugs [37], changes in vaginal microbiota will also improve the efficacy of these drugs.

4. The Vaginal Microbiota and HPV Infection

Infection with HPV is the most common viral infection of the reproductive tract and high-risk (HR) genital HPVs are central etiological agents in the development of cervical cancer and of its premalignant precursor, cervical intraepithelial neoplasia (CIN) [38]. HR-HPV genotypes 16, 18, 31, 33, and 35 are the most diffuse worldwide. Other HR genotypes are HPV 39, 45, 51, 52, 56, 58, 66 and 69 [39]. Generally, HPV infects the basal layer of the cervical squamous epithelium, where viral genomes persist as episomes at low-copy numbers [40]. High copies of virions are produced upon differentiation of epithelial cells and the new progeny of virions may be released from the epithelial surface. Infection of stem cell-like cells of the basal layer ensures persistence of infection [41].

The oncogenic activity of HR-HPVs is based on the functional properties of their E6 and E7 proteins [42]. These proteins inactivate p53 and retinoblastoma protein, respectively, and lead to the inhibition of apoptosis and to cell cycle progression of cells at the basal and differentiated layers of cervical epithelium. Viral integration with genetic alterations ultimately may induce uncontrolled cell proliferation [43,44]. At the histological level, different grades of squamous intraepithelial lesions are the result of persistent HR-HPV infection and, if undetected and untreated, they may lead to high-grade lesions and cancer in an average of 5 to 15 years [45].

The immune response to acute HPV infections is initially mediated by mucosal NK cells [46,47] and by epithelial cells which produce antimicrobial peptides with reported anti-viral effects [48]. However, HR-HPVs have evolved molecular strategies to escape innate and adaptive immunity [49–52]. HR-HPV infection never associates with a marked pro-inflammatory environment [53–55]. A rather high number of CD4$^+$ CD25$^+$ regulatory T cells and the presence of activated TH2 cells were reported in HR-HPV persistent infections and associated with the suppression of cytotoxic functions, induction of T cell anergy [56,57]. Consequently, virus-induced immune suppression may be responsible for increased infection with other sexually transmitted diseases such as *Chlamydia trachomatis* infection [58,59].

Emerging data support the notion that the vaginal microbiome is involved in the natural history of the disease [46].

Since HPV infections, even with HR genotypes, may be transient and more than 50% of them are cleared within six months while almost 90% are cleared within two years, we believe it is critical to consider data obtained in longitudinal studies and to devote special attention to the context in which they were obtained [4,46]. The first longitudinal study observed a cohort of 32 North American sexually active and premenopausal women over the course of 16 weeks using self-sampling at twice-weekly intervals [14]. A total of 930 samples of cervicovaginal mucous were obtained and microbiota studies revealed that women with CSTs III (dominance of *L. iners*) or with a subtype of CST-IV with a high proportion of *Atopobium, Prevotella, Gardnerella* species were most likely to be HPV positive and had the slowest rate of infection clearance.

In a subsequent survey, Di Paola et al. [30] used cervicovaginal samples collected in a study for HR-HPV screening program in Italy. A total of 55/1029 samples were positive for HR-HPV at the baseline screening. The authors used the results of the second HR-HPV screening performed after one year to stratify the baseline sampling in Clearance group, with no evidence of HR-HPV DNA after one year; the Persistence group, HR-HPV+ with at least one of the HPV-DNA genotypes of the baseline sampling after one year. A group of cervicovaginal samples from women negative for HR-HPV (HR-HPV−) infections was included as a control. The results of this study showed that a subgroup of CST-IV dominated by strictly anaerobic species (*Gardnerella, Prevotella, Atopobium, Megasphoera*) was prevalent in the Persistence group, compared with either the Clearance or Control group. Odds ratio analysis confirmed that this CST may be a risk factor for the persistence of HR-HPV infection.

In agreement with previous reports [60,61], a significant enrichment in *Sneathia* and *Megasphaera* was found in the group of HR-HPV+ women, compared to HR-HPV− controls, while the *Atopobium* genus was significantly enriched in Persistence group, compared to the other groups.

Although the association of bacterial vaginosis with higher rates of HPV infection and persistence has been known from a long time [62], metagenomic data revealed that selected microbiota compositions increase the risk of infection, even in the total absence of clinical symptomatology. While it is quite clear that some microbial communities favor HPV infection by modifying the barrier effect of cervical mucus and of stratified epithelium, the effects of microbiota-related immunological changes on the outcomes of HPV infection are not elucidated yet. This may depend on the impact of HPV infection on the host's immune defenses [53,54], and on the mucosal metabolism which can also affect the composition of the vaginal microbiota. Therefore, the immunological signature of HPV infection on vaginal microbiota has to be further elucidated and more data are needed to have a full understanding of how HPV infections are modulated by the vaginal environment.

Persistent infection with HR-HPV is a necessary, but not sufficient, condition for the development of cervical cancer. As soon as the establishment of HR-HPV infection occurs, cellular changes can be observed in the cervical exfoliated cells. Persistent infections can result in different grades of squamous intraepithelial lesions that ultimately lead to high-grade lesions and cancer in an average of 5 to 14 years if undetected and untreated [45].

Recently, much attention has been given to the role of vaginal microbiota in the progression of epithelial lesions up to carcinogenesis. Drago et al. [63] found a strong correlation between *Ureaplasma parvum*-HPV co-infection and CIN1. Mitra et al. [64] have studied a cohort of 169 women with different degrees of cervical lesions and showed that increasing severity of cervical lesions was associated with higher vaginal microbiome diversity and decreased relative abundance of *Lactobacillus* species. CST-IV was associated with increasing disease severity, irrespective of HPV status. [61,65]. In particular, *Atopobium vaginae* and *Lactobacillus iners* were associated with an increased risk of neoplastic progression in HPV+ women [61], while *Sneathia sanguinegens* [54,61,64] and other *Fusobacterial* species [61], *Anaerococcus tetradius* and *Peptostreptococcus anaerobius* [64], were shown to be associated with an increase in disease severity. Novel bacterial taxa (*Shuttleworthia*, *Gemella* and *Olsenella*) and *Streptococcus agalactiae* were found enriched in HPV+ women with low- and high-grade cervical dysplasia (LGD, HGD), invasive cervical carcinoma (ICC) [54]. *Sneathia* spp. was the only taxon significantly enriched both in HPV+ women without lesions of any grade and in women with precancerous lesions and cervical cancer, suggesting that this taxon may represent a metagenomic marker for CIN progression. In particular, *Sneathia* spp. were found enriched in precancerous groups, and invasive cervical cancer, particularly in subjects of Hispanic ethnicity [54].

The molecular mechanisms through which bacteria of CST-IV may favor neoplastic progression are: (a) they produce high levels of nitrosamines which are known carcinogens; (b) they induce DNA oxidative damage [66].

While HPV infection or clearance is not marked by a pro-inflammatory environment, patients with cervical dysplasia and ICC were shown to have an increase in pro-inflammatory cytokines and chemokines (TNF-α, TNF-β, MIP-1α, GM-CSF), as well as an increase in cytokines related to adaptive immune responses (IL-2, IL-4, SCD40L). [67]. Moreover, the concentrations of the immunomodulating cytokine IL-10 were found to be increased in the ICC group. However, no direct association between the increased concentrations of cytokines and chemokines and the microbiota composition was revealed. Only the concentration of IL36γ was always elevated in patients with carcinoma, suggesting a direct or indirect role of this cytokine in the carcinogenetic process [54]. These data strongly suggest that, similar to other mucosal sites, chronic genital inflammation may promote carcinogenesis.

In the future it is highly likely that metabolomic studies, using nuclear magnetic resonance and mass spectroscopy, may better define the association of vaginal microbiota composition in health and disease states. A better definition of the effects of individual bacterial species, such as *L. iners*, *A. vaginae*, and *Sneathia* species, on epithelial and immune cell functions is desirable. In fact, if the responsibility of a single bacterial species in HPV disease is defined, it will be possible to identify patients at higher risk using microchip array or metabolomic technologies. Moreover, it will be possible to develop new therapeutic strategies based on pre/probiotics, in order to manipulate the vaginal microbiota composition.

5. Herpes Simplex Virus Type-2 (HSV-2)

Herpes simplex virus type-2 (HSV-2) is a common STI worldwide and the leading cause of genital ulcer disease [27]. Most HSV-2 infections are asymptomatic, with >80% of HSV-2 seropositive individuals asymptomatically shedding virus. More women are infected with HSV-2 than men; in 2012 it was estimated that 267 million women and 150 million men were living with the infection. This is because sexual transmission of HSV is more efficient from men to women than from women to men [26].

After infection by sexual transmission, virus replication initiates in genital keratinocytes and may spread to thousands of cells. Then, the virus invariably enters the neuron to reach the dorsal root ganglia where lifelong latency is established [68]. Virus periodically reactivates within the ganglia and travels back down the neuron leading to either asymptomatic, low titer shedding, or less commonly recurrent ulcers which are typically associated with prolonged high titer shedding [69–71].

The first two studies examining the associations between HSV-2 and vaginal microbiota were published in 2003 [72,73]. The main data emerging from these studies was that lack of *Lactobacillus* protective species and a history of BV was significantly associated with HSV-2 seropositivity [72]. Additionally, prospective studies confirmed the association between prevalent HSV-2 infection and BV [74,75]. In the case of HSV-2 infection, the association with vaginal dysbiosis is bi-directional. HSV-2 infection indeed seems to increase the occurrence of dysbiosis by multiple mechanisms: (a) the intermittent HSV-2 reactivation also leads to immune activation in the genital environment favouring changes in microbiota composition [76]; (b) increased iron availability which facilitates the growth of *Gardnerella vaginalis* [77]. In the same way, BV increases genital shedding of HSV-2 [73,78,79].

HSV2 infection was extensively studied because it represents a high risk factor for HIV acquisition [80]. This increased risk may occur because HSV-2 reactivation disrupts the epithelial barrier and recruits activated CD4 cells, which are target cells for HIV infection, into the lesion. Moreover, it has been shown that the HSV regulatory proteins ICP0, ICP4, VP16 upregulate HIV replication and increase the frequency and the titer of mucosal HIV shedding. This may occur during both clinical and asymptomatic HSV reactivation. [81,82].

Microbiota-HSV2 interactions and the corresponding changes in vaginal immunity were recently studied through NGS technologies in a group of 51 African Caribbean and other black (ACB) HIV⁻ women [83]. The authors found that HSV-2 infection was associated with an increased number of mucosal CD4⁺ T-cell subsets without significant alterations in local proinflammatory cytokines; selected cytokines or antimicrobial peptides (MIP-3α, IL-6, IL-8, LL-37, and HNP1-3), associated with the number of CD4+ T cells and these were distinct from cytokines usually associated with CST-IV, suggesting that HSV-2 and vaginal CST-IV enhance HIV susceptibility through independent mucosal immune mechanisms.

In murine experimental models of HSV-2 infection, Oh et al. investigated the mechanisms by which commensal bacteria elicit immune protection against HSV-2 infection of the vaginal mucosa [84]. The authors demonstrated that vaginal dysbiosis, like that induced by antibiotic therapy, affects the T-cell mediated adaptive immune response inducing a marked suppression. The molecular mechanisms at the basis of immune-suppression relied on high concentrations of IL-33, an alarmin secreted by damaged epithelial cells in the vaginal environment [85] after antibiotic treatment.

IL33 strongly inhibits the IFN-γ secretion by activated mucosal T cells, limiting the recruitment of T cells which is required to clear viral infection. The suppressive effects of IL33 are also mediated by a recruitment of innate lymphocytes type 2 and eosinophils into vaginal tissue, which contributes to suppression of antiviral immunity against mucosal HSV-2 infection by producing cytokines interfering with a TH-1 response [86]. Interestingly, protease activity by commensal bacteria resistant to antibiotic-treatment is likely responsible for epithelial damage and IL-33 secretion. Thus, in the case of HSV-2 infection a complex interplay among the virus, immune cells, and microbiota occurs, and it likely increases the susceptibility to other sexually transmitted diseases, including HIV.

6. Gaps and Challenges

Despite recent advances, significant gaps in knowledge concerning the vaginal microbiota have yet to be solved. Prevention strategies of sexually transmitted viral infection should be mainly based on the prevention and or treatment of recurrent BV. Treatment with oral or vaginal metronidazole or clindamycin is typically efficacious in the short term (as defined by Nugent or Amsel criteria) but recurrence rates are high [87]. An efficient strategy in the longer term may specifically target pathobionts or BV-associated anaerobs, while sparing *Lactobacillus* species or colonizing vaginal microbiota with appropriate probiotics. Common vaginal strains as *L. gasseri* and *L. crispatus* have been used in recurrent BV with moderate results; indeed, few randomized trials only (all including *Lactobacillus rhamnosus*) showed lower rates of recurrent BV in the probiotic group [88]. Hormonal therapy offers a potential approach to promote *Lactobacillus* dominant communities [89] while treatments to maintain vaginal acidity were not able to promote a healthy vaginal microbiota [90]. Treatments specifically targeting dysbiosis-associated anaerobes or pathobionts while sparing *Lactobacillus* species combined with biofilm disrupting agents, systemic or topical estrogen, and/or *Lactobacillus*-containing vaginal pro- or synbiotics might be more efficacious in the longer term.

The definition of cervicovaginal bacteria which mediate immunomodulatory mechanisms will help to identify molecules and to set up therapeutic strategies for infections that take advantage from a vaginal inflammatory environment. Finally, even when effective diagnostic tools are developed, it will be necessary to define the "harmful" levels of cervicovaginal inflammation, the appropriate "timing" of

Int. J. Mol. Sci. **2019**, *20*, 266

the therapeutic intervention and which women to target. We are confident that the progress achieved in recent years will make it possible to find the optimum solutions for these issues.

Funding: This research was funded by ITT, Regione Toscana, 62042012″ and Ente Cassa di Risparmio, Firenze.

Conflicts of Interest: The author declares no conflict of interest.

Abbreviations

CVF	Cervicovaginal fluid
CST	Community State Type
STI	Sexually transmitted infections
HIV	Human immunodeficiency virus
HR-HPV	High risk human papilloma virus
HSV2	Herpes simplex virus 2

References

1. King, A.E.; Critchley, H.O.D.; Kelly, R.W. Innate immune defences in the human endometrium. *Reprod. Biol. Endocrinol.* **2003**, *1*, 116. [CrossRef] [PubMed]
2. King, A.E.; Wheelhouse, N.; Cameron, S.; McDonald, S.E.; Lee, K.-F.; Entrican, G.; Critchley, H.O.; Horne, A.W. Expression of secretory leukocyte protease inhibitor and elafin in human fallopian tube and in an in-vitro model of Chlamydia trachomatis infection. *Hum. Reprod.* **2009**, *24*, 679–686. [CrossRef] [PubMed]
3. Chen, A.; McKinley, S.A.; Wang, S.; Shi, F.; Mucha, P.J.; Forest, M.G.; Lai, S.K. Transient antibody-mucin interactions produce a dynamic molecular shield against viral invasion. *Biophys. J.* **2014**, *106*, 2028–2036. [CrossRef] [PubMed]
4. Ravel, J.; Gajer, P.; Abdo, Z.; Schneider, G.M.; Koenig, S.S.K.; McCulle, S.L.; Karlebach, S.; Gorle, R.; Russell, J.; Tacket, C.O.; et al. Vaginal microbiome of reproductive-age women. *Proc. Natl. Acad. Sci. USA* **2011**, *108*, 4680–4687. [CrossRef] [PubMed]
5. Kroon, S.J.; Ravel, J.; Huston, W.M. Cervicovaginal microbiota, women's health, and reproductive outcomes. *Fertil Steril.* **2018**, *110*, 327–336. [CrossRef] [PubMed]
6. Ghadimi, D.; de Vrese, M.; Heller, K.J.; Schrezenmeir, J. Lactic acid bacteria enhance autophagic ability of mononuclear phagocytes by increasing Th1 autophagy-promoting cytokine (IFN-gamma) and nitric oxide (NO) levels and reducing Th2 autophagy-restraining cytokines (IL-4 and IL-13) in response to Mycobacteriu. *Int. Immunopharmacol.* **2010**, *10*, 694–706. [CrossRef] [PubMed]
7. Aldunate, M.; Srbinovski, D.; Hearps, A.C.; Latham, C.F.; Ramsland, P.A.; Gugasyan, R.; Cone, R.A.; Tachedjian, G. Antimicrobial and immune modulatory effects of lactic acid and short chain fatty acids produced by vaginal microbiota associated with eubiosis and bacterial vaginosis. *Front. Physiol.* **2015**, *6*, 164. [CrossRef]
8. Fredricks, D.N.; Fiedler, T.L.; Marrazzo, J.M. Molecular identification of bacteria associated with bacterial vaginosis. *N. Engl. J. Med.* **2005**, *353*, 1899–1911. [CrossRef]
9. Gajer, P.; Brotman, R.M.; Bai, G.; Sakamoto, J.; Schutte, U.M.E.; Zhong, X.; Koenig, S.S.; Fu, L.; Ma, Z.S.; Zhou, X.; et al. Temporal dynamics of the human vaginal microbiota. *Sci. Transl. Med.* **2012**, *4*, 132ra52. [CrossRef]
10. Anahtar, M.N.; Byrne, E.H.; Doherty, K.E.; Bowman, B.A.; Yamamoto, H.S.; Soumillon, M.; Padavattan, N.; Ismail, N.; Moodley, A.; Sabatini, M.E.; et al. Cervicovaginal bacteria are a major modulator of host inflammatory responses in the female genital tract. *Immunity* **2015**, *42*, 965–976. [CrossRef]
11. Muzny, C.A.; Schwebke, J.R. Pathogenesis of Bacterial Vaginosis: Discussion of Current Hypotheses. *J. Infect. Dis.* **2016**, *214*, S1–S5. [CrossRef] [PubMed]
12. Kenyon, C.; Colebunders, R.; Crucitti, T. The global epidemiology of bacterial vaginosis: A systematic review. *Am. J. Obstet. Gynecol.* **2013**, *209*, 505–523. [CrossRef]
13. Van de Wijgert, J.H.H.M.; Jespers, V. The global health impact of vaginal dysbiosis. *Res. Microbiol.* **2017**, *168*, 859–864. [CrossRef]

14. Brotman, R.M.; Shardell, M.D.; Gajer, P.; Fadrosh, D.; Chang, K.; Silver, M.I.; Viscidi, R.P.; Burke, A.E.; Ravel, J.; Gravitt, P.E. Association between the vaginal microbiota, menopause status, and signs of vulvovaginal atrophy. *Menopause* **2014**, *21*, 450–458. [CrossRef] [PubMed]

15. Lee, S.K.; Kim, C.J.; Kim, D.-J.; Kang, J.-H. Immune cells in the female reproductive tract. *Immune Netw.* **2015**, *15*, 16–26. [CrossRef] [PubMed]

16. Aflatoonian, R.; Fazeli, A. Toll-like receptors in female reproductive tract and their menstrual cycle dependent expression. *J. Reprod. Immunol.* **2008**, *77*, 7–13. [CrossRef]

17. Hart, K.M.; Murphy, A.J.; Barrett, K.T.; Wira, C.R.; Guyre, P.M.; Pioli, P.A. Functional expression of pattern recognition receptors in tissues of the human female reproductive tract. *J. Reprod. Immunol.* **2009**, *80*, 33–40. [CrossRef]

18. Yeaman, G.R.; Collins, J.E.; Fanger, M.W.; Wira, C.R.; Lydyard, P.M. CD8+ T cells in human uterine endometrial lymphoid aggregates: Evidence for accumulation of cells by trafficking. *Immunology* **2001**, *102*, 434–440. [CrossRef]

19. Wira, C.R.; Fahey, J.V.; Rodriguez-Garcia, M.; Shen, Z.; Patel, M.V. Regulation of mucosal immunity in the female reproductive tract: The role of sex hormones in immune protection against sexually transmitted pathogens. *Am. J. Reprod. Immunol.* **2014**, *72*, 236–258. [CrossRef]

20. Amabebe, E.; Anumba, D.O.C. The Vaginal Microenvironment: The Physiologic Role of Lactobacilli. *Front. Med.* **2018**, *5*, 181. [CrossRef]

21. Olmsted, S.S.; Meyn, L.A.; Rohan, L.C.; Hillier, S.L. Glycosidase and proteinase activity of anaerobic gram-negative bacteria isolated from women with bacterial vaginosis. *Sex. Transm. Dis.* **2003**, *30*, 257–261. [CrossRef] [PubMed]

22. Moncla, B.J.; Chappell, C.A.; Mahal, L.K.; Debo, B.M.; Meyn, L.A.; Hillier, S.L. Impact of bacterial vaginosis, as assessed by nugent criteria and hormonal status on glycosidases and lectin binding in cervicovaginal lavage samples. *PLoS ONE* **2015**, *10*, e0127091. [CrossRef] [PubMed]

23. World Health Organization. *Global Incidence and Prevalence of Selected Sexually Transmitted Infections—2008*; World Health Organization: Geneva, Switzerland, 2012.

24. Weinstock, H.; Berman, S.; Cates, W.J. Sexually transmitted diseases among American youth: Incidence and prevalence estimates, 2000. *Perspect. Sex. Reprod. Health* **2004**, *36*, 6–10. [CrossRef]

25. Saslow, D.; Boetes, C.; Burke, W.; Harms, S.; Leach, M.O.; Lehman, C.D.; Morris, E.; Pisano, E.; Schnall, M.; Sener, S.; et al. American Cancer Society guidelines for breast screening with MRI as an adjunct to mammography. *CA Cancer J. Clin.* **2007**, *57*, 75–89. [CrossRef] [PubMed]

26. McQuillan, G.; Kruszon-Moran, D.; Flagg, E.W.; Paulose-Ram, R. Prevalence of Herpes Simplex Virus Type 1 and Type 2 in Persons Aged 14–49: United States, 2015–2016. *NCHS Data Brief.* **2018**, *304*, 1–8.

27. Looker, K.J.; Garnett, G.P.; Schmid, G.P. An estimate of the global prevalence and incidence of herpes simplex virus type 2 infection. *Bull. World Health Organ.* **2008**, *86*, 805–812. [CrossRef] [PubMed]

28. Nardis, C.; Mosca, L.; Mastromarino, P. Vaginal microbiota and viral sexually transmitted diseases. *Ann. Ig.* **2013**, *25*, 443–456. [PubMed]

29. Nunn, K.L.; Wang, Y.-Y.; Harit, D.; Humphrys, M.S.; Ma, B.; Cone, R.; Ravel, J.; Lai, S.K. Enhanced Trapping of HIV-1 by Human Cervicovaginal Mucus Is Associated with Lactobacillus crispatus-Dominant Microbiota. *MBio* **2015**, *6*. [CrossRef]

30. Di Paola, M.; Sani, C.; Clemente, A.M.; Iossa, A.; Perissi, E.; Castronovo, G.; Tanturli, M.; Rivero, D.; Cozzolino, F.; Cavalieri, D.; et al. Characterization of cervico-vaginal microbiota in women developing persistent high-risk Human Papillomavirus infection. *Sci. Rep.* **2017**, *7*, 10200. [CrossRef] [PubMed]

31. Schellenberg, J.J.; Links, M.G.; Hill, J.E.; Dumonceaux, T.J.; Kimani, J.; Jaoko, W.; Wachihi, C.; Mungai, J.N.; Peters, G.A.; Tyler, S.; et al. Molecular definition of vaginal microbiota in East African commercial sex workers. *Appl. Environ. Microbiol.* **2011**, *77*, 4066–4074. [CrossRef]

32. Martin Harold, L.J.; Richardson, B.A.; Nyange, P.M.; Lavreys, L.; Hillier, S.L.; Chohan, B.; Mandaliya, K.; Ndinya-Achola, J.O.; Bwayo, J.; Kreiss, J. Vaginal Lactobacilli, Microbial Flora, and Risk of Human Immunodeficiency Virus Type 1 and Sexually Transmitted Disease Acquisition. *J. Infect. Dis.* **1999**, *180*, 1863–1868. [CrossRef] [PubMed]

33. Atashili, J.; Poole, C.; Ndumbe, P.M.; Adimora, A.A.; Smith, J.S. Bacterial vaginosis and HIV acquisition: A meta-analysis of published studies. *AIDS* **2008**, *22*, 1493–1501. [CrossRef] [PubMed]

34. Gosmann, C.; Anahtar, M.N.; Handley, S.A.; Farcasanu, M.; Abu-Ali, G.; Bowman, B.A.; Padavattan, N.; Desai, C.; Droit, L.; Moodley, A.; et al. Lactobacillus-Deficient Cervicovaginal Bacterial Communities Are Associated with Increased HIV Acquisition in Young South African Women. *Immunity* **2017**, *46*, 29–37. [CrossRef] [PubMed]

35. McClelland, R.S.; Lingappa, J.R.; Srinivasan, S.; Kinuthia, J.; John-Stewart, G.C.; Jaoko, W.; Richardson, B.A.; Yuhas, K.; Fiedler, T.L.; Mandaliya, K.N.; et al. Evaluation of the association between the concentrations of key vaginal bacteria and the increased risk of HIV acquisition in African women from five cohorts: A nested case-control study. *Lancet Infect. Dis.* **2018**, *18*, 554–564. [CrossRef]

36. Alcaide, M.L.; Strbo, N.; Romero, L.; Jones, D.L.; Rodriguez, V.J.; Arheart, K.; Martinez, O.; Bolivar, H.; Podack, E.R.; Fischl, M.A.; et al. Bacterial Vaginosis Is Associated with Loss of Gamma Delta T Cells in the Female Reproductive Tract in Women in the Miami Women Interagency HIV Study (WIHS): A Cross Sectional Study. *PLoS ONE* **2016**, *11*, e0153045. [CrossRef] [PubMed]

37. Velloza, J.; Heffron, R. The Vaginal Microbiome and its Potential to Impact Efficacy of HIV Pre-exposure Prophylaxis for Women. *Curr. HIV/AIDS Rep.* **2017**, *14*, 153–160. [CrossRef] [PubMed]

38. Fitzmaurice, C.; Dicker, D.; Pain, A.; Hamavid, H.; Moradi-Lakeh, M.; MacIntyre, M.F.; Allen, C.; Hansen, G.; Woodbrook, R.; Wolfe, C.; et al. The Global Burden of Cancer 2013. *JAMA Oncol.* **2015**, *1*, 505–527. [CrossRef]

39. De Villiers, E.-M.; Fauquet, C.; Broker, T.R.; Bernard, H.-U.; zur Hausen, H. Classification of papillomaviruses. *Virology* **2004**, *324*, 17–27. [CrossRef]

40. Doorbar, J. Molecular biology of human papillomavirus infection and cervical cancer. *Clin. Sci.* **2006**, *110*, 525–541. [CrossRef]

41. Egawa, N.; Egawa, K.; Griffin, H.; Doorbar, J. Human Papillomaviruses; Epithelial Tropisms, and the Development of Neoplasia. *Viruses* **2015**, *7*, 3863–3890. [CrossRef]

42. Zur Hausen, H. Papillomaviruses and cancer: From basic studies to clinical application. *Nat. Rev. Cancer* **2002**, *2*, 342–350. [CrossRef] [PubMed]

43. De Marco, F. Oxidative stress and HPV carcinogenesis. *Viruses* **2013**, *5*, 708–731. [CrossRef] [PubMed]

44. Doorbar, J.; Quint, W.; Banks, L.; Bravo, I.G.; Stoler, M.; Broker, T.R.; Stanley, M.A. The biology and life-cycle of human papillomaviruses. *Vaccine* **2012**, *30*, F55–F70. [CrossRef] [PubMed]

45. Woodman, C.B.J.; Collins, S.I.; Young, L.S. The natural history of cervical HPV infection: Unresolved issues. *Nat. Rev. Cancer* **2007**, *7*, 11–22. [CrossRef] [PubMed]

46. Mitra, A.; MacIntyre, D.A.; Marchesi, J.R.; Lee, Y.S.; Bennett, P.R.; Kyrgiou, M. The vaginal microbiota, human papillomavirus infection and cervical intraepithelial neoplasia: What do we know and where are we going next? *Microbiome* **2016**, *4*, 58. [CrossRef] [PubMed]

47. Stanley, M.A. Epithelial cell responses to infection with human papillomavirus. *Clin. Microbiol. Rev.* **2012**, *25*, 215–222. [CrossRef] [PubMed]

48. Yarbrough, V.L.; Winkle, S.; Herbst-Kralovetz, M.M. Antimicrobial peptides in the female reproductive tract: A critical component of the mucosal immune barrier with physiological and clinical implications. *Hum. Reprod.* **2015**, *21*, 353–377. [CrossRef]

49. Guess, J.C.; McCance, D.J. Decreased migration of Langerhans precursor-like cells in response to human keratinocytes expressing human papillomavirus type 16 E6/E7 is related to reduced macrophage inflammatory protein-3alpha production. *J. Virol.* **2005**, *79*, 14852–14862. [CrossRef]

50. Karim, R.; Meyers, C.; Backendorf, C.; Ludigs, K.; Offringa, R.; van Ommen, G.-J.B.; Melief, C.J.; van der Burg, S.H.; Boer, J.M. Human papillomavirus deregulates the response of a cellular network comprising of chemotactic and proinflammatory genes. *PLoS ONE* **2011**, *6*, e17848. [CrossRef]

51. Sperling, T.; Oldak, M.; Walch-Ruckheim, B.; Wickenhauser, C.; Doorbar, J.; Pfister, H.; Malejczyk, M.; Majewski, S.; Keates, A.C.; Smola, S. Human papillomavirus type 8 interferes with a novel C/EBPbeta-mediated mechanism of keratinocyte CCL20 chemokine expression and Langerhans cell migration. *PLoS Pathog.* **2012**, *8*, e1002833. [CrossRef]

52. Hong, S.; Laimins, L.A. The JAK-STAT transcriptional regulator, STAT-5, activates the ATM DNA damage pathway to induce HPV 31 genome amplification upon epithelial differentiation. *PLoS Pathog.* **2013**, *9*, e1003295. [CrossRef] [PubMed]

53. Clifford, G.M.; Rana, R.K.; Franceschi, S.; Smith, J.S.; Gough, G.; Pimenta, J.M. Human papillomavirus genotype distribution in low-grade cervical lesions: Comparison by geographic region and with cervical cancer. *Cancer Epidemiol. Biomark. Prev.* **2005**, *14*, 1157–1164. [CrossRef] [PubMed]

54. Laniewski, P.; Barnes, D.; Goulder, A.; Cui, H.; Roe, D.J.; Chase, D.M.; Herbst-Kralovetz, M.M. Linking cervicovaginal immune signatures, HPV and microbiota composition in cervical carcinogenesis in non-Hispanic and Hispanic women. *Sci. Rep.* **2018**, *8*, 7593. [CrossRef] [PubMed]

55. Shannon, B.; Yi, T.J.; Perusini, S.; Gajer, P.; Ma, B.; Humphrys, M.S.; Thomas-Pavanel, J.; Chieza, L.; Janakiram, P.; Saunders, M.; et al. Association of HPV infection and clearance with cervicovaginal immunology and the vaginal microbiota. *Mucosal Immunol.* **2017**, *10*, 1310–1319. [CrossRef] [PubMed]

56. Bordignon, V.; Di Domenico, E.G.; Trento, E.; D'Agosto, G.; Cavallo, I.; Pontone, M.; Pimpinelli, F.; Mariani, L.; Ensoli, F. How Human Papillomavirus Replication and Immune Evasion Strategies Take Advantage of the Host DNA Damage Repair Machinery. *Viruses* **2017**, *9*, 390. [CrossRef] [PubMed]

57. Bonin, C.M.; Padovani, C.T.J.; da Costa, I.P.; Avila, L.S.; Ferreira, A.M.T.; Fernandes, C.E.S.; dos Santos, A.R.; Tozetti, I.A. Detection of regulatory T cell phenotypic markers and cytokines in patients with human papillomavirus infection. *J. Med. Virol.* **2019**, *91*, 317. [CrossRef] [PubMed]

58. Smith, J.S.; Munoz, N.; Herrero, R.; Eluf-Neto, J.; Ngelangel, C.; Franceschi, S.; Bosch, F.X.; Walboomers, J.M.; Peeling, R.W. Evidence for Chlamydia trachomatis as a human papillomavirus cofactor in the etiology of invasive cervical cancer in Brazil and the Philippines. *J. Infect. Dis.* **2002**, *185*, 324–331. [CrossRef] [PubMed]

59. Alberts, C.J.; Schim van der Loeff, M.F.; Papenfuss, M.R.; da Silva, R.J.C.; Villa, L.L.; Lazcano-Ponce, E.; Nyitray, A.G.; Giuliano, A.R. Association of Chlamydia trachomatis infection and herpes simplex virus type 2 serostatus with genital human papillomavirus infection in men: The HPV in men study. *Sex. Transm. Dis.* **2013**, *40*, 508–515. [CrossRef]

60. Gao, W.; Weng, J.; Gao, Y.; Chen, X. Comparison of the vaginal microbiota diversity of women with and without human papillomavirus infection: A cross-sectional study. *BMC Infect. Dis.* **2013**, *13*, 271. [CrossRef]

61. Audirac-Chalifour, A.; Torres-Poveda, K.; Bahena-Roman, M.; Tellez-Sosa, J.; Martinez-Barnetche, J.; Cortina-Ceballos, B.; López-Estrada, G.; Delgado-Romero, K.; Burguete-García, A.I.; Cantú, D.; et al. Cervical Microbiome and Cytokine Profile at Various Stages of Cervical Cancer: A Pilot Study. *PLoS ONE* **2016**, *11*, e0153274. [CrossRef]

62. Gillet, E.; Meys, J.F.; Verstraelen, H.; Bosire, C.; De Sutter, P.; Temmerman, M.; Broeck, D.V. Bacterial vaginosis is associated with uterine cervical human papillomavirus infection: A meta-analysis. *BMC Infect. Dis.* **2011**, *11*, 10. [CrossRef]

63. Drago, F.; Herzum, A.; Ciccarese, G.; Dezzana, M.; Casazza, S.; Pastorino, A.; Bandelloni, R.; Parodi, A. *Ureaplasma parvum* as a possible enhancer agent of HPV-induced cervical intraepithelial neoplasia: Preliminary results. *J. Med. Virol.* **2016**, *88*, 2023–2024. [CrossRef] [PubMed]

64. Mitra, A.; MacIntyre, D.A.; Lee, Y.S.; Smith, A.; Marchesi, J.R.; Lehne, B.; Bhatia, R.; Lyons, D.; Paraskevaidis, E.; Li, J.V.; et al. Cervical intraepithelial neoplasia disease progression is associated with increased vaginal microbiome diversity. *Sci. Rep.* **2015**, *5*, 16865. [CrossRef] [PubMed]

65. Oh, H.Y.; Kim, B.-S.; Seo, S.-S.; Kong, J.-S.; Lee, J.-K.; Park, S.-Y.; Hong, K.M.; Kim, H.K.; Kim, M.K. The association of uterine cervical microbiota with an increased risk for cervical intraepithelial neoplasia in Korea. *Clin. Microbiol. Infect.* **2015**, *21*, 674.e1–674.e9. [CrossRef] [PubMed]

66. Piyathilake, C.J.; Ollberding, N.J.; Kumar, R.; Macaluso, M.; Alvarez, R.D.; Morrow, C.D. Cervical Microbiota Associated with Higher Grade Cervical Intraepithelial Neoplasia in Women Infected with High-Risk Human Papillomaviruses. *Cancer Prev. Res.* **2016**, *9*, 357–366. [CrossRef] [PubMed]

67. Mhatre, M.; McAndrew, T.; Carpenter, C.; Burk, R.D.; Einstein, M.H.; Herold, B.C. Cervical intraepithelial neoplasia is associated with genital tract mucosal inflammation. *Sex. Transm. Dis.* **2012**, *39*, 591–597. [CrossRef] [PubMed]

68. Thellman, N.M.; Triezenberg, S.J. Herpes Simplex Virus Establishment, Maintenance, and Reactivation: In Vitro Modeling of Latency. *Pathogens* **2017**, *6*, 28. [CrossRef]

69. Beyrer, C.; Jitwatcharanan, K.; Natpratan, C.; Kaewvichit, R.; Nelson, K.E.; Chen, C.Y.; Weiss, J.B.; Morse, S.A. Molecular methods for the diagnosis of genital ulcer disease in a sexually transmitted disease clinic population in northern Thailand: Predominance of herpes simplex virus infection. *J. Infect. Dis.* **1998**, *178*, 243–246. [CrossRef]

70. Johnston, C.; Corey, L. Current Concepts for Genital Herpes Simplex Virus Infection: Diagnostics and Pathogenesis of Genital Tract Shedding. *Clin. Microbiol. Rev.* **2016**, *29*, 149–161. [CrossRef]

71. Brankin, A.E.; Tobian, A.A.R.; Laeyendecker, O.; Suntoke, T.R.; Kizza, A.; Mpoza, B.; Kigozi, G.; Nalugoda, F.; Iga, B.; Chen, M.Z.; et al. Aetiology of genital ulcer disease in female partners of male participants in a circumcision trial in Uganda. *Int. J. STD AIDS* **2009**, *20*, 650–651. [CrossRef]

72. Evans, B.A.; Kell, P.D.; Bond, R.A.; MacRae, K.D.; Slomka, M.J.; Brown, D.W.G. Predictors of seropositivity to herpes simplex virus type 2 in women. *Int. J. STD AIDS* **2003**, *14*, 30–36. [CrossRef] [PubMed]

73. Cherpes, T.L.; Meyn, L.A.; Krohn, M.A.; Hillier, S.L. Risk factors for infection with herpes simplex virus type 2: Role of smoking, douching, uncircumcised males, and vaginal flora. *Sex. Transm. Dis.* **2003**, *30*, 405–410. [CrossRef] [PubMed]

74. Kaul, R.; Nagelkerke, N.J.; Kimani, J.; Ngugi, E.; Bwayo, J.J.; Macdonald, K.S.; Rebbaprgada, A.; Fonck, K.; Temmerman, M.; Ronald, A.R.; et al. Prevalent herpes simplex virus type 2 infection is associated with altered vaginal flora and an increased susceptibility to multiple sexually transmitted infections. *J. Infect. Dis.* **2007**, *196*, 1692–1697. [CrossRef]

75. Masese, L.; Baeten, J.M.; Richardson, B.A.; Bukusi, E.; John-Stewart, G.; Jaoko, W.; McClelland, R.S. Incident herpes simplex virus type 2 infection increases the risk of subsequent episodes of bacterial vaginosis. *J. Infect. Dis.* **2014**, *209*, 1023–1027. [CrossRef] [PubMed]

76. Van de Perre, P.; Segondy, M.; Foulongne, V.; Ouedraogo, A.; Konate, I.; Huraux, J.-M.; Mayaud, P.; Nagot, N. Herpes simplex virus and HIV-1: Deciphering viral synergy. *Lancet Infect. Dis.* **2008**, *8*, 490–497. [CrossRef]

77. Piot, P.; Van Dyck, E.; Totten, P.A.; Holmes, K.K. Identification of Gardnerella (*Haemophilus*) vaginalis. *J. Clin. Microbiol.* **1982**, *15*, 19–24. [PubMed]

78. Cherpes, T.L.; Melan, M.A.; Kant, J.A.; Cosentino, L.A.; Meyn, L.A.; Hillier, S.L. Genital tract shedding of herpes simplex virus type 2 in women: Effects of hormonal contraception, bacterial vaginosis, and vaginal group B Streptococcus colonization. *Clin. Infect. Dis.* **2005**, *40*, 1422–1428. [CrossRef]

79. Cherpes, T.L.; Hillier, S.L.; Meyn, L.A.; Busch, J.L.; Krohn, M.A. A delicate balance: Risk factors for acquisition of bacterial vaginosis include sexual activity, absence of hydrogen peroxide-producing lactobacilli, black race, and positive herpes simplex virus type 2 serology. *Sex. Transm. Dis.* **2008**, *35*, 78–83. [CrossRef]

80. Looker, K.J.; Elmes, J.A.R.; Gottlieb, S.L.; Schiffer, J.T.; Vickerman, P.; Turner, K.M.E.; Boily, M.C. Effect of HSV-2 infection on subsequent HIV acquisition: An updated systematic review and meta-analysis. *Lancet Infect. Dis.* **2017**, *17*, 1303–1316. [CrossRef]

81. Heng, M.C.; Heng, S.Y.; Allen, S.G. Co-infection and synergy of human immunodeficiency virus-1 and herpes simplex virus-1. *Lancet* **1994**, *343*, 255–258. [CrossRef]

82. Mbopi-Keou, F.X.; Gresenguet, G.; Mayaud, P.; Weiss, H.A.; Gopal, R.; Matta, M.; Paul, J.L.; Brown, D.W.; Hayes, R.J.; Mabey, D.C.; et al. Interactions between herpes simplex virus type 2 and human immunodeficiency virus type 1 infection in African women: Opportunities for intervention. *J. Infect. Dis.* **2000**, *182*, 1090–1096. [CrossRef]

83. Shannon, B.; Gajer, P.; Yi, T.J.; Ma, B.; Humphrys, M.S.; Thomas-Pavanel, J.; Chieza, L.; Janakiram, P.; Saunders, M.; Tharao, W.; et al. Distinct Effects of the Cervicovaginal Microbiota and Herpes Simplex Type 2 Infection on Female Genital Tract Immunology. *J. Infect. Dis.* **2017**, *215*, 1366–1375. [CrossRef]

84. Oh, J.E.; Kim, B.-C.; Chang, D.-H.; Kwon, M.; Lee, S.Y.; Kang, D.; Kim, J.Y.; Hwang, I.; Yu, J.W.; Nakae, S.; et al. Dysbiosis-induced IL-33 contributes to impaired antiviral immunity in the genital mucosa. *Proc. Natl. Acad. Sci. USA* **2016**, *113*, E762–E771. [CrossRef] [PubMed]

85. Cayrol, C.; Girard, J.-P. IL-33: An alarmin cytokine with crucial roles in innate immunity, inflammation and allergy. *Curr. Opin. Immunol.* **2014**, *31*, 31–37. [CrossRef] [PubMed]

86. Ebbo, M.; Crinier, A.; Vely, F.; Vivier, E. Innate lymphoid cells: Major players in inflammatory diseases. *Nat. Rev. Immunol.* **2017**, *17*, 665–678. [CrossRef] [PubMed]

87. Bradshaw, C.S.; Brotman, R.M. Making inroads into improving treatment of bacterial vaginosis—Striving for long-term cure. *BMC Infect. Dis.* **2015**, *15*, 292. [CrossRef] [PubMed]

88. Anukam, K.C.; Osazuwa, E.; Osemene, G.I.; Ehigiagbe, F.; Bruce, A.W.; Reid, G. Clinical study comparing probiotic Lactobacillus GR-1 and RC-14 with metronidazole vaginal gel to treat symptomatic bacterial vaginosis. *Microbes Infect.* **2006**, *8*, 2772–2776. [CrossRef]

89. Van de Wijgert, J.H.H.M.; Verwijs, M.C.; Turner, A.N.; Morrison, C.S. Hormonal contraception decreases bacterial vaginosis but oral contraception may increase candidiasis: Implications for HIV transmission. *AIDS* **2013**, *27*, 2141–2153. [CrossRef]
90. Decena, D.C.D.; Co, J.T.; Manalastas, R.M.J.; Palaypayon, E.P.; Padolina, C.S.; Sison, J.M.; Dancel, L.A.; Lelis, M.A. Metronidazole with Lactacyd vaginal gel in bacterial vaginosis. *J. Obstet. Gynaecol. Res.* **2006**, *32*, 243–251. [CrossRef]

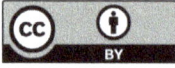

MDPI

St. Alban-Anlage 66

4052 Basel

Switzerland

Tel. +41 61 683 77 34

Fax +41 61 302 89 18

www.mdpi.com

International Journal of Molecular Sciences Editorial Office

E-mail: ijms@mdpi.com

www.mdpi.com/journal/ijms

www.ingramcontent.com/pod-product-compliance
Lightning Source LLC
Chambersburg PA
CBHW051849210326
41597CB00033B/5833